Is This Book for Me?

This book is for you if you are ready to work with your vagina/vulva/womb/ root/pelvic bowl/pussy/cunt/yoni . . . to find happiness.

And if you don't think you can find happiness through your vagina, this book is definitely for you.

In Your Vagina Lies the Key to Your Happiness

In Your Vagina Lies the Key to Your Happiness

Five Steps to Unlocking Joy, Pleasure and Happiness

Naomi Gale

In Your Vagina Lies the Key to Your Happiness:
Five Steps to Unlocking Joy, Pleasure and Happiness

© 2023 Naomi Gale

Published by Aphrodite Athena Publications

Aphrodite Athena Publications Margate

Paperback ISBN: 978-1-7392058-3-6
Ebook ISBN: 978-1-739058-4-3

Cover design by Priscila Barbosa and Rebecca Thomas ©
Interior design by Rebecca Thomas
Illustrations by Author ©

Author Photograph by Artemis Szekir-Rigas ©

For hope

Naomi Gale

Vaginologist, educator, guide, speaker, content creator. Naomi Gale is a highly qualified, nervous system-led, somatic-focused, root-healing mentor, guiding people back into connection with their wombs, vaginas and vulvas.

As a former classroom-based teacher, Naomi educates with ease, making everything accessible. Her primary focus is on people learning the tools needed to live a more rooted nervous system-led life.

Naomi's work has been featured widely, from BBC podcasts to sex-positive influencers' YouTube channels, to articles in *Cosmopolitan* and elsewhere.

She lives in Margate, England, with her husband and three children (a result of IUI and IVF treatments).

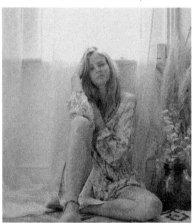

You can find Naomi online at
www.thisisnaomigale.co.uk

She's also on Instagram:
@thisisnaomigale
TikTok: **@thisisnaomigale_**
and YouTube: **@naomigale**

In Your Vagina Lies the Key to Your Happiness is Naomi's first book.

You can find this book's website at
www.thisisnaomigale.co.uk/books.

Education for All

From eighteen-year-old Hope:

I see your TikToks quite a lot and idk what to do.

I have had bleeding during and after any form of penetration, including with fingers and penis, by another person.

I feel embarrassed because I don't have a BF etc. It's hard to tell people when it's a casual thing, and the whole relationship is based around casual sex.

I was raped when I was 15. Idk if it's because of this unhealed trauma (which consciously I don't feel is unhealed), idk if this is vaginismus or if my body is just built narrowly . . . as after a while, my body adjusts. When I don't have penetration for a while, it goes back to square one with all this pain. Any help or advice? Thank you <3

From Naomi:

Hey Hope,

So glad you reached out. I am sending love with this vulnerable share. I can't imagine how challenging this all must be. I presume you've been to the doctor with your bleeding post-penetration?

My advice can only be from a holistic standpoint. I encourage people when they are ready to engage with a vaginal massage. One session won't 'heal', but one session will bring you some comfort and support. It will give you the tools you will need to continue this work to support you further. This may be linked to your experience of rape and the fact you are likely still processing this. The root is a gentle soul who just wants to protect you. You've been through a lot. x

From Hope:

Thank you so much for getting back to me. I haven't been to the doctor about this, but I think I will. For now, I will look into how to heal my root and practice the massaging as you said. Naomi, thank you so so much. <3

From Naomi:

When you go, be clear on your boundaries around speculums etc. Bleeding at times between periods should always be taken seriously by doctors, and everything checked. x

From Hope:

I'm on the arm implant, so bleeding is random for me.

From Naomi:

The videos pinned explain how to do the massage.

From Hope:

Does it make things more sensitive—the implant? X

From Naomi:

Yes, this can create random bleeding. It could be best to ask for alternatives to the arm implant if you're randomly bleeding .x

From Hope:

Yeah, I'll look into it! It's not random/often enough to bother me! I love it compared to the pill. I'm going to look into pelvic floor exercises too and poses to help relax my body. X

March 26, 2022 3:04 am

From Hope:

I did some relaxations and used your massage technique, and I was able to have sex after a fair few close times!!!

I feel so much better.

Thank you for always being here to help; I really appreciate it. <33 I will stay consistent with massages and work on using more foreplay! <333

Navigate the Flaps

Do you know how I view my vagina?
I see it as a cactus.

Do you mean a Venus fly trap? I asked.

Yes. As if it has sharp spikes.

A relatable vision of many, I think
to myself.

—The Spiky Fanny

Preface
The Birthing of This Book

In 2021, I shared a video on TikTok entitled: 'Working with your vagina is the key to your success'. I shared this one afternoon when I was frustrated about the lack of reach my work was getting. I was genuinely starting to believe no one wanted to hear my message on social media.

I had been on TikTok for all of eight days at this point. A thirty-three-year-old on TikTok, fumbling around, trying to work out how to remove the lip-filler effect I'd tried out for shits and giggles the day before.

While standing in the school queue on Friday, 17th November 2021, collecting my twin girls, I did what any other parent does: feeling the daily grind of preschool pickup, I flicked open the TikTok app. I had 99+ notifications. My heart started racing while I wondered what had happened to suddenly get to the dizzy heights of any notifications, let alone 99+. I noticed that one of my videos, which I mentioned above, was getting a lot of views. I watched the video, in real-time, reach thousands of people.

As I cycled home with my three children scooting alongside me, I realised my life would never be the same again.

Of course, I thought, 'Why the fuck did I share that video with no concealer on?' But to be honest, I couldn't even remember what the content of the video was.

Safely home, I sat with my husband, flicking through hundreds of comments. Some were brutal, some were kind, and others had taken the time to follow me. I rewatched the video. I'm not quoting verbatim here but in the video my words were along the lines of, 'You're going to reach your full potential if you're working with your vagina. Your vagina holds the key to your success. You spend your life sitting on your root, sitting on your own vagina. What happens is all your wounding, any traumas that arise, any stresses—they go right down and sit in your root, sitting in your vagina. In the walls of your muscles'. And I continued in this vein for a full three minutes. I thought nothing of this kind of share on social media, but I quickly realised this had become a very controversial video.

All weekend my account went wild. I went from twenty followers to 10k followers in two days. The video reached and eventually surpassed one million views. Over the weekend, I shared another video: 'How to massage your vagina'. This video also went viral and eventually hit and surpassed two million views.

TikTok continued to go wild when people began finding their own keys in their own vaginas. You see, because I had said the key to your success lies in your vagina, people began finding the keys to their success . . . in their vaginas. Keys were dropping into their hands in duets through humorous videos where they would exclaim, 'Found 'em'—you know, the keys to their success. I had apparently started what TikTok users call a TikTok trend, where people follow the same video format on their own feed in slightly new, creative ways. I eventually lost my sense of humour with this video after seeing the same gag for the hundredth time. You know you've really made it when viral videos spill onto Instagram. Huge accounts followed this new 'keys in the vagina dropping into hands' trend I'd somehow created. Not that they tagged me, of course. It was all fun and games . . . and content.

As I write this on 26th June 2022, my account has slowed and sits at around 40k followers, with several videos surpassing one million views.

It has taken a lot of nervous system work, finding further support from a therapist and additional inner work for me to cope with what unfolded on this app. I received a lot of abuse and a lot of frustration. I have had many duets and stitch responses (this is where people use your video on their own, to either chat further about your video, make a joke about it, use it as inspiration or repost what you're sharing). Sometimes these shares have been abhorrent.

People talk about growing a thicker skin on social media, learning to ignore the 'haters', and knowing you have 'made it' when you get hate. But we don't talk enough about social media's impact on the person, their nervous system, their family and the people who know them. I have been featured in others' videos, which have also surpassed millions of views, not often getting credit and generally being mocked.

The thing is, I share this work not because it is humorous (though it's taboo, so a little humour is of use here and there) but because I am passionate that my rounded approach to pelvic work is necessary for all. There are, of course, people who get it, those who feel like seeing my videos has been a godsend.

Since joining TikTok, I have received a constant stream of DMs from people looking for support. Sometimes, these people have been as young as fifteen.

I work with people in workshops, ceremonies, and one-on-one spaces. Of course, not everyone can access these spaces, due to a variety of factors. Most people can access a book. When I was messaged by Hope, I realised I could provide hope to more people if I expanded beyond social media.

Everything has changed for me since the early days on TikTok. My account was tiny when I first went viral. Now, every single video I post is reviewed before it goes live—even if I post a video about how blue the sky is. Many of my videos have been taken down because they supposedly breach TikTok's rules. I have to click the 'Please Review' button to summon the TikTok video reviewers, hoping they will allow them back onto my page. The system doesn't want you to hear the words empowerment and vagina in the same sentence. I have shared this with my audience before, and the responses have been mixed. Some people say, 'It's just bots, Naomi' or 'You're overthinking it, Naomi'.

Am I?

I tell you what. If my email newsletters land in your junk folder because I use the word vulva, then I am overthinking nothing. You may be reading this with a 'Hell yes' or a 'Meh, I dunno'. As I wrote this preface, the Roe vs Wade ruling was overturned in the US. Another reminder of how little control we have over our bodies and how our needs are continuously shut down.

As I wrote the book, Andrew Tate, a man under investigation for sex trafficking, had garnered millions of followers for selling misogynistic propaganda. Dubbed the king of toxic masculinity, he's spouted such things as, 'If you put yourself in a position to be raped, you must bear some responsibility'. His videos were shocking. And yet, his videos reached millions. It took pressure from other social media influencers to have him removed from all the major platforms. TikTok was the last to remove him because they were conducting an investigation into his account. The same platform which silences me. How dare a woman share the importance of working with the feminine while stating the stats on rape? Removed. Silenced. Reviewed constantly.

This book has been birthed in the face of a constant uphill battle to share what I believe is life-changing, necessary and incredible support for people. What does it look like to put up a fight in this situation?

This book. A 'fuck you' to the system that continues to suppress.

In the words of Rick Astley, I am here to tell you how I am never going to give you up or let you down. This is my gesture to show you that I won't desert you. I am all about beating the system that binds us. It's my life work. Nothing will change unless we use our voices for good. So here I am using mine.

Introduction:
Not a Single Swimmer

'The count was zero'. My husband asked the doctor to repeat and clarify what he meant by zero. After this, I recall the next few minutes being a blur. My husband dropped his phone, clutching his chest. I reached to pick up the phone and asked the doctor to repeat the news to me.

'But I don't understand what that means; he ejaculates, so how can there be zero?' I questioned.

'Your husband has azoospermia, but don't worry, there are plenty of things they can do nowadays. We will check again in a few weeks'.

And that was that. Poof, he disappeared off the call and left us sitting on the sofa in the lounge in complete shock at 7:00 p.m. on a Friday night. I kinda thought when a doctor in a movie delivers news like 'You're completely infertile and will never bear a biological child of your own', this was done in their office with a box of tissues and a caring pair of eyes. A pair of eyes that say, 'Gosh, yes, this is shit news, and I am so sorry I am the one delivering this to you both'. Instead, this doctor was chipper AF, making out as though there was plenty we could do. I don't know if he knew of a magical unicorn that flew around to those with azoospermia, injecting them with a whole load of motile, perfectly formed sperm, but we certainly never found it.

We learned early in the journey that we'd been thrown into a system that just doesn't get it. A system that places those on a challenging fertility journey next to pregnant people in a waiting room for hours. A system that determines the financial support you'll receive as you try to conceive based on where you live in the UK. A system in which consultants have a poor bedside manner with very little trauma-informed training, if any.

A second jizz into a cup later, to sticky porno mags in the local NHS hospital, confirmed that my husband had one non-motile swimmer at the bottom of the tube. Bless its little soul.

When we sat wide-eyed and feeling as positive as any pair of late twenty-somethings can in a fertility consultant's office, I realised this was going to be a maddening experience.

The first part of this journey meant going to an appointment in the local NHS hospital with a gate-keeper-style consultant who would assess whether we could step foot into a fertility clinic with NHS funding to support the financial costs of having a child under fertility treatment. We were told, 'Unfortunately, you won't receive any NHS-funded help. Anyway, there's no help with the donor sperm aspect, so you'll have to find that yourself'.

Find sperm? Like it's something you add to your food shop basket. Anything else we need this week? You know, alongside the bananas, lube and digestive biscuits.

One day in a bank, the manager asked me if I'd considered nipping into a hotel room in one of those 'under-the-radar sperm donor scenarios'. I had. Research gathered data from over sixty English-language websites and social media pages worldwide reckons an estimated 350,000 people have received unregulated sperm.[1] Unregulated sperm donation is also known as 'informal', 'self-arranged', 'DIY', 'non-clinical', or 'private' donation, which involves receiving sperm from a known or unknown donor. Unknown donors can be found via social media platforms, advertisements or 'connection websites'. The insemination then takes place away from clinics and is all done as a DIY job. The sperm is inserted by the recipient, the partner or through sex with the donor. It's currently a huge issue due to how the system manages donors and donor sperm, particularly in countries like the UK. This is without discussing the costs of going to clinics, making unregulated sperm a positive prospect as it can save people thousands of pounds. But I digress.

This same NHS hospital-based consultant who delivered the news that we would not receive funding with such compassion and understanding also said things like, 'Your BMI is too low, so it's more likely you'll miscarry' and 'That's why the NHS won't help you, because you will cost too much money with all the potential complications'. After leaving her room feeling like we'd been gut punched, she grabbed me back into a photocopying side room, telling me she had decided to refuse a retest on my hormone levels as they currently weren't meeting the NHS criteria, which would have given us one last chance at receiving some free NHS fertility support. Said news was delivered as an afterthought. I imagine that photocopying room was where the staff enjoy a bitch about the latest protocols. I was expecting some fun gossip as she dragged me in there, rather than, 'You will never, ever get help from the NHS to have a child of your own'. I made a complaint to the hospital where she worked, and it was bulldozed. Of course. She never said any of those things . . . I made it all up.

Gaslit, silenced, shamed, ignored.

I spent hours researching azoospermia, and we swanned off to another hospital to meet with a top London urologist. Finally, some hope.

Oh, except he turned out to be a complete wanker. This is a recurring theme with those placed on pedestals. It's as if they are essentially God. They literally have our futures in their hands, and they know it. It was just wanker after wanker on our journey.

I'd managed to get our doctor to refer us to this urologist's office, as he said he offered free NHS appointments to those he thought would be great for his 'portfolio'. When we met inside his plush Harley Street office, he seemed like the nicest guy. We thought we'd finally found someone who wanted to help us and explore why there was a count of zero. He could help. Handing over a sheet, he gave us a list of some tests to get at a clinic down the road. We left feeling as though we may actually be getting somewhere.

My husband dutifully got his tests, and we were asked to pay.

Pay.

Pay for the tests.

Now, it was swanky.

But six hundred pounds? That's what it cost for these tests.

We started to piece it all together and realised none of this was free. Not the appointment with this urologist, Dr Wanker, or the tests or the smiles.

After a while, the fees from that appointment with this consultant were waived, but those six-hundred-pound tests remained on a Natwest credit card.

We were then due a follow-up appointment with this consultant to discuss the tests and whether there was any chance of increasing my husband's sperm count. At this next appointment, we went to yet another hospital in London. This office was next door to a prison rather than on Harley Street. We sat in a tiny room with Dr Wanker on a swivel chair. His first words to us were—I quote verbatim—'This is what free looks like'. He just loved clarifying that he'd had to waive his previous fees and that, if we wanted to be here under the NHS, we were deserving of an appointment, only minus kindness and plush seats to sit on while he chatted all things sperm.

After the tests, we realised that my husband's azoospermia wasn't obstructive, and there weren't any options except to donor or adopt. Azoospermia refers to having a complete absence of sperm in the ejaculate. It's important to distinguish between someone's azoospermia being obstructive and non-obstructive. In some cases, a count of zero sperm is due to an obstruction, giving hope, but when it is non-obstructive, it's due to abnormal sperm production and there is really no hope of conceiving a child.

Eight months after the first phone call diagnosing my husband's azoospermia, we reached out to yet another hospital, Guy's Hospital, again in London, which we hoped could help us decipher his blood results in more detail, as there was something very strange about one of his blood tests. We later found out it would mean even if there was sperm, trying to conceive a child would have been risky genetics wise, which is a whole other story we wouldn't have discovered without going on this wild journey. This consultant at Guy's Hospital looked at me as tears uncontrollably poured down my face. She asked whether we'd been given any emotional support. Of course, we hadn't. She kindly said we would be once we were referred to a fertility clinic. I explained that it had been eight months, and we hadn't so much as wiped our feet on a clinic's mat, let alone had any clinic support.

'Oh, but you will get that', she confirmed.

'When?' I asked, sobbing.

'When you increase your BMI. Have you considered eating loads of cake and then weighing yourself again?' She smiled.

I got up, slapped her across the face in a rage and stormed out of the appointment.

Jokes. I actually just sat there like I had every other time someone told me to eat cake, agog. As twenty-something, it still baffled me as to how people believe it is acceptable to make such personal, off-the-cuff remarks about others' weight.

At every appointment and in every conversation, the doctors and consultants would flippantly chat about my husband's lack of sperm. I dunno if you know how it works, but just in case you weren't sure—believe me, I began questioning this many times during this journey—to make a baby, you need one egg and one motile sperm at the very least. Now, I had wonderful eggs, and there were ways to get that sperm. But apparently, I didn't eat enough cake.

My BMI (or body mass index, derived from calculating mass and height) has always been an issue with those in the medical profession. BMI means nothing. Most athletes are deemed 'obese'. BMI was started by an insurance company in the 1940s, proving it is complete bullshit.[2] But anyways, my weight has been an issue. I suffered from body dysmorphia from a very young age. I refused to wear skirts or dresses as soon as I realised I hated my body. I wore cardigans all the time to cover my 'skinny' arms. Here I was on a fertility journey, thrown between doctors in my late twenties, when just before this journey I was just beginning to move through my body dysmorphia issues, mainly as a result of feeling loved and grounded in a healthy relationship with my husband. This journey where my BMI was being questioned was all too much for me to cope with. No amount of cake would help. But I did spend most of this nine-month journey to nowhere with a personal trainer. I figured that was a start. One day the PT sat with me and told me I just wouldn't get to the minimum BMI number they wanted me to be at to start any kind of fertility treatment there; it was too far out of reach, and then maintaining my weight while undergoing fertility treatments would be difficult. I knew they'd be weighing me during the process. They categorically told me if I dropped below the BMI threshold, they'd cut the funding wherever we were in the process.

After this last appointment at Guy's Hospital, I came home and couldn't move from my bed. I was helpless. I felt as though there was nothing I could do. My husband could not have children, and I could not give him a child in this system. It was honestly heart-breaking.

One day in the staff room of the school where I was teaching, a fellow teacher told me about a Greek clinic a friend had gone to and said the owner, Penny, was a real-life angel. We'd discussed donor sperm plenty, but we'd not chatted about going abroad much. My husband said the words anyone would dream of hearing in this scenario: 'I just want to be a father, so have a call with them'.

A few days later, I answered a call from Penny. 'How are you?' she asked.

I cried.

What I realised at this moment was that no one had asked me how I was for nine months. I think back to this moment often.

'Darling, you just need some sperm; come over when you're next ovulating'.

Turns out, I was ovulating the following week.

'It probably won't work', I told my husband when we discussed the conversation. 'I know you can't come then, but I'll be absolutely fine'.

Standing on the tarmac of Gatwick airport at 5:30 a.m. with a load of cruise ship-goers, headed to Athens so I could be inseminated by a stranger's sperm, was a wild ride. Though the only physical ride for this whole process was the plane in case your mind wanders to the how-tos of how I was inseminated with sperm.

I was going to do IUI, intrauterine insemination. With this treatment, they simply check your follicles, time the insemination perfectly and allow the swimmers to sniff out the egg.

While in Greece, I finally began to breathe. The clinic was loving, kind and understanding. The others I met in the waiting room took me under their wing and showed me what sisterhood looked like. They showed me Athens and what gyros are, and shared their own stories of pain, sorrow, loss and indescribable battles to get to where they were when I met them.

After I returned home, one day I placed a seatbelt across my chest, and the pain in my breasts shot through my body. I'd felt twinges and pangs for days. I knew.

One positive test later, I was pregnant with my first babe from my first round of donor sperm, via IUI. My son was eight pounds and four ounces when he was born. It was the easiest, breeziest pregnancy.

I would love to stop there and say that was it. We all lived happily ever after as a family of three. The end.

Except. We wanted a sibling. I panicked. Fuelled by fear, I threw myself back into the fertility journey when my son was six months old. This time, it took round after round of treatments. I had a hysteroscopy in Greece on my own, giving my phone and rings to the security guy and hearing the doctors talk about Brexit and how 'maybe the UK had got it right' as I fell under anaesthetic. Twenty-five thousand pounds stretched across credit cards, and a loan later, we decided to switch from IUI to IVF. IUI means the sperm are inserted when you ovulate, and IVF is where they remove your eggs, placing them in a dish with the sperm, growing the fertilised eggs for a few days before placing an egg back in.

Once I did become pregnant again, the news was delivered at the first private ultrasound. We were having twins and my family would be complete.

During my fertility journey, singleton pregnancy and then twin pregnancy, something changed for me. I realised that my story to that point was the same story many have had. So many people sit through appointments where bad news is shared with no humanity. Where doctors focus on someone's 'lack' instead of celebrating their progress. Many people aren't cared for or treated with the respect they deserve as human beings navigating a hard path. This isn't just the case in the world of IUI and IVF. This happens for those in pain every cycle, those feeling lost, those who have been through trauma and who are out of touch with their rawest needs.

The pages of this book follow my own story of how I empowered myself to come back into a deep relationship with my body so I can in turn support others to find empowerment through their rooted system.

She knew she was made of stardust
Except she forgot she was made of magic
The dull days dimmed her light
Until it was simply a spark in her womb space
Untapped potential
Untapped power lying within
Ready to be stirred when she remembers
She's made for it all

—Sacral Power

Things to note: The Metamorphosis Journey

My Metamorphosis

I was searching for a fucking missing shoe . . . again. Except I couldn't look for missing shoes, lost keys or missing worksheets for a class I was teaching the next day without feeling like I was having a heart attack.

Once this started to happen three or four times a day and I began to question whether jumping onto the railway line right outside my Cheltenham flat window would genuinely end it all, I went to the doctor. A few numbers next to some statements later, I was diagnosed with PTSD, depression and panic attacks.

A tablet a day keeps the feelings away. Numb. That's how I felt on antidepressants, and as soon as I could decrease and come off those bad boys, I did. They did wonderful work for me at the time. I got my panic attacks under control, and I didn't quite look at the train line in the same way.

I went through a lot of trauma growing up. It all came out when I left home to find safety at twenty-one. We think that leaving will be the silver bullet: 'If I get out of here, if I leave them, if I finally get my own place'. Except what I learnt and have seen many times with clients is that once we find safety and grounding, our bodies feel safe enough to bring whatever is ready for healing to the surface. We finally then have to deal with some pretty challenging experiences.

I've suffered from many issues, but they all link up: body dysmorphia, IBS with Accident and Emergency trips, painful ovulation, period pains I wished I just had morphine for, depression, panic attacks, seasonal affective disorder and a debilitating lack of self-belief.

After the antidepressants, I truly felt at the age of twenty-one that there must be more than just tablets and masking the pain. So, I started yoga. But once I felt 'cured', I just dived into my career as a primary teacher. I didn't look back until I collapsed in a toilet on the strip of my local town, Haywards Heath after being handed a date rape drug. I surrendered to burnout, went through a breakup and decided to go it alone without my immediate family.

Truth is, I wasn't really sure where to turn or whom I could turn to.

I was never truly, sincerely all that happy. Even after meeting my now husband, who gave me all the love anyone could ask for. Even after buying the cutest kitten. Even after knowing how excellent I was in my job as a primary teacher. Even after purchasing the most perfect skinny jeans from French Connection and thinking, 'Yeah, my arse looks incredible in these'. Even after having my three children.

It was always as though I was looking through slightly shit-smeared spectacles.

Nothing ever felt like it was enough. I never felt like enough.

It was when I was in a doctor's room when my periods returned after my twins that something changed in me. He lifted his hairy toes out of his sandals onto his desk to tell me that if I was going to continue refusing the pill to deal with my out-of-control period pains post-three children, then the best option was a hysterectomy. I realised it was the final time I was going to sit in a clinical setting asking for this kinda support with my body, womb, vagina or ovaries. I was done.

I remember feeling as though I was about to surrender. I could feel a hard shell forming around myself, and I sat in darkness until the answers came.

And still, to this day, this is what I do.

I often sit in my safe space, my chrysalis. Once I feel I have moved through whatever is ready to be carried through, I emerge. I flutter my bright wings to all, feeling as though I am all over the next chapter of my life until the darkness calls again.

The journey to this point: Me sitting in my cabin at the bottom of my garden, deciding I would write a book unfolded because I knew I deserved better. I have seen how many people also feel they deserve better. I know you deserve better.

I shared my IVF journey on my Instagram account, and I still have followers who remember it all. We shared it all in real-time. After this, I got request after request to help people. I could give them informal support, but I knew there was more to all this.

I've been through plenty; I have come through the other side in a way I could only have dreamed of.

I used to listen to P!nk, screaming the lyrics to 'Runaway' into my pillow when I was growing up at home. Wondering what that would feel like to run.

But running doesn't help.

Grounding and sitting with it all does. But that's much harder.

In my late twenties and early thirties, that's what I have done.

In the years since that hairy-toed doctor's appointment, I've learned a tremendous amount. I funded my training myself and went through course after course, all focused on womb healing, root healing, vagina healing and working with the feminine.

On a personal level, levelling with you here at the beginning of this book and potentially at the beginning of your journey, I have found working with my root genuinely transformative. I don't say this lightly. And honestly, I ain't the type of gal to sit writing a long-ish book on something that 'works a little bit' or 'may help'.

I came home to my body through nervous-system-led tools and support through my pelvis, and I'll share some of these techniques and strategies with you.

I invite you to come home to your body. That's where the long-lasting transformation takes place.

The Bodies

With my approach to my work, I marry up all the bodies: the physical body, the emotional body, the spiritual body and the mental body.

What does that mean in this book when it comes to the way I write?

Well, it means I will be referring to our physical challenges: discomfort, pain or basic needs.

I will discuss the emotional body: how we feel and what we need. What the nervous system desires to unravel.

The mental body: our subconscious, our ego, and how these play an essential role in our journey.

Then there's the spiritual body: the universe, our higher selves, a version of God (insert whatever aligns for you), Mother Earth, and how we are all interconnected.

Switching between the bodies through my writing gives healing an integral and rounded approach. We live in a society where things, in general, have to be proven in some way, where they have to be tangible and black-and-white. In my opinion, there's more to it. So in these pages, you may sometimes have to open your heart and mind to some of my approaches. But in my experience, that's when we truly begin to heal.

Your Mufty, Your Noo-Noo, Your 'Downstairs Region'

In a study by Eve Appeal,[1] only 1 percent of parents who completed a YouGov study used the term vulva. In fact, 44 percent of parents used euphemisms like 'fairy', 'flower' or 'tuppence'. If you have been using other language with yourself, friends, cousins, nephews, nieces, within your immediate family, with your own children, and, after reading the book, you switch to the anatomical language to describe the 'bits down there', then that's plenty. This book has had the impact it needed to have.

Here's why: One day in school, on a teacher training day, we were told a story about a four-year-old child who was coming into school telling her teachers her dad was playing with her fairy. She would explain this more than once and in many different ways but always said 'fairy'. Now, you can imagine that in a classroom of thirty-plus children who all live in their own fantasy lands, a child saying that a father was playing with her fairy would likely not register in a teacher's mind. A classroom is a busy place. But if the child described the same scenario and said he was playing with her vulva, you'd be able to act instantly. This child's meaning was eventually understood, but many children won't be, and many will have shared and then felt shut down because no one heard what they were saying.

Use the correct language; it's a child protection issue.

In this study, 22 percent of parents never even referred to any parts of the pelvis, and if you don't label anything, it's almost as if they don't exist. Or, at least, awkward conversations won't have to be engaged with.

I use the anatomically correct language for your 'downstairs' area: vagina, vulva, labia, ovaries, fallopian tubes and more. You'll also see me use the term *pelvic bowl*. I'll use *pussy* and even sometimes work on reclaiming the word *cunt*. Sometimes, I'll refer to your *root*; I use chakra language here.

I also use the word *yoni*. This is a more rounded word when describing our root space, our vulva, and our pelvic bowl. It encompasses it all: the vagina, womb, shakti life-force energy (*shakti* means divine feminine), source, temple. *Yoni* is a Sanskrit word that describes the power between our thighs. I acknowledge that I am using a term here that is a Hindu word, and I am not Hindu. I use it because I trained as a yoga teacher, where yoni is often used and where the yoni is honoured for its power. I am a yogini, and I am in deep devotion to the yogic path.

Pussy is a word we will be claiming back here in these pages. *Pussy* doesn't land lightly with people. Most of the time *pussy* feels pretty confrontational. Why? Well, when we use *pussy* in society, it tends to be used in a derogative way: 'What are you, a pussy?!' 'Don't be a pussy'. 'I'm gonna go out tonight and find me some pussaaaay'. You get it. What we want is to hear the term *pussy* used in celebration. Regena Thomashauer, author of *Pussy*, reminds us of how someone may smile, laugh and giggle when using the word *pussy*. They may feel a little bit risqué using it. Regena talks of how using it can feel like a naughty secret loaded with an inner knowing of exactly what we are talking about. The word *pussy* brings us closer; there's a reclaiming of what is rightfully yours. It's not something to be downplayed or ignored, nor should you be made to feel like it's someone else's to claim on a night out after three rounds of Jägerbombs.

Knowledge for All

One thing I feel strongly about is that we all deserve the same support. I worked and continue to work hard to listen and hear what everyone has to say on inclusion when I was writing about the pelvis.

This book focuses on the challenges that bind, gag and keep us quiet. This book was birthed because society makes it unnecessarily difficult for us to access what is rightfully ours—the wisdom that comes from the pelvis.

Sex and gender continue to be seen not as fluid but static. The standard relationship between the genitalia and the fixed gender identity leaves little room for your actual feelings about your own body. Consider that a baby is born with a penis and thus is recorded as male at birth. This baby is raised as a boy; when this child becomes an adult, they are a man. OK, actually, I missed a part. The twenty-week scan reveals a penis, and a blue baby shower rains down over the growing baby, and then they are raised as a boy. A baby born with a vulva is recorded as a female. This child is raised as a girl, and as an adult becomes a woman.

You've picked up this book because you are fighting the same fight everyone who feels drawn to this book is part of. We all want to have full bodily autonomy. We want sexual freedom and freedom from sexual violence. Therefore, this book is for anyone ready to reclaim the power housed in their pelvis in order to experience long-lasting happiness. It includes every single person who has been disempowered in some way.

Regarding gender inclusion, I am doing the best I can, given that I am a cis white woman in a relationship with a cis white man.

I will not simply replace 'woman' with 'vulva owners'. I understand that feels degrading. When I refer to relationships, remember that the relationship may take many forms. Penetrative sex isn't about P in the V. It's so much more than that. So it is unnecessary to refer to relationships with any kind of specifics.

Most research separates men and women, which is why you will hear the word women used when referring to research. And gender-neutral stances will not automatically support a gender-equal approach either. Sex-disaggregated data would also make it much harder for women's needs to be heard. So I've seen that we cannot just be gender neutral all that much when it comes to research if we want to truly acknowledge specific challenges we encounter with the pelvis with hard-hitting stats.

I want you to know that all I am doing is the very best I can while I continue to learn and educate myself. I am a trans-inclusive feminist. And if that doesn't sit with you, I suggest you don't disregard the book. You'd be cutting off ya nose to spite your face. I have a whole section on why this book is inclusive. It's worth reading and sitting with, particularly when discussing the pelvis. We are all on the same page.

What I want to ensure is that your access to this—in my opinion—life-changing information isn't impacted by my lack of inclusion. Because, unless you have lived experience, all you can do is your best and be as open-hearted/minded as possible.

Here are some words from a community member to reinforce why I am approaching this book inclusively.

> As a transmasculine person, gender dysphoria and years of confusion about my gender identity had caused me to hate my body. To feel like I'm living inside of an enemy. Something that is not me. And I felt so ashamed of all the parts of my body most associated with femininity. It took me a long time to realise it was not my body's fault. And there's nothing wrong with being trans. Trans people have existed for as long as humans have, and there must be a good reason for us being here. These days I'm slowly growing into the understanding that what makes me a man is not any part of my body. I can be a man with a womb. And since that's my reality, I want to start feeling and enjoying its power. I want to learn more about how having a womb connects me to parts of the divine that I would otherwise not be able to communicate with.
>
> I think every type of body, whether female or male or intersex, gives us certain powers and certain types of access to divinity. And that can be explored with the help of a safe practitioner like Naomi who has space for gender-diverse beings.

Don't Swear, Bitch

You'll see profanity in this book. I am a prolific swearer. I've always been told that it signifies a lack of intelligence. 'Stop swearing', people will say to me.

Fuck-ooooooff.

I cannot stand this kind of societal suppression. Makes my skin crawl as much as when someone turns to someone else and says, 'Smile, love'.

In fact, knowledgeable people can fling expletives into sentences effectively. Science—and we know some people love things to be proven—shows how swearing has a vast list of benefits and is not a sign of dishonesty or lack of anything; it's the opposite.[2]

Some people in the world of all things spiritual may say that swearing lowers your vibration. Listen, I don't really worry all that much about it. I believe that inserting a swear word every now and then simply shows passion.

By some miracle, I didn't swear in the classroom while teaching. Yet, I continued to swear like a trooper outside school. So we all know we can help ourselves. I simply choose not to.

Cunt is also an underused word. I would have written a whole book about it, but it turns out there is one on this called *Cunt: A Declaration of Independence.* Maybe next time. There is a powerful back story to this word that society ignores because that would mean giving people back more power. *Kunthi* refers to female genitalia in Sanskrit. Kunthi/cunt/kunt will also be used in this book. There's also a Hindu nature goddess called Kunti. There have been findings of *kunt* in Egyptian writing, referring to women as a term of respect.[3] I decided to explain all things cunt in the swearing section. Notice that was on purpose.

The vagina is really the passage between the uterus and the vulva. The path between the internal and external. But *cunt* describes it all: the labia, vulva, clitoris, vagina. It's a more rounded term which really, when we think about it, includes everything that involves pleasure. If we bring in the G-spot, clitoris, vagina, vulva, and labia, think of the power that houses. The argument is that if we are to truly claim back our power, we must reclaim the word cunt.

Something to ponder.

Hun, Hunz, Babe, Loves

The other type of language you will see in this book are terms of endearment. Not everyone loves these, I get it. I use them genuinely and to be sarcastic at times. Is it a flaw? Maybe sarcasm can be confusing at times. It's why a head teacher categorically said I shouldn't apply for a teaching post lower than year 3 (seven-year-olds). I was best placed with the eleven-year-olds, after all. I don't use sarcasm to offend. It's a flourish here and there. It's to make a point at other times. But mostly, I use it in these pages and off them because I genuinely care, babe. Sorry if it offends—that's not the intention.

Your Journey through These Pages

I hope you grabbed this book by both hands because you know you deserve more in your life as someone with a cunt. OK, OK, I'll stop . . . for now.

We all deserve more happiness, that's the truth of it. Society has shut down your pelvic bowl for so long. You can see this journey as an awakening of your root, voice and deepest needs. You are never too old or young to awaken the power within your centre, though this book is definitely not aimed at children. It's for anyone ready to dive deeper into the knowledge and happiness that comes from being in connection with their pelvis. I have a wide range of ages working with me as clients, from fifteen to seventy and beyond.

When I work with clients, I remind them that I am here to simply share tangible tools they can take away and implement for the rest of their lives. We live in the Aquarian Age; gone is the idea that we learn from gurus, and we don't subscribe to the theory that anyone is deemed a 'healer'.

You will follow the unique metamorphosis process many of my clients have been through when working with me at a 1-on-1 level. This book makes this work accessible to all. Between the chapters, you will find the voices of some of my previous clients, whom I reached out to for this book, to simply inspire you to try these steps yourself. This is a thank-you to each and every one of them for sharing their experiences with you. Stories are powerful. Rooted stories have extra weight, I feel.

To begin with, we will be exploring our foundations and our current knowledge of the pelvic bowl. We will be exploring how we got here in the first place, with some much-needed words around society today vs our actual needs.

This book is split into five steps that I feel you should go through to truly experience it all. However, if you just want to skip specific steps, go ahead. The tools can be brought in separately; I have written this as if we were working together on a one-to-one basis. If we were about to go on one of my metamorphosis journeys, I'd ensure you gently implemented these five steps.

Step one focuses on your foundations and what they were built on. This step navigates the knowledge you should have been given and how your voice may have been shut down. This step also introduces you to some of the topics we will be diving into more deeply as we move through the rest of the steps. It begins to fill in these cracks.

Step two is all about mothering. You likely didn't receive enough mothering, or you now, as an adult, don't receive enough or give yourself enough mothering. This step is all about connecting to the seasons of life, your cycle seasons and how we connect to Mother Earth for further holding. We discuss how we can genuinely bloom into all that we are.

Step three is where we will be exploring 'mirrovulva' work, a term I have coined to integrate yoni worship, mirror work and the work of Francesca Woodman known for her self-portrait mirror photography. The idea of this step is to allow you to begin to work with your whole body, exploring the relationship you have with your body and then specifically with your vulva. You will be given many tools, tasks and affirmations to work with daily. We will also be working with the themes of consciousness and assessing where you find yourself in these themes. Is there shame, fear, guilt or maybe just a lot of love?

Step four focuses on pleasure and joy in daily life. Together we will find the things that bring you warm feelings daily and discuss how this can bring you more happiness in every aspect of your life. We will explore living an orgasmic life without the need to directly discuss orgasms. If you are here because you feel you haven't had an orgasm, or you used to orgasm plenty, but now they are aloof, or you feel you want more of 'em, I want to share with you the importance of orgasms being seen as a beautiful side-effect rather than the main focus.

Step five is all things somatic touch. How can you explore the landscape of the vagina to find what truly lies in the subconscious? Here you will be bringing in all the previous steps to begin to bring in touch externally and then internally. Yes, an internal vagina massage. When I started my journey with clients and vagina massage, I popped a Facebook post out in my local area looking for anyone who would be keen to be case studies. A well-meaning man replied that I clearly didn't mean internal as that would mean a 'very different thing'. No, I literally mean an internal massage for reclamation and healing.

We end these above five stages with **further rooted support**. How can we then bring these tools in so they actually stick? So this work doesn't become another 'healing fad' we tried? We examine how we marry up all the keys in this book to find happiness through the pelvic bowl.

Finally, there's a chapter on the physical challenges that may show up for you in your pelvis. I believe that physical manifestations begin as emotional challenges. I also believe these may not be yours; these could have been passed down through your lineage. But this section may be a helpful chapter for anyone looking for further support with something that is showing up physically or if they have been diagnosed with something particular. The manifestations are explained, and I share helpful tools to support whatever may arise for you.

This book is intended to start conversations and provide tangible tools. Let me tell you, hun, you and your pussy deserve so much more. You both always have. I know what a difference this work makes to people. I have seen it many times. I truly hope this book is everything you need right now.

Know that this is a process. You are undoing years of oppression. This is enormous work. Thanks for showing up for us all. As you read these pages, you aren't just changing your life. You are changing the lives of those around you. Every person who reads this book engages in our silent protest against the binds placed on us. Here's to you.

You'll notice as you move through each section that there are keys:

· **Key practice:** These are practices I believe are a must-try at some point. Preferably in order.

· **Try these keys:** These are practices you may want to try but that aren't absolutely necessary.

· **Key affirmations** are affirmations to read aloud, write down, share on socials for others, and write on your mirrors. Daily reminders for you to fall back on as and when needed.

· **Unlock your answers:** These are questions you can use as prompts for your journaling practice. If you haven't found journaling ever lands with you, treat yourself to a new journal. (And just like that, you've started working on finding little pockets of joy because a new journal is a gift.)

Holding you exactly where you are as you begin.

Let's dive deep into it. Together. Just you and I. Exploring whatever's ready to be explored.

You've got this.

You are loved. You are held.

Let's begin.

I was never fully loved as a child in a way a child needed love

In the way anyone really needs love.

And now I don't know whether my love for my own children is enough

Because

What does love actually look like?

And what feels enough when it comes to love?

-Re-parenting myself as a parent

Kirsty's Love Story with Her Discharge

I have had a mixed relationship with my vagina. When it birthed my two children (large children I love dearly, though I wish they were smaller and came out a little easier), the neutral relationship I had with it took a nose dive. I didn't feel like I knew it or that it was even mine anymore. To be honest, I didn't want to get to know it.

I started to learn the fertility awareness method (FAM) with Naomi. It is something I would have never really considered before, but Naomi's passion sparked a curiosity that I couldn't ignore. Although initially, I did, scrolling past her offering. But something niggling in my brain kept bringing me back. I messaged her and haven't looked back.

I haven't ever really had any open discussions about my vagina or cycle. Not even with my husband. Even to the point I did not know that you could only get pregnant during certain times of the month until I was trying to conceive, at age twenty-nine. We were fortunate to fall pregnant with little difficulty, so I didn't need to explore this further at the time.

During my initial meeting with Naomi, she was so open in her manner, and I felt instantly at ease and also, in a way, liberated. It was good to talk about it all; it's part of life, right!?

Since tracking my cycle and learning about my body, I have started a journey of acceptance and feel we understand each other more. I know why my body is doing what my body is doing.

I was an avid panty liner user. I hated my discharge and saw it and my period as a huge inconvenience. In a way I thought of it as dirty. I realise this is not the case. It is the total opposite. Every bit of discharge is my body doing what she is designed to do and doing it perfectly!

I have ditched panty liners and now don't worry about discharge. I understand it fluctuates with my cycle. This saves me financially and means I'm not walking around with plastic and goodness knows what next to my most sensitive parts all day.

I wish I could tell my younger self to learn more about her body and explore, explore and explore. It's nothing to be embarrassed by. I hope that future generations find themselves a Naomi Gale.

Someone to spark their curiosity. Have enough curiosity to explore a bit more and learn much more than any mainstream outlet or school will teach, which is such a shame.

My vagina and I are a team, and I wouldn't have it any other way.

Step One
Holding onto the Cracks in Our Foundations

It's Only a Vulva

Love or hate her, Gwyneth has put our pelvic bowls under the metaphoric limelight. She's got what I would call clout. She can get spots in newspapers and push her blog posts to page one of Google. She's got the monnneeeyyyy, celeb status and a general 'no shits given' approach.

Gwyneth and Goop, sharing the wonders of vaginal steaming on a blog post. If you google it, you'll see it sits between articles from certain newspapers about why steaming is an alarming trend to get on board with. (It ain't no trend, hun.) Goop sells a 'This Smells Like My Vagina' candle for £83 (which apparently has tones of geranium, citrusy bergamot, and cedar absolutes juxtaposed with damask—my kind of candle). They've shared jade eggs, which I am not a big fan of as a pelvic health specialist. Still, there's an argument for how they are used (yes, she may have ever so slightly gotten sued for making big claims instead of promoting the possibilities of connecting energetically with these said eggs). There are not one but two Netflix series featuring sex, love and what Western society would deem 'out there' approaches to wellness. Then there are the 'It's Only a Vulva' tees. Oh, and plenty of blog posts on all things vagina. Gwyneth recently invested in a menopause start-up alongside Drew Barrymore and Cameron Diaz. A trio of 90s women I grew up with and adored. Why did they invest in a menopause start-up? Well, I think she is a very clever business-woman. I am not here saying she doesn't share information with a lack of care at times (she's already been sued for that). I'm approaching Gwyneth here regarding how she's used her power to push all things vagina chat.

She quite literally smells what sells. Being controversial over on Goop is why she has made such a success of it. She knows that coming back into connection with our roots will be where it's at, and she's getting ahead of the game. Trailblazing the way she approaches it. This is precisely why she invested in all things menopause when HRT (hormone replacement therapy) chat kicked off across the media. Anyone talking about menopause was paving the way for thousands of people who have felt ignored for far too long.

In the words of Hadley Freeman in a Guardian article that made me snort when researching, 'Gwyneth no longer has just her head up her vagina; she has crawled all the way inside'.[1] Good for Gwyneth. And look at her blooming into all that she is, huns. Actor, singer, lifestyle writer and business gal with a net worth of $200 million.[2]

Really deep (very deep) down, Gwyneth knows it's more than a vulva.

Now, here you are. Ready to explore why you should be getting on board with the 'trend' that is celebrating our vulvas.

Our Fanny (Funny) Education

Your sex education

His shoes squeaked. Same pair of shoes every day. Same squeaky noise back and forth, from one side of the classroom to the other. He was also a very heavy mouth-breather as he squeaked along the floor, which now I realise would have done very little for his overall health.

Post squeak from the back of the room to the front, he plonked a box on the front table filled with polystyrene cocks.

My geography teacher was one of the teachers I landed with for years in secondary school. I was utterly shook when I realised he was about to teach me how to place a condom on a penis. A mixed class of titters, lols and snorts.

If I am brutally honest, I only remember this cock-based fear-mongering lesson. Oh, and I remember when my form tutor told us how she loved to place her knickers on a radiator to dry up her discharge so she could sit and peel them, giving her endless satisfaction. Something that to this day I haven't tried but always think of when I see my own discharge dry and flaky when removing my knickers for the evening.

Our sex education is below par. Some teachers genuinely hate teaching it. I used to adore teaching it, but after primary school, they leave for secondary (here in the UK, that happens when kids are eleven or twelve), and it just doesn't get taught well. They recently tried to improve our UK RSE curriculum (relationships, sex education) in schools in September 2021, but I don't foresee much changing.

In our society and education system, we mainly teach people one thing: If we look a sperm in the eye, we will likely get pregnant . . . so don't have sex. Those with a uterus then believe that they are fertile all the time, and sex is something you definitely don't want to dabble with.

We instil fear and further disconnect from what it means to be sensual, sexual beings.

Some of us likely go on to binge-drink at a sixth-form[i] party and forget whether we actually did use a condom with sexy James from upper sixth. So, we then panic-buy the morning-after pill. Two weeks later, we decide it's probably best to go on the pill. We stick to the pill for fifteen years and then wonder why we don't understand or cannot answer questions like 'When is day one of your period?'

It's time to settle down and unzip your new WHSmith fluffy pencil case of dreams with new Paper Mate pens, because class is underway.

Spreading Your Legs for Those in the Medical Profession

We must go to doctors and gynaecologists to rule out anything that could be underlying. This book is a holistic approach to all things vulva/vagina/womb/periods. If you have any symptoms that are out of the ordinary, then you must get everything

---

[i]   Sixth form is the equivalent to 12th grade in America

checked. Any random bleeding, pain, changes to discharge, mood changes when using hormonal contraceptives—anything you just aren't sure about. Get it checked.

The issue is many of us (not all, but lots of us) sit opposite people with challenges. One challenge is they lack much understanding of the pelvic bowl. The second is that they lack any bedside manner. In a US 2006 review of schools that train medical professionals, it was found that 9 out of the 95 medical schools who entered in data offered any type of course that they'd describe as a 'women's health course'. In fact, 2 out of 9 of these gynaecology and obstetrics courses (taught only in the second or third academic years of medical school) were actually even mandatory.[3]

I spoke to a doctor who recently underwent his training in the UK.

One balmy September evening, we jumped on a Zoom call. Sam was currently in his second foundation year here in the UK, and I was in my cabin looking out at my apple tree, which was beginning to lose leaves to the autumn as the sun started to go down.

We chatted for over an hour. It was enlightening and shocking. It left me feeling a range of emotions. Buzzing that I could include Sam's words in this book but upset for the thousands of us with no answers. The thousands of us left to feel abnormal or pathologized. Here is Sam's story.

Dr Sam and Years of Handwashing-Based Training

My training took place over the last few years, where I qualified in 2021. In the UK, you complete five to six years of medical school with two years of foundation years after this, where you explore a small range of different areas, but the choices come in packages of three medicine specialities. After the foundation years, you specialise in your chosen fields.

During these years, I'll be honest, gynaecology was ignored. They roll obstetrics and gynaecology into one. Obstetrics and gynaecology (O&G) incorporates care for pregnant women and unborn children and looks after women's sexual and reproductive health. There were around four weeks of obstetrics and gynae in my third year of training. In the final year, there were around six weeks. This is placement based. However, I would say the actual focus on gynae would be about one-fourth of this overall.

I remember doing a gynae clinic one afternoon, and an IVF clinic placement morning. That was it. There were also a small number of lectures, but these were not compulsory. There were no specific exams on either area, though sometimes the odd question on gynae or obstetrics could appear in final exam papers.

In the foundation years, the jobs are in groups of three, so in three rotations, three areas per year. So six overall across the two years. However, you can't choose the specific areas you want. The groups are the groups. So you land in the areas you are given. You can rank the groups for yourself, but what you'll be given is never apparent until you approach your foundation years. This means you wouldn't be able to specifically choose obstetrics, gynaecology and the third area of choice if this was your area of interest.

O&G exposure in GP training is minimal to none unless they specifically choose an O&G placement, and even then, it is subject to availability. A GP could land in GP training with minimum to no gynae and obstetrics training. I can't speak for GP training myself, but from my understanding, it's very minimal training for this area before they become a GP. I agree; this is terrifying when you think about it this way.

Obviously I can only speak for the curriculum of my medical school. However, having spoken to colleagues, it sounds like they had similar experiences regarding gynaecology. Curriculums vary a fair bit, surprisingly.

It's important to note that, from what I have seen, anything like vaginismus was glossed over. In our training, delivering babies or treating cervical cancer would always be discussed. Vulvodynia and vaginismus weren't deemed as important. Anything linked to psychiatry will mostly be ignored and downplayed, or a patient will be discharged with the challenge because they haven't a solution. Consultants and doctors are often scared of these challenges because they know they can't give patients the support or solution they need.

I feel that most of the time, everything is dealt with so insensitively. I find it frustrating that we generally lack the ability to treat patients like they are human beings. So often, patients are spoken to with a dismissive approach.

I am wondering if the issue is the training process. You are taught what critical analysis and critical training are, as a scientific 'thing'. But then, in the job, you are brainwashed not to critically think. Essentially you are led to think a certain way and not challenge. You are told that research is 100 percent correct and accurate. Even though anyone barely looks into how the research was collated or what was excluded. So I think it's partly fear. They've not been taught this far down the ladder. Perhaps they want to avoid feeling out of their depth. Knowing they don't have the answers but not wanting to say that . . . blatantly. From what I have seen, I don't think that's really ever heard in these scenarios: 'This is out of my depth of knowledge, and I am sorry'. If they are a specialist in this area, there's no harm in apologising for not having all the answers. So yes, ego often gets in the way.

One example that's burned into my memory as it was so awful was when I was with a doctor who was a gynaecologist. This doctor was leading the gynaecologist clinic. The woman in the room was around twenty-six and had endometriosis. She'd had the laparoscopies and many other tests at this point. He was delivering the news that he thought she would never get pregnant after she'd been trying to conceive. There were no warning shots; she hadn't even sat down when this news was delivered. The aftercare carried on in the same vein. No extra time was given; he was repeating the need for the appointment to end as he had another patient. It was all about how she simply needed to 'move on'. There was no extra time or advice on where to go next. It was like she was on a cliff edge. There was nowhere else for her to go. He was making it clear that he felt she'd reached the end of her road—and 'it's done' kind of thing. To be in this appointment felt awful. I felt as though I shouldn't have been in the appointment, but I was so young at the time and didn't challenge any of it.

A growing number of doctors and nurses in the NHS are quietly challenging the system. But yes, it's still hugely ingrained, this difficulty many have with admitting they don't have the answers. This is also a very hierarchical profession. For example, juniors don't challenge seniors. Even as a medical student in the first year, you think by the fifth year you'd know it all ... and then that doesn't happen. So essentially, it comes down to the feeling that we all need to appear as if we know our stuff. This is a big part of passing practical exams—how do you come across? Based on this, saying you don't know will appear unprofessional.

When you have experienced other forms of brainwashing—for example, I have been in the church—once you come out the other side, you are cued into when another organisation is doing a similar thing. This is definitely what's happening within medicine and the NHS, even.

One of the main things ingrained into us, in the pre-clinical years, in preparation for speaking to patients, was that in challenging situations, we should show empathy, not sympathy. So the point they were making was don't ever show emotions on your side, but try and convey that you're feeling for them. They repeated, 'Show empathy, not sympathy'. Appear that you care, but don't take it as yours to deal with. Of course, this is so that we aren't taking anything on.

The system 100 percent needs to be better for feminine healthcare. The issue is that the profession as a whole has got it wrong.

The profession needs to change, and then the training will change. There is very little support for people as a whole within feminine healthcare, especially when we know they will be breaking the kind of news that completely changes the trajectory for someone. There should be psychologists and mental health support.

We need to be aware that there is a divide between psychiatry and medicine. It's an unspoken 'thing' that psychiatry isn't real medicine. Psychiatry is labelled almost as if it's not real science. So if psychiatry and psychiatrists are treated in this way—something that can't be defined by tests or imaging they already have—then whatever is being presented can't be real. Perhaps it's even seen a joke.

The majority of doctors are burned out and/or stressed and are constantly thinking of how much they have got to get done, and that they don't want to miss any urgent pathology/diagnoses. A large number of doctor and nursing posts are unfortunately unfilled, and this sadly has an impact clinically.

For those reading this book and looking for support around going to a doctor or consultant with a current challenge, my advice would be to find someone you can take with you into the ten-minute appointment. Someone who is supportive and understands what you are going through. When we are discussing something painful, we forget what has been said. If you have someone with you, they can help go over what was discussed. Or you can ask if the appointment can be recorded. Having a dictation of the appointment can be very useful so you can go over what was said at home in your own time.

It's helpful to be upfront with what the concerns and expectations are from the appointment. Hopefully, a doctor will draw this out of you, but if you're in with someone who doesn't decipher what your main concerns are or what you hope to get from the appointment, you can be proactive as the patient. Be transparent with what you know already. Some patients will go into an appointment knowing way more than the doctor, even as they've lived with whatever is presenting for so long—for example, a chronic disease they've had for their whole life. You can be clear with what you know and areas you've already looked into.

During this call, I asked Sam what else you learn in five or six years. What else exists? Ya know, I am so far up my own vagina I forget the NHS deals with many, many areas. I was joking . . . kinda. He said: 'Mainly handwashing; we are very good at washing our hands'. We both sat there laughing, but of course, we were well aware of what his words will mean to those reading this book.

We discussed the lack of knowledge around specific challenges doctors may see. For example, Sam mentioned the speculum issue he saw: 'Literally, many aren't aware that there are different speculum sizes'. I exploded right there and then. Can we just, for a moment, discuss this? Helpfully, I explained to Sam that if there were a line-up of cocks and I could choose which size I had to engage with for the rest of my life, I wouldn't go for the largest. Each to their own, babe.

Many of us need smaller speculums—except this is never explained to people. I know because many clients experiencing pain look at me in shock when I explain they must ask for a smaller size when going into appointments. 'A big part of this', Sam explained, 'is because they just aren't educated on it all. Genuinely'.

How Does Your Garden Grow? With Silver Bells and Cockleshells

That's as far as some of us get. We know we have a vagina . . . somewhere. We know there's a uterus. Many of us will be all over this knowledge, armed and ready for any question at a local pub quiz. But for some of us, we may feel that we haven't a clue. Later in this book, we discuss exploring our vulvas in a mirror. I believe this should be done in a ceremony, with a more nervous system-supported lead-up, so don't feel pressured to grab a mirror just yet. This will come.

Externally

Your vulva. This is your external area; the entire area externally is your vulva. Here we include your labia majora (your flappy flaps or not-so flappy flaps). Your mons pubis (the mound where your pubes flow in the wind as you run naked on the beach). The labia minora: your inner flaps, which may flap about externally or may be in hiding behind your majora flaps. The one and only clitoris, peeking out at the top of your curtains (labia), though it may not be visible externally for some. The clitoral hood exists because every badass needs a hood for extra badassery. Your vulvar vestibule is the area around your two holes, your holes being, ya know, your urethra and vaginal opening holes. It includes the perineum, the space you can feel just under your labia majora and before your anus. The hymen is the somewhat famous area of our pussy which is essentially a ring-shaped piece of tissue covering the entrance to the vagina that often wears down over time.

We often get confused between the vulva and the vagina. I often receive comments on social media: 'Er, don't you mean your vulva . . . LOL!!' when referring to a vaginal massage, for example. No, babe, I am referring to touching your body somatically internally.

Your vagina is the internal area; it is a muscular tube that connects the external places mentioned above to your inner landscape. It connects the vulva to the opening of the uterus. If you part your magical labia, you will begin to reveal your vagina. But you cannot see your vagina externally.

Let's explore your outer landscape in a little more detail.

Mons pubis (wave your hair back and forth)

That mound at the top that waves at you in the form of pubic hair is your mons pubis. If you are without said pubes, it's the area where the hair grows back as soon as you make it back home after your waxing appointment.

Clitoris (ya clit)

We all know that the clitoris has been ignored for far too long. Not anymore. It was only in 1998 when a urologist, Helen O'Connell, first shared the whole internal structure of the clitoris.[4]

Can we even wrap our heads around that? The organ packed with ten thousand nerve endings (double that of a penis) has been wholly ignored in science. This organ is nestled deep within your root, here only for pleasure. It is the most sexually sensitive part of your body. Ignored, hunz.

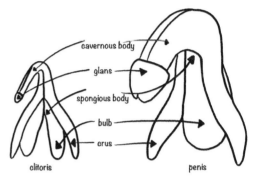

The clitoris is basically the equivalent of a penis. The penis or the clitoris develops from the same tissue in utero. This is why both engorge with blood when aroused. We just don't need to windmill it around with one hand while our other hand waves in the air to get all showy about how incredible our clitoris is.

We all know why people get all 'showy'; I don't need to go into that, do I?

Instead, our seat of pleasure is nestled under a hood, just doing its thang. Fun fact for pub quizzers everywhere: this type of structure, which develops from the same tissue in males and females, is called a homologue.

As with everything else with your body, your cunt is your own and will look very different to your friend Sarah's or Heather Cumhither's from that porn site.

Labia (rebrand underway to be thus labelled as labia majorca and menorca)

Labia is Latin for 'lips', and if you were to cock your head to one side, some vulvas look like a mouth's lips. Everyone's labia are different; no one has symmetrical labia. No one. The outer skin folds extend from the mons pubis and are called the labia majora. Your outer lips are plumper because they are there to cushion and protect. They also have hair follicles. Perhaps while we are here, let's take a moment to share some fun pubes-loving facts, as I have many clients who worry they are a little hairy. Personally, I am all for full bush myself, but it's whatever brings you the most comfort, joy and happiness when working as a team with your vulva:

· Your pubic hair reduces friction during sex and for other activities . . . such as wearing those very 'in' fash-hun bike shorts. You can think of it as a dry lubricant.

· Keeps genitals warm, which is essential with all things sexual arousal.

· And my personal fav, just like when we discuss all things discharge later on, pubes protect from bacteria and other pathogens. They trap dirt, harmful microorganisms and such like. In actual fact, hair follicles even produce oil to prevent bacteria from reproducing to protect from STIs, UTIs, vaginitis and yeast infections.

So if you've got 'em and you're into them . . . flaunt them. And if you hear any remarks about your pubes peeking out on either side of your bikini bottoms, hit them with all the pube facts. Don't hit them; I'm not condoning violence, but I'm into protests filled with facts. *Free the Pubes* signs at the ready. And seriously, can all bikini and swimsuit designers consider how uncomfortable it is when the crotch is designed to simply house the labia? I want the crotch a little wider. Just a personal whinge.

The labia majora has loads of sensory nerve endings, too, which is why it's imperative to include the labia during sexual experiences before diving anywhere near the vagina. If this feels uncomfortable, this is why you're reading this book. I've got you.

The inner labia, called the labia minora, don't have fatty tissue and are much thinner than the labia majora. These begin at the clitoral hood and flow below the vagina. The colour of your inner lips also varies from dark brown to pink. They can be super smooth or super wrinkled. Sometimes you may also see raised dots as there are oil glands here; this is entirely normal. For most of us, the labia minora are obvious and extend past the labia majora; for others, you can hardly see them. The inner labia are way more sensitive due to the blood supply they get, as they also swell when you are feeling aroused.

Labiaplasty is one of the fastest-growing plastic surgery treatments. Across the world, there were 164,667 labiaplasties performed in 2019, a 24.1 percent increase compared to 2018 and a 73.3 percent rise compared to 2015. Labiaplasty was the fifteenth most popular plastic surgery procedure in 2019.[5]

Once you explore your vulva in the mirror in ceremony later in the book, it may prompt you to go on and explore other vulvas. There's a PDF you can search online by popping 'gynodiversity classification of the anatomical variation in female external genitalia' into a search engine. Your vulva is yours and is an incredible source of all that is. You and your vulva deserve to be celebrated and loved as you are. We will explore this further. Until then, let's discuss the rest of your root's anatomy. Holding you, wonderful soul.

Perineum (the bit between your flaps and anus)

This is the area between the vaginal opening and the anus. This is the area you sit on; therefore, we will be working with this area when connecting to Mother Earth 'cause you are literally sitting on the earth on your perineum.

This area can tear during childbirth, so you may have heard of or even worked with that often uncomfortable perineal massage I frequently get asked about when I mention a vaginal massage. It's not the same thing or the same technique. I had an episiotomy in one of my births, and I get this chat on a deep, deep level. I discuss how tears and episiotomies can impact your root and create challenges in the back of the book in the 'Dear Vagina' section.

Urethra (a separate hole)

'There's one hole'.

'I thought the penis went into the pee hole'.

We all know there's plenty of confusion around the number of holes one has in their root. There are three, hun. The urethral opening is the tiny hole where your pee flows from. This is just below your clitoris, while the vaginal opening is directly underneath your urethral opening. The urethra tube carries urine from the bladder to the outside of your body. Then, of course, there's the anus.

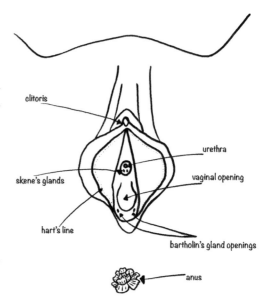

When I am waiting in a queue to use the female toilets, while the urinals are without a line, I wonder whether it is worth buying a Shewee. I know I am not alone in these thoughts. Can I get a noise of understanding about female toilet queues and the need to squat to pee?

Vulvar vestibule (no man's land)

When spreading the inner labia apart, you will see your vestibule, which extends from Hart's line to the opening of the hymen. It's the bit between your labia, your vaginal opening and your urethral opening. See it as the landscape, the no man's land, that wraps around your two holes. It's important to note because opening into the vulvar vestibule are the major and minor glands.

These major glands are called Bartholin's glands. They open into the vestibule, and, if you picture a clock, open at 4 and 8. I bring these up because sometimes these glands can develop into cysts and cause pain, so it's essential to have at least heard of them.

Another significant point to note is that the Skene's glands in your vaginal wall that extend out on either side of the urethra make up around one-third of the fluid you produce when aroused. If you've ever squirted, then this is where the squirt originated from.

The penis has an equivalent, the Cowper's glands, which release pre-ejaculate. you may have felt this during sex. (We should still avoid this fluid during our fertile windows when we track our discharge.) Initially, the vestibule developed from the urinary system, not the vagina or the outer parts of the vulva. Many kinds of sexual and vulva pain can originate from the vulvar vestibule.

Hart's line (named after David Berry Hart)
Hart's line can be seen on the inner labia minora and marks the transition between two body parts. The tissue actually changes, and this is important to note.
We are about to crawl à la Gwyneth inside our vagina.

Hymen (nothing to do with society's made-up term)
The hymen is at the entrance to the vagina and is a thin mucous ring. It has a minimal role within the overall scenario here, but it has been written about more than anything else listed in this section. There are so many myths about the hymen.

But ya know, does it really surprise us that the part of the pussy that plays a small role in the pelvis has had the most attention? We end up focusing on the hymen, getting ourselves entangled in the logistics of the hymen, until the focus is removed from the magic and power we house in our pelvis. I see that this focus from society is on purpose. So let's debunk some myths so we can move on.

Some hymens can cover the whole of the vaginal opening and then require support medically so menstrual blood can leave easily, but most have a hole or lots of holes. Some hymens only partially cover the vaginal opening. Hymens naturally tear and decrease in size over time. Tears can occur from sports, tampons or general movement. Over time, the hymen will become a perforated ring around the vaginal opening. That's literally it. Sometimes we are born without one. It is simply a piece of tissue that does its thang to move into the place it needs to be.

It has nothing to do with virginity. Virginity is heteronormative, meaning society focuses on the P in the V scenario as superior to everything else. Sex is more than all things penis in the vagina. Virginity cannot be tested. It has nothing to do with the hymen being 'intact'. It's all been made up. Wild.

All these myths around the hymen have been made up to keep you small, to prevent you from truly trusting in your body's wisdom. For example, blood from the first P in V experience could likely be a lack of lubrication. You weren't lubed up enough but instead accepted that you had something literally 'broken' in your body in order to experience pleasure. We then subconsciously associate pleasure with something that breaks and bleeds. It's just not what happens, and this language leads to more confusion. And yet the penis is free to experience pleasure.

Let's imagine if we said: 'Your penis will break a little and bleed a little when you first have penetrative sex. That's just the way it is, enjoy hun'. Imagine the new narrative.

Vagina (the key to your happiness lies in your vagina)

You cannot see your vagina, as it is an internal tube that connects your external areas (genitalia) with your womb space (uterus). It stretches from the hymen to the cervix, the mouth of the uterus. The bladder sits at the front, and the anus at the back. This is why sometimes we confuse a UTI (urinary tract infection) with vaginitis when we feel sore around the vagina.

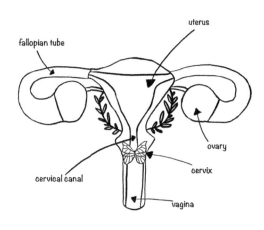

The vaginal walls often touch unless we insert something. The vagina has few nerve endings, which is why we often don't realise we have an infection until it reaches the vestibule, which is filled with nerve endings. Suddenly we feel pain or get itchy.

The walls of the vagina are made of muscle and covered with a mucus membrane. I like to remind clients that the vagina comprises the same tissue as the mouth. It's super stretchy due to it being covered in ridges called rugae. Sometimes the rugae disappear through experiences like childbirth. Rugae are like pleats of extra tissue that allow the vagina to expand. Our vagina will feel drier or wetter depending on where we are in our cycle and at certain times in our lives. I've got a whole section on all things lube for this reason. The tissue of the vaginal wall changes as hormones fluctuate in the menstrual cycle. Cells in the outer layers store glycogen to help maintain the PH level and protect the vagina from bacteria and fungi. The vagina acts as a physical barrier to the uterus, protecting it from pathogenic microorganisms.

The bladder, urethra, vagina and uterus are attached to pelvic walls by a complex system of connective tissue called the endopelvic fascia.

Understanding and then exploring the fascia in the walls of the vagina has a massive impact on the whole of your pelvis.

Cervix (here's a big mwah for the cervix)

You'll likely be most familiar with the cervix after hearing about it with all things smear test chat. It's the area they collect cells from to check for any changes. There's more support for smear tests and tools to help you get yours, as they save lives, in the 'Dear Vagina' section of this book.

The cervix is the lower part of the uterus that moves up and down and opens during birth. If you have given birth, your cervix will never close tightly again.

You can feel your cervix, although not everyone can find it with fingers. It feels a little like the end of a nose or like your lips are puckered for a kiss.

There are a couple of good positions to try to find your cervix. One would be to place one leg on a ledge, such as the edge of a toilet seat, and reach inside with two fingers. It can often be felt by placing the fingers up to the knuckles. The other position is to lie on a bed and reach around, lying flat on your back or side. As you move through your cycle, your cervix shifts.

Note: always wash your hands before rummaging for your cervix. Not everyone will feel comfortable doing this, so only do so if you are interested. I'd also recommend waiting to discover yours when you know how to enter with intention, safety and love, which we'll discuss later in the book. I'm simply sharing how you can find yours in this section.

The closer you are to ovulation, the harder it will be to locate your cervix. Essentially, your cervix lifts; it becomes soft and open as you reach ovulation and changes back to being low, firm and closed outside of this window. The difference is fascinating, and we can rely on our cervix right through perimenopause when discharge is less reliable. This is because the cervix will continue to move as it needs to if we go to ovulate in our perimenopause, whereas our body often won't produce reliable discharge at this stage in our cyclical life.

The cervical canal passes through the cervix to allow blood and babies to move from the womb to the vagina. Sperm travel along the cervical canal through the uterus and into the fallopian tubes to the ovum (egg).

I like to think of our cervix as a flower, the way it opens and closes during our cycle, allowing the sperm to easily reach the egg. Essentially the cervix moves higher to make the journey shorter for the sperm. In our discharge section, you will learn more about the plethora of support our body gives sperm.

I ran an in-person event in my hometown, Margate, and shared this. One participant snorted, 'Is there anything we don't do for men?' This is something many feel. Society has set the limelight on sperm. How powerful they are, how not to look at them else, poof, you will be with child. But we have tiny windows where our bodies do everything they can to help them survive and sniff out the egg.

The cervix produces discharge which you could also call mucus or your nectar. Whatever fits.

Uterus (also known as your womb)

This pear-shaped organ sits in the middle of your pelvic bowl, gently guided into the centre by ligaments. Considering it can accommodate a baby, it is mind-blowing to know it is only the size of a fist. The average size is around 8 cm in length and 5 cm in width. It stretches from this fist-size space to the size of a watermelon during pregnancy. Mind-blowing.

Your womb isn't just here to grow a baby. Many of us do not become pregnant. Some of us feel let down by our wombs or as though they are a hindrance.

But your womb is a magical portal tending to your creativity. It plants and grows seeds of intentions. It also allows you to have a wonderful monthly cleanse. Shitty months can be moved through and out with the power of small contractions expelling the blood that has built up.

The uterus has 'laaaayeeers'. I cannot not think of Mary Berry[ii] when I hear *layers*. Let's think of the womb as a jam doughnut.

The perimetrium is the protective outer layer (the crusty, sugary housing). The myometrium is the muscly middle, which contracts (the spongey bit of the doughnut). The endometrium is the lining of the uterus that sheds during your menstrual cycle or builds up for a growing babe (the jam bit of said doughnut).

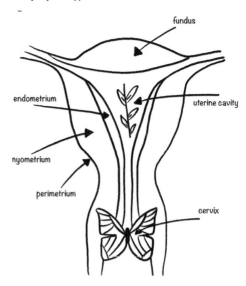

There are sections to your womb space; the fundus is the widest part at the top. Then the main body is where we plant a fertilised egg or idea. The cervix is the lowest part of the womb, where the cervix opens into the vagina.

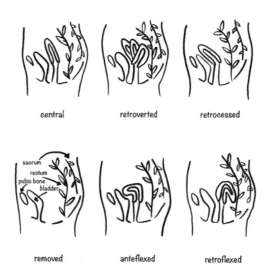

Generally, you will find that a uterus sits in an anteverted position, which means it sits forwards with the fallopian tubes slightly waving (OK, not actually waving, but you get the idea) behind. The positioning of your uterus adjusts due to things like posture, genetics, menopause and endo, to name a few examples. Some of us have a retroverted uterus, which may also be called a tipped or tilted uterus. This means

---

ii   Famous baker with many cookbooks who used to cut into cakes on *The Great British Bake Off*.

it curves back toward the spine rather than leaning forwards toward the abdomen. There's also a chance a uterus can be anteflexed, which is where it leans forwards, or retroflexed, tipped back and bent backwards.

The womb is supported by your pelvic floor muscles, perineal body, those ligaments we've mentioned already, and the lower back and hips. They keep it all in place. Working with a trained womb massage specialist can gently bring the womb back into your 'normal' position, depending on the severity of any scarring or adhesions, which can alleviate period pains or pain during sex or recurring UTIs, for example. The idea of this support is to manually release the ligaments and holding patterns of the muscles. Here are some tangible examples of how this helps.

The uterus is between the bladder and the rectum; this actually explains a few thangs when it isn't sitting slap-bang in your centre. If you feel pressure on the rectum, especially towards your period, then this is because your womb doubles in weight as it approaches menstruation. There's a chance your uterus is retroflexed. Internal organs need this fluid ability to move, but if there's a shift or if something is not quite aligned, it makes sense for their functions to be challenged.

When I see clients in my space and support them with their womb love, they often report less painful, generally easier bleeds. But we must remember that life still occurs; we must always be in tune with our womb if our body starts to speak to us and lets us know that there may be some kind of misalignment again, even after this support.

We must also remember that if we have our womb removed or anything else removed, we still hold onto the energetics of this space. We call this space, energetically, our hara. Hara is a Japanese word that hasn't an equivalent in English, which literally refers to the lower abdomen, however it also has a psychological and spiritual meaning in the Japanese culture. It is often a term used to discuss bringing our spiritual, physical and psychological bodies together as one. Everyone has a hara, whether you were assigned male or female at birth. This is the centre of our body. It's referred to as the centre of one's true nature.

Fallopian tubes (teamwork makes the dream work)

There's a right fallopian tube and a left fallopian tube—arms, if you will—that extend from each side of the uterus near the top. The tubes really are tube-like and extend roughly 10–12 cm, where they open at the ovaries; however, they aren't directly attached. They have fimbriae, Latin for fringe, to sweep any eggs into the tubes and down towards the uterus. The egg (ovum) is fertilised in the fallopian tube. It then carries on to the womb before getting nested in the uterus lining.

The tubes use a wave-like motion to move the egg, plus they have cilia hairs to support chivying the egg along. We also have cilia hairs in our noses and cervix. Gosh, our body is incredible.

OK, actually, this next fact blows my mind.

Minus a fallopian tube? No worries, hunz. The fallopian tube will move to the other ovary and get the egg. It literally moves over, picks it up and moves it along. The kind of sidekick we all deserve.

I just want to mention something I share with clients on a conception journey. I feel here would be the perfect place. If the tests show the sperm is excellent (while your other half is patriarchally peacocking around as a result of having super sperm), we should always have our fallopian tubes checked. The number of people who do not have their tubes checked by professionals blows my mind. An aqua scan, a HyCoSy, uses clever 3D ultrasound technology to check fallopian tubes. You will likely have to pay for it here in the UK; it isn't something you'd receive in the NHS (highly unlikely), but having one can save people a lot of money and emotional pain in the long run.

Ovaries (a pair of walnuts)

The size of walnuts, they house more than 100,000 eggs when we are born. We develop around 8,000 follicles, but know that these don't all become the dominant follicle that then releases as an egg.

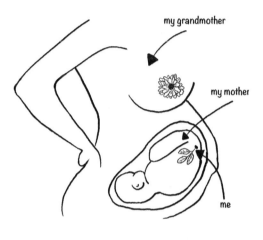

We can form a beautiful image here in our minds of being a cup in our mother's cup. Then your mother is a cup in your grandmother's cup. Think of it like a Russian doll if that helps with this image. The egg that made you was inside your mother when she was growing in your grandmother. This can lead down a path of ancestral holding patterns that we carry in our womb spaces. Often clients may say that they don't feel the pain they are holding is theirs. And it may not be.

Think of your ovaries as equivalent of testicles. A pair of balls with a lot of gumption produces eggs in most cycles. They produce oestradiol, progesterone and testosterone, hormones that are all part of the menstrual cycle's monthly dance-off.

The biggest cycle event occurs with your ovaries. The egg literally bursts from your ovary. Some people feel this pang or get a small amount of pain, but this should be a short blip out of the day. It's called *mittelschmerz* (German for 'pain in the middle of the month'). Some of us don't notice this occurring at all.

Coccyx (your tail bone's connected to your)

I wanted to mention the coccyx here because it often goes unnoticed yet plays an essential role in all things experiencing pleasure.

If you ever had a hard fall on your bottom, such as when you were a child, skiing, snowboarding or horse riding, there can be a lot going on in the coccyx.

It's a triangular-shaped structure at the very bottom of the vertebral column.

There are three to five bony sections held in place by joints and ligaments. We can experience more injuries due to a broader pelvis; thus, the coccyx is more exposed.

Impacts on the coccyx can create further tightening throughout the rest of the pelvis and within the pelvic floor. It makes sense, as it is all connected. In a study by Meloy in 1998,[6] he showed how in his female patients, if he placed electrodes in the 'right place' to stimulate pleasure, they interacted with various nerve networks, including nerves from the pelvis that then entered the spinal highway near the tailbone. This stimulation shoots pleasure signals up to the brain, which processes incoming information from the root (genitalia).

There's also evidence of a sacral orgasm, which is a way of stimulating the nerves in the lower back area.

So you see, the coccyx does deserve love and attention, and as a side effect, there will likely be the ability to move through holding patterns and find more pleasure.

Pelvic bowl (the whole lot)

I will often refer to the pelvic bowl in this book because it is a beautiful way of bringing rooted presence to our centres.

Our pelvic bowl is home to all of the above, as well as the root chakra and mula bandha lock.

All spinal and hip joint movement comes from the pelvis, using a network of muscles that form your pelvic floor. Visualise the edges of the bowl. This would be from the hip points across and down to the tips of the labia and back around. Imagine your bowl is filled with magical liquid gold contained by bringing in awareness and excellent posture.

The pelvic bowl houses our delicate rooted system, and we all know the roots' importance to any organism. This is why working with our roots first and foremost is the key to thriving and blooming into all that we are.

Throat and vagina (open your vagina, voice your needs)

While diving into all things bowl, let's also take a moment to tune into the connections our root has with the rest of the body.

Our vagina is linked to our throat. A vocal vagina correlation. The cervix means neck, and the throat has a very similar structure to the vagina. Singing, orgasming, and childbirth are powered by muscular pulsations. If our voice or vagina is shut down, then we have also turned away from finding what it is we truly need on our path to long-lasting happiness.

The vagus nerve links the throat with the pelvis. This is the largest nerve in our body and connects the brainstem to the sacral nerve plexus. About 80–90 percent of the vagus nerve is sensory, responding to movement and stimulation. Vagus means 'wanderer', which makes sense as the nerves wander through the body. The vagus does, in fact, go to the cervix, uterus and vagina. Impulses from those regions travel up through the abdomen, diaphragm, chest, neck and brain.

When you think about it, people will flippantly say, 'Dig deep to express your needs', 'Take in a deep inhale and then speak your truth', etc.

We want our breath to utilise our lung capacity every time we breathe. If our breath is taken deeper, it activates the parasympathetic nervous system (the nervous system that brings in rest and restore). Breath brings power to the voice, and our voice's vibrations stimulate the vagus nerve, sending relief through the body. As we vocalise our needs, we allow ourselves to bring more comfort to any tension or anxiousness we may be holding. And as we learn to understand our needs, we drop into our bodies and into pleasure more. The side-effect of all of this is a vagina-throat connection which works in tandem.

Jaw and pelvic floor link (grindin')

To deepen into the pelvis one final time before we finish up and explore more of the above content, later on, there's also a link between our jaw and pelvic floor.

Fascia is the connective tissue connecting up everything, including muscles, organs, bones, and nerve fibres. Holding everything in place. A fascial line runs from the pelvic floor to the muscles in the jaw. When talking or toning, this can impact the pelvic floor. Low tones and humming can relax the pelvic floor, while high tones can contract it.

Often those in childbirth are reminded to unclench the jaw so the root relaxes.

So if you are a clencher, consider whether this clenching is in the jaw, root, or maybe both.

But for now, you've made it. You've explored all of your bowl, your inner landscape. You likely need a break. So break (or recess, if you're American) has begun.

After your break, when you've finished queuing for the toilets (because even schools forget that we sit down to pee), we're diving into all things discharge.

Wet, Wet, Wet

I feel it in my fingers ... no, *you* heard Marti Pellow singing, 'Love is All Around' when thinking about the title of this section on all things discharge. Still a classic, though, isn't it?

Cervical discharge is the liquid you feel in your knickers, at your vulva or when you insert your fingers into your vagina. We also call it mucus or just discharge. You can call it magical nectar. Whatever suits. But essentially, your discharge offers you a lot of information.

So my advice at this point in the book is not to skip. Read it all, take it in and try these keys given to you on these pages.

This is a gift from you to you.

When people turn their noses up at all things cervical discharge, it's simply a lack of education about the topic. I posted pictures of discharge on my social account, and the uproar! How dare I post a picture of water on my page? How weird. She's, like, so gross. *Immediately hits the unfollow button*.

We don't mind a bit of snot chat. We watch sports players snot-rocket all over the pitch and don't bat an eyelid. Imagine if we started snot-rocketing from our cunts all over the pavements. We don't mind a dribble of snot leaving someone's nose; we may simply say something like, 'Oh, got a bit of dribble there, babe'. If we had a bit of mucus running down our legs while waiting for the bus, would the reaction be as meh? Nope.

It's just another bodily fluid.

Though, if we all truly understood the importance of this vital sign, we would feel empowered, more at home with our bodies and able to find our fertile and infertile days. We'd be able to time sex perfectly to avoid or achieve pregnancy. We'd finally sack off any panty liners we wear and feel the moist love from within.

Not understanding our discharge paves the way for patriarchal control. It does. Plenty of things are linked to our lack of knowledge on all things root-based liquid that brings money to someone somewhere. Some examples include panty liners, ovulation tests, contraceptives, morning-after pill, etc. These all have a place, but they'd be less necessary in a world where we were all educated about our discharge.

This information is still for you even if you are on contraception and don't have the usual discharge dance. This chat aims to empower you with the knowledge you need to feel in awe of your discharge rather than feeling frustrated or even disgusted by what you find in your knickers daily.

We are going to dive into it, goggles on, hunz (I joke . . . kind of):
· What is discharge?
· How our cycle works
· The different kinds of discharge we have monthly
· How to monitor your discharge

It's time to return to your root-based liquid love language, darling soul.

Discharge is made up of water and mucin. Mucin is glycoprotein, sugar and salts. It comprises water: 90–95 percent rising to 98–99 percent before ovulation. Seriously—it's mainly just water. Who knew? Not many, unfortunately. We are here to normalise it, and just you reading this chapter supports this. Thank YOU for being here. Seriously. You are a mucus cheerleading hero (at least you will be cheerleading it by the end of this section).

Give me a D-I-S-C-H-A-R-G-E . . . go discharge, go discharge pattern, go mucus, go cervical crypts. You're amazing. We love you. Yay!

Have I ramped this up enough yet . . .

Too keen? I don't care.

My own children will be learning all about theirs from the get-go.

I want you to be empowered to find your cervical discharge pattern. If you are ever unsure about yours or are concerned, you must raise this with your healthcare provider. Equally, if you have bleeding which seems out of sorts, again, this should be checked. You should also get checked out if your mucus shows odd signs, such as being particularly smelly or lumpy, or you are generally itchy. You can read more about this on Eve Appeal's website for further support.[7]

The Monthly Dance

The HPO axis is absolutely key here. The conversation between the components of your HPO is so essential for your overall fertile health.

The hypothalamus, pituitary gland and ovaries are the three organs which secrete hormones and interact with each other; this interaction is known as the HPO axis. The menstrual cycle is controlled by this interaction.

The information here is *a lot*, and it can seem overwhelming. The idea of this is just so you have an idea of how the hormone dance works.

Glossary:

- **GnRH:** Gonadotropin-releasing hormone
- **FSH:** Follicle-stimulating hormone
- **LH:** Luteinising hormone
- **TSH:** Thyroid-stimulating hormone

Your monthly cycle goes like this, bear with:

- **Hypothalamus:** supports body-regulating functions, e.g. temp and appetite; produces GnRH in short pulses. The GnRH then stimulates the pituitary gland.
- **Pituitary Gland:** This produces FSH and LH. Your FSH stimulates immature follicles in the ovary and the secretion of oestrogen.
- Your oestrogen reaches a peak. Sixteen hours after this peak oestrogen moment in blood levels, there will be a surge in LH.
- This surge of LH means the biggest egg (most mature follicle) leaves, and the corpus luteal left behind stimulates progesterone. This progesterone that is produced inhibits FSH. Progesterone also stops the production of LH. Oxytocin, anti-diuretic, and thyroid-stimulating hormone (TSH) are also being produced.
- **Ovaries:** GnRH is inhibited by the ovarian hormones oestrogen and progesterone.
- You bleed if there hasn't been any fertilisation.

And so the cycle repeats every single month.

- In other words, your body tickles itself to produce hormones.
- These hormones tickle the ovaries (think feather duster/magic hands) to grow
  the egg.
- The egg reaches its peak size and is pushed out of its little nest.
- Your body stops the original tickle, so no more eggs are grown.
- Hormones drop, you bleed, and the tickle begins again, providing there hasn't been any fertilisation.

- When this conversation runs smoothly, your oestrogen stimulates the production of your cervical mucus, which plays a crucial role in getting the sperm to the egg. Hence the need to produce fertile mucus.

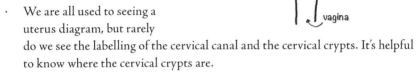

- We are all used to seeing a uterus diagram, but rarely do we see the labelling of the cervical canal and the cervical crypts. It's helpful to know where the cervical crypts are.
- These crypts are where we find our cervical mucus. They are like little folds through which the mucus flows in and out.

In our cervical canal, we find different cells which have two functions.

Secretory cells:
- These secrete mucus in response to oestrogen
- They are covered in finger-like membrane protrusions called microvilli which increase surface area

Ciliated cells:
- These beat in a wavelike motion to propel sperm upwards towards the uterus to find the mature egg
- They are covered in hairlike structures known as cilia

Think how your snot is similar to your discharge, and you totally get how it all works. Also, a reminder of how our root matches our throat. It makes sense that it all works very similarly.

So now that we are a little more aware of the monthly hormone dance, let's discuss the monthly dance and your discharge.

As we move from our period towards ovulation, our mucus changes from infertile to fertile. It then switches back to infertile after ovulation as we move back towards our period again.

Ovulation, where we reach our peak mucus day, is the biggest event of our cycle and should be honoured and celebrated whether you aim to use it or don't.

Our bodies are magical, cyclical and incredible. We should always take time to rest and honour this big event where we can.

The diagram on the next page shows the cycle of moving from dry to fertile and back to dry again. I'm using the term 'dry' loosely. For some, you may never feel dry like the Sahara; you may always feel a little damp, wet, moist.

For example, you may always produce mucus every single day. We are all different, but the key is to tune into how it changes over your cycle.

As you will have already noted, I try to clarify that everyone's mucus pattern is individual. No two people will match exactly, which is why I firmly believe in carefully making your own daily mucus sign notes using language that works for you.

Here's what happens.

Start of discharge production directly after your bleed:
- · You may feel dry or none
- · Scant or sticky means this is the start of the fertile stage
- · Any sign of any discharge means you are fertile from that moment on until post ovulation

ripening follicle · ovulation · corpus luteum

oestrogen · progesterone

period · dry · fertile phase · dry

p123

As the discharge increases towards ovulation:
- · Fertile mucus showing to be stretchier/tackier
- · Feelings of being damp. Maybe even wet at the vulva ('sensation at vulva')
- · Dense in appearance. The swimming lanes in your discharge are opening up.

Being super close to ovulation day means discharge will be increasing and becoming clearer:
- · There's more water content
- · Discharge stretches and becomes clearer
- · Likely to be much wetter at the vulva

Your peak discharge stage:
- · Wet, clear, stretchy, slippery
- · Not necessarily always clear but more transparent (and sometimes you may miss this stage, so keep a beady eye on your tissue and knickers)
- · Sometimes even reddish if blood is lost at ovulation (you know, it literally bursts from your body)
- · Ovulation is very close. You are looking for your PEAK day.

Post ovulation:
- · Mucus dries, becomes thick, sticky and may even disappear altogether.

As you move towards your bleed, your discharge may be dry, or there will be a BIP (basic infertile pattern) for you to track, which means your discharge will remain the same each day from now on until the next cycle begins.

Why the different types of discharge, though? Let's explore them.

Infertile mucus

We can categorise infertile mucus as the mucus that happens after confirmed ovulation. Any sign of mucus pre-ovulation is considered fertile, even if it is white and thick. This is because sperm can live for up to six days in mucus; thus, if you ovulate and sperm are present, it is important to time it all correctly. This is why working with a gal like myself, a certified fertility awareness practitioner, can help you navigate your discharge. Believe me, I offered my support to a sex influencer for an upcoming video on tracking her cycle when I saw she was using 23,445 apps for comparison's sake. Post-chat, I lost count of the times she emailed me to ask questions. I loved every question, as it shows us we deserve this support. Apps aren't all that useful when genuinely getting to know your infertile and fertile patterns. But they are a great starting point. I advise exploring the 'Read Your Body' app as another option if apps feel the most accessible to you. This is currently the most editable app out there. It's the best of the best by a long shot.

To confirm you are post-ovulation, there is a 0.2 degree rise in your body temperature over three or four days when using the symptothermal method. Each person's confirmed post-ovulation infertile mucus will present itself differently. Usually, post-ovulation infertile mucus is thick, creamy, white mucus where you generally feel moist at vulva, dry or Sahara dry.

When someone is in the menopausal years, post-contraception or breastfeeding, we look for their BIP (basic infertile pattern). This is when we look at the daily mucus, which is classed as infertile because it is their BIP. It doesn't change from this for weeks or months. However, when we know the BIP, and one day there is a change after eight weeks of no changes, we know something is occurring, i.e., there's a chance of ovulation.

Fertile mucus

Fertile mucus is classed as such as soon as you see any at all after a period. Any mucus is considered fertile until you have confirmed ovulation.

However, you will find your discharge changes as you move towards ovulation. The changes you experience are personal to you. For some, they will find they experience stretchy egg white discharge. Others feel super wet, and it's slippery, transparent, or both. Your pattern is just that—yours. No comparison is needed, but you are looking for a change.

As FAM (fertility awareness methods) practitioners, we are trained to discuss 'highly fertile mucus'.

You can use any kind of language that you feel suits you, but in general, I teach my clients to use adjectives: tacky, stretchy, wet, stretchy, transparent, clear, and egg white. Stick to the same adjectives each month.

Key practice:

Even if you are on hormonal contraceptives, your first key task in the book is to begin to peruse your discharge. Simply take time to be more aware of your discharge. That's all. No need to write anything down yet. Just become aware of the 'sensation at vulva' and what lands in your pants.

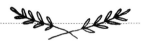

Mesh mucus vs motorway mucus

There are two types of mucus, and it's important to note there is a difference.

Acidic, mesh-type mucus, which we commonly describe as white and thick, is like a barrier, your personal gatekeeper, your 'no thanks, hun' discharge. It prevents further sperm from entering further into the cervix and also kills sperm off. How clever. Once you have ovulated, your body relies on any sperm already present to reach the egg. After this, if the egg isn't fertilised, what's the point of more sperm coming in? The cycle will now produce progesterone, and the LH surge has been and gone. Things have changed, so oestrogen is no longer being made, and the mucus changes back to infertile, mesh-type alkaline mucus.

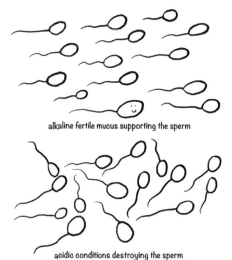

alkaline fertile mucus supporting the sperm

acidic conditions destroying the sperm

When you are super fertile, you have motorway mucus. The lanes open (if you looked under a microscope, it is like open lanes vs a mesh-type appearance). The sperm are welcome to zoom straight through. It's the M1 down there,[iii] and nothing can stop them now. The mucus feeds the sperm with fructose, keeping them alive while checking for the best little swimmers and supporting them only. Survival of the fittest. Your discharge is magical, babes, like seriously clever stuff.

A note on pregnancy mucus

Many who get pregnant find they have lovely discharge in their pants but sometimes panic because it can sometimes feel like A LOT. Some may not feel much at all. Either way, it is essential to note that mucus is absolutely normal (unless you think it itches, smells in a particular way, or you just feel it has changed for you in a way you

---

[iii] One of the clearer UK motorways.

aren't sure about, in which case it's always worth asking your midwife). It could be sticky, white, or pale yellow. It often begins early in the first trimester and continues throughout pregnancy. There's more blood going to your vagina, and your hormone levels—for example, oestrogen—rise; thus, you may experience extra discharge. It also has an essential job of preventing infections while your cervix and vaginal walls get softer for birth prep. Honestly incredible.

Liners

Some people feel wet and wear liners. It is entirely understandable to feel this way. The best advice I can give is to avoid them if you can. If you feel you need liners, grab some reusable or 100 percent organic cotton ones because mainstream brands include chemicals in theirs. Said chemicals create a potential hotbed for infections, further disconnect you from your natural magic and also add to the list of endocrine disrupters you are in contact with (pesky hormonally active agents that mimic your natural hormones).

BBT

BBT stands for basal body temperature and is included when using the symptothermal method. So there are a couple of primary cycle tracking methods. One is the Billings Method, where you only track your discharge, nothing else. Then there is the symptothermal method, where you take your temperature after a minimum of three hours of sleep, upon waking. You are looking for a 0.2-degree rise to prove ovulation. This rise is a result of the production of progesterone. Apps are based on the symptothermal method. You don't need a fancy thermometer for this, just a thermometer that goes to two decimal places. You can then track your discharge alongside your BBT. This can be of use if someone is on the path of welcoming a babe into their womb. Before a period, your progesterone drops, so your basal body temperate drops back to pre-ovulation temperature. If you were tracking and your temperature didn't fall and your period didn't arrive, you'd know you had a successful cycle—there was implantation. But if you saw it drop a couple of days or the day before your period was due, you'd be able to see what was going on when on the conception journey. This saves taking three million pregnancy tests and looking for every sign of a successful cycle.

Before your bleed

You may also note that before your bleed, you get an increased amount of discharge. Again, this is entirely normal when the progesterone starts to drop.

Key practice (how to track and actually remember the changes):
Another daily task, similar to the last one, is to tune into your discharge, but this time to wipe before you pee. Yeppers. If you wipe before ya pee, you'll tune into how you're feeling at your vulva. Remember, it's the 'sensation at vulva'. No

need to rummage.

We suffer from cycle amnesia. So though you think you will remember you had thick, white, creamy mucus on day six, you will not remember this in your next cycle.

Note down your changes daily. Create a daily habit. Utilise a diary, notepad, calendar or app that allows you to note down your discharge. Every day write down what appears in your pants or how you feel at the vulva. After around three months, you will begin to see your discharge pattern and tune into your magical mucus.

My recommendation when teaching FAM is to simply watch throughout the day and then note down your observations just before bed.

You can see changes in your pants, at the opening to your vagina or on the tissue as you wipe. Whatever works best for you. (But no rummaging.)

Utilise the words below to help you describe it each day, and if none of those words helps, make up your own. This is so that when you look back at it, you will remember what you were describing so you can be consistent each month.

My advice is to keep in mind SCAT:

- Sensation
- Colour
- Amount
- Texture

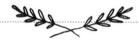

Facts for your next pub quiz and a round-up of all things discharge

The mucus is a fluid secreted by the glands in the cervix lining under oestrogen influence.

It is whitish to clear and made up of water and mucin. Mucin is glycoprotein, sugar and salts. It's 90–95 percent water rising to 98–99 percent water before ovulation.

When we observe a change of sensation from dry to moist, we know our fertile phase has started.

Mucus is essential for achieving pregnancy as it controls the transportation of sperm.

Sperm survive three hours in the air and six hours in the vagina but seven days in fertile, alkaline mucus.

During the infertile phases of the cycle, the environment in the vagina is acidic, and sperm cannot survive in this environment.

When the cervical mucus is alkaline in the fertile phases of the cycle, it neutralises the acidic environment in the vagina, which is why sperm then survive in the vagina under these conditions.

Mucus acts as a filtering system. It has its own built-in Tinder. Not every sperm is perfect due to the speed at which they are produced. Cervical mucus will sift out the sperm that are less likely to fertilise the ovum (egg). It acts as quality control. Clipboards at the ready.

The mucus is a magnet for sperm. If genital contact occurs during the fertile phase, the sperm will be taken in without full penetration. In fact even the sperm at the tip of the penis in the alkaline lubricative fluid from the Cowper's glands can be taken into the vagina through the cervix and into the uterus.

Thick mucus is hostile to sperm. It blocks the canal, and sperm cannot enter.

Sperm are nourished by fructose in fertile mucus.

When oestrogen stimulates the cervical crypts to produce fertile mucus, it acts as a motorway mucus so the sperm can zoom straight in and towards the egg.

The egg is only receptive to sperm for ten hours. (And we wonder why we shut down our cycles completely, yet sperm are consistently produced and always fertile.) Those assigned male at birth can have around two hundred children in their lifetime. Two hundred. Women and those assigned female at birth can have between fifteen and thirty depending on recovery time.

That's a whole quiz round right there. You're welcome.

Hello, it's you you've been looking for.

Celebrating you and your discharge.

Looking after number one

When I refer to number one. I mean your vagina.

Let's consider some vagina love right now. If you are tuning into your beautiful vulva, then let's look after your number one.

Some dos and don'ts advised:

Liners: Let's try and ditch them. Let me explain why. They pop chemicals in liners, and these upset the delicate PH balance of your vagina. Though, of course, many feel they need liners. I get it. You can feel very wet, and it can almost feel uncomfortable. But it's best to change your knickers or invest in reusable liners or even light-period pants. Liners from big brands include chemicals. Here's a statement from a large brand's website: 'All our products meet rigorous safety and effectiveness standards, regardless of what they are made of. Our panty liners are designed to provide high levels of protection and comfort. The materials used in our panty liners better enable us to deliver these performance needs'. They essentially disregard the ingredients they use. Though they could be 100 percent organic cotton (and this is an option), they choose to not include these in their mass-produced liners, so they include things like scent because, apparently, our vaginas need to smell like roses. All in all, it's best to look around for other options and try and empower yourself to let your mucus free-flow in your knickers so you can monitor it easily. You could also transition to some organic or reusable ones to begin with, as a stepping stone.

Douching: Don't douche. Giving your pelvis a rinse with some water is absolutely fine. But some people clean theirs with chemicals. Such washes can upset the PH balance of your vagina, which can then increase the chances of an infection.

Feminine washes: Avoid them. They are marketed to tell you that you need to clean and rinse. To be odourless. In actual fact, as mentioned above, these alter your delicate balance and should just be avoided. Simply wash with water, and you could grab the shower head and focus on that area for a deeper clean.

Use organic or reusable if financially possible. When it comes to tampons and liners from those non-organic brands, they are filled with chemicals. These aren't looked into enough. To make these products even more absorbent, they often use rayon, a chemical without a safe exposure limit. So it is advised to always go organic, i.e. 100 percent organic cotton or reusable. Save your vagina and the planet. Win-win. But granted, they are pricier. However, if you often suffer from infections, painful periods, bloating or heavier bleeds, you must try to see if you can make a change. Use organic options or reusable options, or you can even free-bleed into a designated towel on the floor. This may sound like a wild concept, but on those heavier days, if you can be home to do this, try it.

Change your tampons every 4–6 hours. Tampons aren't supposed to be in for hours on end; you all know that because they talk about toxic shock. No reported cases of toxic shock with an organic product have been reported. But to keep your vagina happy, you should change every 4–6 hours. If you simply can't afford organic and are using absorbent tampons from mainstream brands, then it is super essential you change more regularly than you think, following these guidelines. In fact, the biggest problem is not the length of time. It's the fibres that are left behind from the non-organic tampons. These little fibres contain chemicals, creating a breeding ground for bacteria in your vagina. Organic tampons don't shed. You must also try and use the correct absorbency. When removed, your tampons should be filled with blood, as they are less likely to leave said fibres behind; they should not be dry where possible.

The Big Shutdown

Over the years, our voices, needs and bodies have been shut down. I am not beating around anyone's bush here when I speak to the shutdown of the feminine. There are many ways in which the feminine has been shut down. Still, we continue to find it challenging to advocate for our rights. From fourteen-year-olds being told the pill is their best option before their HPO axis has fully matured at twenty-one, to those being told hospital birth is safer than home birth. We need you. We need you here reading these words because the way I view it, this book is a silent protest. You are reading this book with its bold front cover daring to splash the word *vagina* for all to see; you go, hun. You are a modern-day hero. An activist. Just think, you will go through the steps and create a new relationship for yourself with your pelvis, which will have a ripple effect on all those around you. This is you changing the narrative as you open your heart and soul to this work. Here's to you. I am celebrating you for being here.

This pilgrimage into the yoni makes us more deeply rooted into life. See this as an awakening of your root. See this as a slow but necessary awakening for the generations coming through. The older generation may sometimes mock the Gen Zs coming through. But I absolutely can't get enough of the generations coming through asking, 'What the fuck? No, seriously, why?' This current age of TikTok proves that we are asking critical questions; there's a thirst for knowledge because I believe the generations will know there's more to life than what has been presented. My reference to TikTok will date this book in time. But the age of TikTok will go down in history as the time when younger generations were asking questions we weren't asking. I'm not advocating for TikTok—I'm advocating for those wanting answers.

I write this chapter as I approach my thirty-fourth birthday. I seriously feel bereft that I didn't know this. I took those purple pills daily, slapped on the moisturiser that did nothing for my skin for years, and was numb to sex and the joys of life. Genuinely. I am in my thirties, feeling alive. I don't say this to sell my work. I say this because I feel it, and those around me think this for me too. Maybe it's because I moved from my maiden to mother years too, but moving into the power that lies in my centre has brought me from feeling shut down to an awakened state I can't put into words. I just feel alive . . . finally. This was triggered by the fact that I began questioning life. Questioning the options laid out for me previously. I knew I wanted more for myself, finally.

Bertrand and Bertrand write how the remembrance of womb consciousness is as vital to men as it is to women.[8] We were all created and birthed through a womb and within womb consciousness. This primordial and transformative energy flows within every part of our being, regardless of gender.

We all house a centre; even without a womb, we have our energetic hara. If there has been a hysterectomy, we speak of the blueprint of the womb. This work, as you know, is more than just working with our physical organs. We are working with the creative, sacred magic that lies within our centres. It's this that has been shut down.

The research into feminine health is minimal. It's piss-poor. Society knows it. I mean, we only have to look at the uproar over the Covid-19 vaccine. This isn't a for or against it paragraph. Don't close the book on me just yet.

What happened was that they ignored the necessity to check for the gender differences involved with how Covid-19 behaved in the wild and in the trials for the injection, which is crucial when developing a vaccine.[9] Case fatality rates were higher for males vs females. A quarter of the studies included twice as many males as females.[10] What then occurred was confusion galore. Pregnant women were left perplexed: Do I, or don't I? There were over thirty thousand reports of changes in the menstrual cycle, with people left with heavy periods or AWOL periods.[11] Honestly, as someone in this field, it was a wild ride to watch it all unfold. I had scared clients trying to conceive, googling what it all meant. The point is there was a ridiculous amount of ignorance, yet again.

People were turning to socials for the facts—brilliant—creating more confusion.

Newspaper articles squashed these fears. Panic not. 'Everyone needs to calm down; it's in your head'. Or, 'Ya know, hunz, these changes are likely because you're a little bit stressed'. Were our voices shut down during the pandemic jab crisis? Of course.

Meanwhile, it was all kicking off on socials when articles were circulating about the risk of blood clots; people were up in arms. Suddenly many were refusing to get the jab altogether because of this blood clot risk. In April 2021, one in 250,000 were at risk of getting a blood clot as a result of having the Covid-19 vaccine, while 1 in 1000 are at risk of getting a blood clot when taking the pill. So yeah, of course, there was backlash around how people for years have been risking blood clots while on the pill, and no one had taken a moment to notice until both men and women were subjected to a vaccine with a much lower blood clot risk.

Native Americans honoured the bleed through the red tent ritual of placing those bleeding into a separate space. They were listened to for their dreams, and insights were taken and heard. They considered this to be a more creative time and when they were more in tune with the spirit world. And this happens to us if we can pause, communicate and listen to the wisdom of our bleed. Except in general, we are either on contraceptives (there's zero judgement here, but know this does, of course, shut down the natural rhythm of a cycle) or life is busy, and we don't have the time or know-how to start to tune into our bleeds like this. We have jobs that require us to crack on (though, of course, some workplaces honour periods more, whether for the kudos or because they actually care).

Once, the birther to all was known as the Great Whore. In the Middle East, in the Semitic languages, *hor* means cave or womb. The birther was known as the 'Womb of Light' or the 'harlot'. We are here to reclaim our inner harlot, the womb of light, our inner whore. Great whores, unite. This is the kinda club I wanna be part of.

To be honest, this is why many people land in my space or on my socials. This is likely what brought about this book. Your light may have been dimmed in some way, and you may be ready to claim back your inner power, which stems from a deeply rooted inner knowing. In your centre, the dimly lit light is calling you, ready to be turned all the way up to the full beam.

You may be ready to claim back little pieces taken from you from flippant comments, disregard for your needs or traumas to your body from the hands of others. I hear you.

I'm going to dive into a few of the ways you may have been silenced.

Sanitary Wear

The fact shops have signs for sanitary wear, and we've all grown up asking, 'Have you any spare *sanitary towels*' under toilet cubicle doors, is enough to show us how problematic period products have been and continue to be.

What's the word *sanitary* got to do with being silenced? I hear you silently question while simultaneously running through the current products you use in your mind. Well, sanitary means to be clean, right? So to be hygienic, clean, and to dispose of something. You get the idea. So every time you use the word, you subconsciously believe you need to be clean during your bleed. Bleeding is clearly a dirty act.

This explains why Ted didn't text you back when you started bleeding on one of your date nights all over Ted's bed.

Our bleeds are a wonderful cleanse; they aren't dirty. But what we believe, and how 'they' share all things menstrual bleeds, is that it is a dirty act when we bleed. This results in us shutting down from our cycles, ignoring the power that comes from our bleeds, and indeed ensures we continue to throw money at some potentially below-par period products. Some organic companies or hard-working beings are on a mission to bring you reusable organic cotton period products. But some companies pile a whole load of chemicals into their products.

Pre-2017, if you were watching period company adverts, they were pouring blue liquid onto a pad. Hun, I don't know about your period, but mine certainly isn't the colour of those blue men bobbing their heads in the Eiffel 65 'Blue (Da Ba Dee)' music video. Or the colour of the blue sanitary cleaner residue left in public toilets worldwide.

Obviously, we continue to create more shame and taboo around the bleed by using blue food colouring instead. We all know the media won't be there catching someone's bleed in a cup to prove to you how absorbent their (chemically filled) pads are on a TV commercial going out when Brenda is about to sit down for her afternoon scone with red jam. But it genuinely was revolutionary when they started using the colour of blood on the tele in 2017. I'll let that sink in: this only began in 2017. They wrote newspaper articles all about it and everything. The cynic in me celebrates those companies who got on the bandwagon to make a few more sales for 'breaking taboo'.

Menstrual blood was revered in ancient societies before we replaced it with blue liquid to avoid offending the patriarchy's eyes. Healing properties, history, birth and renewal are all held within menstrual blood.

We can refer to menstrual blood as our feminine wisdom. It's associated with Mary Magdalene, the prophet of all prophets, ya know, the woman torn out of the Bible. After Jesus's death, Magdalene went on to teach and guide us through love and womb renewal. This only further suggests the understanding that menstruation is the gateway to God. And when we refer to God, we mean however you refer to God: your guides, lightworkers, higher self, ancestors, the universe, Mother Earth. Let's not close our minds off when we hear 'God' thanks to previous experiences; let's rewrite this and open our hearts/minds to the idea of support from our greater selves/guides in whatever form they take.

To really tap into the energy of our blood, we must take the time to consider a womb space as a portal of renewal. We come from the dark and into the light, renewed. A resurrection, if you will. We talk about going into the belly of the earth and coming out changed. The list is endless when it comes to comparisons.

Witches have been persecuted for using their knowledge and traditions around the power of menstrual blood.

Stem cells held within the womb were believed to only be activated with pure love, which gave rise to courtly love. Ya know, the kind of love from knights, troubadours.

I am trying to clarify that those bleeding should be honoured and cherished. Instead, the power has been misused over the years or minimised.

'Virgins' have been sought after, believed to have the 'perfect womb spaces'. Those with their first menstruation are told they are suddenly ready for marriage. In some communities, they are taken out of education and forced into motherhood as young as ten.

Wombs and bleeds hold such power. This is ripped from young menstruators.

Periods are seen as a portal to the higher realms, the path to heaven. We aren't often aware of this. Menstruators are instead abused, gaslighted and silenced.

It all makes sense when you consider how lucid we are during our periods. Where we can literally birth creativity and love in ways we can't do the rest of the cycle. Our hormones are at their lowest, and we are the closest we ever are with spirit during menstruation.

And if you think some of the above sounds far too wild for you right now, just consider that menstrual blood is only now being looked into for its ability to heal with menstrual blood stem cells. Stem cells really do respond to love, desire and intention.

We often feel disconnected from our bleed, body and pelvis due to subliminal messages. We aren't learning about how incredible our bleeds are. Nope. Instead, we are presented with a white advert, a white pad lying on a white table with one of those glass jugs that look similar to the ones in our science lessons, pouring blue food colouring onto said white pad.

And don't forget, hun, you can get the scented pads, so your fanny smells freshhhhh.

Don't underestimate the power of this kind of shutdown.

I advise all to check the ingredients of their pads, tampons and pants moving forward. If you can afford 100 percent organic cotton (not just wood pulp in the centre, which some organic companies have), switch. Find inclusive brands that use terms representative of your cycle and who care about your body and the planet. These exist. You likely won't find them in supermarkets or big healthcare shops.

The pill

You do not have a true period, true bleed, when you are on the pill.

The pill shuts down your cycle, so the monthly dance no longer occurs. This means you do not release an egg. If you don't release an egg, then there isn't anything for the always fertile, loaded with sperm penises to fertilise.

Nothing is perfect; I have had clients who have gotten pregnant on the pill. Plenty of them, in fact.

There are no guaranteed contraceptives. OK, except one: never, ever have sex near sperm again.

For some of you, that is entirely possible, but for others, the reality is you'll have to find a method that works for you.

The pill has a place for some of us. It also has a dark side, and I believe, in a book sharing all things finding your happiness, if you are already questioning the pill and its impact on your body, I think it is necessary to disseminate this information. It's not to shame anyone; it's simply to highlight how shut down our voices have always been when trying to regain control of our bodies. As always, we simply need to be informed when the pill is offered.

At the end of this book, the aim is that you will have taken away some tangible tools to take back this control.

A few years ago, during Black History Month, I shared the pill's history on my Instagram page; one person who had followed me for years felt ultimately attacked by it all. I understand how challenging reading the below may feel. Sit with it, feel into it, and allow it to land. It's up to you what you then do with it.

I am damning of the pill here, but take what you will from this section. It's your body, your rights, your choice.

Margaret Sanger marketed herself as a women's advocate. Women's reproductive rights start here, hunz. She opened a clinic and got arrested in the face of trying to support women. She coined the term 'birth control' . . . except Mags was really in it for eugenics.

On the surface, Sanger pushed for people to have autonomy over their bodies. But we know now that contraceptives are used to take away our power and control in so many respects. Many of us have asked for help with period pains, endometriosis, or AWOL periods, only to be handed a prescription with a smile: 'You need to help yourself; here's the pill'. We often shut down our cycles because that is hella easier than actually diving into our needs. Or at least, easier for the doctor.

Essentially, the pill acts as a silencer in some cases. It's like, 'Aw, you got some little period-based issues you are struggling with, here's the pill'.

Nine out of ten people who ask for contraceptives end up on the pill. It is the most prescribed form of contraceptive in England.[12] Why? Because handing over a piece of paper is much easier than anything else.

The pill is used as a tool to 'deal with' our emotional experiences. Younger people are placed on the pill to control their moods and emotions. The pill has some adverse and severe side effects for some. Despite this, the pill is given to children and teenagers as they get their period, way before their HPO axis fully matures (the monthly dance-off we discussed earlier in the book). When people decide to come off the pill, finding a rhythm with their cycle may take a long time. Of course, that's because it was shut down before it found the groove. A 2019 study in the Netherlands found that sixteen-year-olds on the pill were significantly more likely to show depressive symptoms than those who were not. There were more reports of crying, challenges with sleep and eating issues. Wonderfully, the published article concluded that those who more likely to be depressed were more likely to take the pill.[13] A generalised, manipulative, victim-blaming conclusion to come to. But at least they are looking into it, hunz. Do you see my point in how awful research into pelvic healthcare truly is?

Sanger was very into all things controlling who actually had children.[14] Only those outside her 'undesirable' groups were to have babies. The undesirable groups were labelled as 'mentally and physically defective' or 'those in extreme poverty'. She was pro birth-control wiping out the 'greatest present menace to civilisation'. Some historians argue that she didn't promote controlling who had children when it came to the colour of their skin, but I always like to say that there isn't any smoke without fire, and I have read plenty that would point to this being true.

Eugenics is all about 'planned breeding' and 'racial improvement'. Eugenicists were about 'breeding' the perfect human being.[15] Sanger and Gregory Pincus, a controversial biologist, were very much into all things eugenics.

Now Gregory Goodwin Pincus was the one who developed the pill, but after a while, he needed a larger clinical trial. So he went to Puerto Rico. It had a population that was rapidly growing, and there was widespread poverty. It was also the perfect place because there were birth control clinics that were once funded by the government. However, this had changed, and they were then sponsored by a Procter & Gamble heir, eugenicist Clarence Gamble. Perfect, right? (I am referring to Procter & Gamble, the American multinational consumer goods corporation that owns such brands as Always and Bodyform.) Gamble was all for wiping out those in Puerto Rico living in poverty. These so-called birth control centres were the perfect places to find those willing to try the pill. One red flag (I mean, if I haven't already listed a fair few) was that those in the trial were not told it was a trial. The pill contained much higher doses of the hormones than are in the current pills, so those in the trial experienced significant adverse side effects. But they ignored those who complained of nausea, depression, oh, and the five women who died in the trial. It went on the market with the large clinical trial ticked off the list.

The trials were very secretive; they were unethical and unsafe. Those who took this pill did so because they were desperate. If they weren't given the pill, they would be sterilised without full consent through the same clinics. However, Pincus found the pill to be a huge success: people didn't get pregnant. So Gamble funded a second trial, using people in mental asylums—you guessed it, without their consent.

It was approved in 1957 and was a hit. The marketing was very clever. The posters represented women by depicting them as being ready for men sexually now that they were on the pill. Actual text on the posters included, 'Birth control babe; pill-poppin', penis lovin' and 'Satan's girl who votes democrat as a free-thinker'.

These kinds of messages haven't changed all that much when it comes to the pill. Lemme prove it. One of my community members told me a doctor said these very words to them: 'At your age, boys will look at you and get you pregnant; you should be using condoms and the pill'.

At times, the pill is exactly what someone needs, gives them space to breathe when it comes to avoiding pregnancy, supports those in chronic endo pain at times. But if we actually educated ourselves from the beginning and poured this money into people understanding how cycles work (I am talking about everyone), then we wouldn't feel as much pressure to take the pill overall. We'd all be making more informed choices. There'd be less disconnect from our wombs and perhaps fewer physical manifestations.

This is why at the beginning of this section on the pill, I said that being on the pill means you aren't having a true period. Many of us aren't even aware of this fact.

It's all about being informed. So next time you are handed a prescription for the pill, make sure this is your choice. Not theirs.

If you are with your child and placed in this position, the position of what to do with their contraception or period pains for example, do your research and feel rooted in any kind of decision when it comes to the pill.

Menarche

When I first bled at the late age of seventeen (I lacked body fat which is why I started later), I was sitting in my psychology class, feeling horrendous pain. I asked to use the toilet and dragged myself through the school to the bathrooms. When I got there, I gripped the edges of the sink and looked up in the smeared mirror; I genuinely had never seen my face so pale. I felt horrific. I was beginning to panic. I realised I had the slightest bit of blood and decided my only option was to try and cope just like everyone else. I had no idea why I was in so much pain, but at one point, I remember lying on the floor in the empty corridor because lessons were in session. I literally began at one point to drag myself along. Ridiculous when I look back. I didn't know what else to do or who to turn to. I found my way back to psychology, sat down, and the lesson was about to finish. People were looking at me, and the teacher commented on how awful I looked.

Once everyone left, I told her I was on my first period, and she laid me down on the psychology classroom floor. Later, my mother came to collect me. I was skipped off to the doctor with my mother commenting on my low pain threshold, the doctor handing me the pill with some ridiculously-sized pain-relief style tablets and the words 'You have to help yourself, Naomi'. I used to look back with all the 'fuck you' feelings around this. But I have done some inner work, hun. In fact, my first-ever breathwork journey relived this memory in such detail. We underestimate the impact of our first bleed (menarche).

Menarche, pronounced men-ar-ki, simply means your first period. The first time you menstruated. The average age for a menstruator to get their first period is around twelve and a half, though this varies greatly, and many girls are finding that their periods start much earlier. Some say this is due to the hormones our young girls are in contact with. For example, the hormones from the pill in the water system. Some say it is endocrine disrupters in general.

Menarche is symbolised by the number thirteen, the age of physical and spiritual initiation worldwide. This is the age when we become sexually awakened. It's our sexual coming of age. We suddenly bloom fully in our springtime.

Let me just clarify this for you. The UK does not celebrate first periods on the whole. The UK doesn't acknowledge such a transition. If you google 'Menarche celebrations, UK', you get results about the recent abolition of the tampon tax and free period products for schools. (I feel deeply honoured, celebrated and blessed.)

So let's look at a few places that do celebrate menarche.

In various areas of Japan, the family celebrate with a traditional meal called Sekihan, which includes rice and adzuki beans. The red dish represents the period and symbolises happiness and celebration for this magical time.

Some areas of Fiji acknowledge the milestone on day four of someone's first period, which they call 'tundra'. They celebrate with a feast.

Though periods are still widely shamed in India, in some south Indian communities, a girl's first period is welcomed through a coming-of-age ceremony called Ritusuddhi or Ritu Kala Samskara, or a half-sari function. They will receive gifts and wear an outfit called langa voni, known as a half sari.

In some cultures, they offer baths. In others, such as Greece, there are celebratory gatherings.

The point here is that this moment, the first period, is celebrated in some cultures. In others, it is shamed; in some, it is ignored; in others, it's weaponised.

In *Yoni Shakti* by Uma Dinsmore-Tuli,[16] she writes how Sodasi (one of ten Hindu Tantric goddesses) is associated with menarche as Sodasi is seen as a beautiful sixteen-year-old. Sodasi is unaware of her power but has an incredible force. Uma explains when we hit our menarche we come into a new phase with a new kind of power. Except, we are unaware of our power as menstruators. This is the same for Sodasi, she is an incredible force but unaware of the power she has. This is why Sodasi is used to represent our menarche.

There is a vulnerability, full receptiveness and openness. A beautiful raw innocence with power beyond comprehension.

Such power found through menstruation is closed down by our society and patriarchal system.

We will be exploring your menarche in step two.

Social media

I have a love/hate relationship with socials. One year I broke up with it, turning to my newsletters. I allowed them to creep back into my life and worked on better social media boundaries. I still dream of not using socials. I also dream of getting a Nokia 3310 circa 2000 and using it only for text messages, phone calls and Snake.

But without social media, of course, I likely wouldn't be here doing this work. I wouldn't have found as many people in one go who wanted to hear what I have I say. It is mind-blowing to think you can start a whole business from a social media account, where you no longer even need to have a website. All for free. Where petitions can garner a whole lot of support and where body positivity has a home.

Now I love body-positive accounts. There are loads of wonders doing this work on behalf of us all. But there is always going to be a gap. If you are plus-size or owning the word fat once and for all, you will find solidarity in fat-positive accounts. If you've grown up slim, finding those who get what it's like to be called anorexic even though you eat 3,456 slices of bread will bring you solidarity. Accounts sharing vulva diversity are a huge win; despite the risk of them being shut down, they continue to fight the good fight.

I try not to be in an echo chamber on my socials. I follow a diverse range of accounts to ensure I am always learning. To ensure I am pushed to constantly remember the white privilege I have and what I can do with that for good. To learn from those in the LGBTQIA+ community. I won't get it all correct, but I am willing to learn. The beauty of socials is just that: we really do learn from a diverse scroll. Every day is a school day, hun.

The problem we have, however, is that comparison is the thief of joy. Finding happiness isn't gonna be found via endless scrolls on socials.

Any appearance-focused media, even that of body-positive posts, can lead to self-objectification. Those plus-size or slimmer size, or those just showing how they give no shits size and don't even place themselves in any sized bracket, or those sharing diversity in any way, may lead people to self-objectify. A 2019 study conducted on 195 women aged 18–30 showed they experienced a slight boost in mood when looking at diverse bodies. Those who saw their 'ideal body' found their mood plummeting. However, researchers noted that both groups made more appearance-related statements after being on socials.[17]

Studies have found that Instagram is linked to lowering body satisfaction and increasing the need to diet. They have shown that such changes happen quickly. One undergraduate took just seven minutes to begin feeling a little bit shit once on the gram. One social company slide showed leaked documents: 'We make body image issues worse for one in three teen girls'.[18]

So the point I'm making is that though it feels like some people have found a voice on these accounts, it continues to shut down many of us.

If we are to indeed find security, safety and love from within, then we must be able to go within. It feels exceptionally challenging to even find the head space when the scroll is very real for us all.

Not just this, plenty of people have their accounts (voices) shut down on socials. I can't find you hard facts to prove the numbers (the suspicious part of me wonders why), but I know that being 'shadowbanned' is very real. Getting threats from platforms with 'You will be permanently shut down' happens all the time. I found one example where a TikTok influencer focusing on body positivity shared her sexual assault story. She got shut down by TikTok because she continued to speak up in the face of adversity. I've seen other accounts doing the same and disappearing.

The witch wound and social media

The witch wound is an intergenerational trauma that we see passed down through our lineages and ancestors. Many were hanged and persecuted if they were deemed 'witches'. In the sixteenth century, hundreds of 'witches' were hanged during the 'witch hunt'. It was particularly common in Scotland. They hanged anyone who could have been accused of being slightly 'witchy'. But most of the evidence didn't even exist. If you had something to say and stood up for yourself, you were the perfect candidate to be . . . hanged. Most of those who were hanged were simply standing up for themselves or for the others being hanged: 'Oh, you think she was hanged for no reason, then you too must be part of this witchlike behaviour, so you too will now be hanged' kinda vibe.[19] The witch hunt can be seen in today's society, especially on social media.

It feels, at times, like those speaking out are being strangled. Ding dong, the witches are alive and kicking. The witch wound is very real.

It wasn't until 2008 that Parliament scrapped the latest saucy—I mean sorcery-based—law.[20] Anyone sharing the healing love in any form could be considered a witch. If they decide to bring it back, I am fucked. But they won't be able to burn all these books. Once finished, maybe hide yours in a vault for safekeeping, just in case. Or pass it on so we keep the information in our minds and bodies for safekeeping. Once everyone reads this book, there's no going back.[iv]

We don't talk about the witch wound because that would mean having to sit with it; it's uncomfortable. But we must talk about it. I have been called many names on social media in the comments on most of my viral videos. I've deleted as many as possible and blocked those users. But fuck, the collective wound is pervasive. And to prove my point, adding a final nail in the coffin here, Nicola Sturgeon, the then Scottish prime minister, apologised for the hanged witches. On International Women's Day 2022, she called it a colossal misogynistic injustice that we still have to live with.[21]

And the easiest way to keep silencing the witches would, of course, be through social media accounts.

Including the T in LGBTQIA+

'You're having a boy!' I could see that my child would be assigned male at birth, as all I could see was an arse and the unmistakable outline of a penis. We had a few more scans when I was first pregnant that we'd paid for privately, as the care was much kinder, as I was consistently presenting as 'small'. This was based on the presumption that a tape measure can tell you the precise weight of a baby, which is wild given how different we all carry and how our bodies are so different. Having these scans turned out to be a godsend when my private scanner appeared in the NHS hospital, swapped her appointments and saw me over anyone else, preventing them from unnecessarily inducing me two weeks early. But the penis was confirmed at each scan.

---

iv   She cackles, toad next to her, wart at the end of her nose, turning the wooden spoon in her cauldron.

My child was indeed born with a penis; it wasn't simply engorged labia. We did our very best to navigate the world of babies and gender. I researched, read books, and worked on creating a gender-neutral house.

Then one day, everything changed when preschool began.

We have always used the pronouns he/him and she/her for our children. I now realise how challenging it is to bring up a child with they/them pronouns in our society. School and new friends undo your hard work. I keep saying to my four- and six-year-olds as they land in school now and cry that they have to have 'boy talk partners' or 'that's a boy's toy' or 'only girls wear skirts', 'Gender is a construct, babes'. They don't understand, of course, but it makes me feel better. I buy picture books, and I ensure we always get a book out at the library that discusses topics we need to discuss in the home environment to support them with removing these shackles placed on them due to societal oppression.

They've watched drag queen performances, and more recently, when attending Gay Pride here in Margate, they could not get over how incredible this 'girl dancer' was. I kept explaining to the twins as they danced like her in the kitchen, high-kicking and demanding sparkly dresses for Christmas, that she was assigned male at birth and now is expressing herself through sparkly outfits, high-heeled boots and twerks to Shakira. Wasn't she amazing?! We continue to do our best as parents. I can see now, as a parent, why ignoring the T in LGBTQIA+ is easily done in the home environment.

My son is a gentle, grounded, loving child who loves to twirl in a skirt sometimes and ignores the girl/boy chat. He isn't into football or Spiderman. He enjoys being creative.

'He's probably gay, then'. Legit, do you know how many times someone has made this comment to me? A close friend of mine, while they were in the bath, could not believe I would let him grow his hair long if that's what he wanted. 'He'll be bullied'. This was said right in front of him.

A plumber working on our avocado-green 1960s bathroom conversion (renovation life) saw his skirt one day and questioned how on earth I could 'let him out like that'.

Is society OK? Do we all need a minute here? This child, under age six, tells us that he feels he is a boy, he enjoys using the pronouns he/him, and here we are, removing his choices around his body. Telling him how to behave because he has a penis. 'You have a penis; behave as you should in our society'. This right-and-wrong lens is based on penises and vulvas. For what? To crush his expressive personality so you feel comfortable because you are a slave to the patriarchal binds that exist to keep us small. Sad. Oh, so fucking sad. We must hold him through the confusion in our home whenever he hears a comment. Every time. Over the years, we have seen this expressive personality be slightly less expressive through how he approaches life as someone assigned male at birth.

It's unsettling for people to acknowledge gender variance. Human sexuality is complex, and we are aware of this now. OK, some of us are aware, some are waking up to this, and some don't agree.

Cis means cisgender. Thus, if you are born with a penis, were raised as a boy, and still call yourself a man, then you would be a cis man. Or a cisgender man. And, of course, the same applies to those who were born with a vulva and raised as a girl; they still label themselves as women; thus, they are cis women or cisgender women. Some ain't into this 'cis' label. Why would we need to label the majority? The kinda chat that arises from the term 'cis'. If we utilise the term in the way I understand it, cis means we allow women to be nonconforming with their gender or ignore the sexist norms that exist but still be categorised as women.

When we refer to trans people, these individuals defy the binds placed on them being assigned male or female at birth. Trans women will have been assigned male at birth, and trans men will have been assigned female at birth. Some are nonbinary and don't feel the need to categorise themselves this way. To them, there are not just two categories. Cue gasps, horror and confusion from society. This section focuses on trans people, trans men, trans women and nonbinary people.

I have had so many people come at me on socials when I include trans and non-binary people in my work. Commenters would ask why I would erase the voice of most of my audience in favour of 1 percent of the UK population. Based on an estimate, it is said that trans people make up 200,000 to 500,000 people in the UK.

There's so much confusion here. My spaces are inclusive because we are all fighting for the same thing with our bodies. I am in awe of the fight trans people put up in the face of the most significant amount of ignorance. They inspire me to keep on keeping on. If there's one thing I have learnt as a cis white woman, it's that I need to be aware of all my privileges and use my privilege to amplify the voices of those who are not heard.

Trans people have been mainly erased from the world of pussy work until now. I do not feel they are heard, yet we must open this conversation. We must be aware of the overlap with the fight we are all fighting. There is no them and us. Do you want more happiness, more joy in this world? You've picked up a book on finding more happiness. Then you need to understand more about compassion and solidarity in a world that insists on creating a war to perpetuate pain and confusion. And as I write this book, there are huge arguments on the internet about this. Huge. Sometimes the arguments miss the education in the original post, perpetuating further pain and confusion.

Suppose you think the education system will explain everything to your child or the children you interact with in your life. In that case, you're mistaken. Twenty-one MPs in 2019 voted against LGBTQIA+-inclusive education in our RSE curriculum. Then there were parent protests as the new 2021 RSE curriculum started to be shared. There was uproar. And this was not just for the inclusive aspect, this was on educating our children on their bodies.

Thanks for being here and listening to the conversation.[22]

The health service and trans people, well, it's pretty appalling. Evidence shows that the NHS is letting down trans people with an approach deemed discriminatory and in breach of the Equality Act.

That's why I feel books like this should be accessible for all, especially when we often get little support from the health service with our pelvis.[23]

We must acknowledge the impact genitals have on a trans person's feelings around their body. Dysphoria is characterised by generalised discontent and agitation. Dysphoria exists for some trans people around their genitals. When discussing the reproductive organs in this book, it isn't just women who have reproductive organs. This ignores trans and nonbinary people. And yes, some people reading this will be outraged at this comment. Yes, they were assigned female at birth, and in your minds they are technically women, but they do not view themselves as women now—that's only your perception. It is more accessible for people to understand phrases such as 'women's reproductive healthcare' and to use the term *women* in a book like this one. Historically and predominantly, reproductive healthcare, including abortion, contraception and fertility, has affected women in a society that has ignored the nuances of gender and sex. Society acknowledges that it's women who birth children, so politically, we understand reproductive healthcare to only affect women.

We all deserve access to the necessary information, support and help. Except we know this doesn't happen. Many of us will find friends who were given much better support and help with a similar challenge. Or the postcode lottery found in the UK, for example. It is frustrating that where you live in the UK dictates how much fertility support you will be given, which can vary between absolutely no support to three chances of trying for a baby in a clinic. Our rights to receive the healthcare we need should not be determined by factors wrapped up in a political system with an agenda that doesn't put patients first.

Access to healthcare should be about taking control of your own body and using your rights for your mental health to find freedom from any current binds. Except in trans healthcare, the ability of trans folk to access contraception support, smear tests, abortion and medical transitions is challenged because they challenge society's gender roles. Therefore, you are reminded once again that you are simply here to make babies as a woman. That is your role. You're reminded of that many times through the way healthcare approaches your reproductive organs. The patriarchy relies on separate male and female sex roles; trans people are seen as a threat to this separation.

It's abundantly clear through careful media messages that if you get an abortion, you may regret it. Those hellbent on taking away your abortion rights focus on many reasons for removing these rights and always include regret. Society does the same for trans healthcare. Focusing on the regret. Politicians who ain't into you having any reproductive rights will also be anti-trans. There are many examples, including David TC Davies, an MP from Monmouth. Davies is not into trans rights and same-sex marriage. Also, he wanted to limit the abortion timeframe to 4–12 weeks from 20.

Thanks to the Roe vs Wade being overturned in the US, we are now more aware than ever of how much of a struggle it is to remain in your power and keep body autonomy. This challenge is real. Having an abortion in the UK is still a serious criminal offence. The procedure must be completed under the guidelines of the strict 1967 Abortion Act, which entails that two doctors must approve why the person wants the abortion. Only then can it go ahead. This abortion act only existed because the number of deaths in 1967 from backstreet abortions was out of control, with 50–60 women dying yearly. The law wasn't passed to give people their rights back. It was passed to prevent as many deaths as possible.[24]

Transphobia stems from the prejudice that a person's identity becomes more trustworthy if it aligns with their 'natural' human reproductive role. Cisgender women's reproductive freedom is the first thing to be controlled. Misogyny, homophobia and transphobia stem from patriarchal oppression in society.

If you want full rights to your body, then you are doing it all wrong in the patriarchy's eyes, hun.

This book is a transfeminist book written by a transfeminist; this isn't feminism against any other feminism. It includes all who suffer from our patriarchal system.

The patriarchal system gives us roles at birth due to our specific organs. If we are all to be liberated, then we must liberate all. Otherwise, you will only ever be able to use people's sex organs against them to prove a point. Whatever point that is. For example, those who are anti-trans will always use the penis as a weapon to prove their points; they rely on biological essentialism. One idea perpetuated is that anyone born with a penis is more aggressive. 'Penis', anti-trans movement feminists will shout, to prove their point. Or anti-trans feminists place penises onto stickers to be placed around toilets: 'Women's sex-based rights are not for penises'. Biological sex and anatomy, then, are about gender.

These pages discuss the balance of the feminine and the masculine energies. This isn't a woman against the whole-world feminist approach. This approach, I believe, is dangerous. When men's mental health matters are discussed on social media, there can be found a plethora of comments such as 'good', 'they deserve it', or 'finally'.

Social media pulled apart the text of a recent *Glamour* magazine article on women's dating standards being higher than ever, which included lines about men feeling lonelier than ever. Comments again were 'at last' and 'deserved'.[25]

This men-over-women patriarchal bind we find ourselves in will not be removed if we continue to reinforce men vs women and the binary model of sex and gender.

Feminist and LGBTQIA+ philosopher Robin Dembroff shares that the patriarchy is based on 'male' and 'female' being binary. Feminine = females, and masculine = men. Through this lens, masculinity is superior to femininity. Therefore, Dembroff explains, your genitalia dictates how you must comply with society, which can never be changed. You must follow the rules for how you process your emotions, for example, your work/job choice, clothing options, the behaviour we expect from you and your role within the family. Femininity is anti-masculine, and masculinity is more valued than femininity.[26]

Regularly I get comments on socials like, 'Rather than us having to work through things like shame, we should just be dismantling the patriarchy'. Such enthusiasm.

Sure, let's dismantle the patriarchy by empowering ourselves to understand how it fully manifests itself.

In 1972, 'Transsexual women of the UK Gay Liberation front' in their *Come Together* newsletter wrote that a women's revolution would be more joyful when it includes all.

We also cannot simply say that we are trans-inclusive if we are only including trans men either. You are ignoring their experience of their bodies.

Essentially, I shouldn't have to even label myself as a transfeminist. I did so to ensure you were clear on where I stand regarding inclusion and reproductive rights. 'Cause the system loves a label. I don't care what lies between your thighs. This isn't what this book is about. Don't be misled here.

There's so much to be done in these pages. There's so much to be done outside of these pages. It would be best if you simply preserved this energy to fight for everyone's rights to make their own choices and have their own experiences with their bodies.

Enough already.

The TERF war was over before it began.[v] That isn't even a war.

The actual war is the one we are having with our own bodies. It's creating so much pain and sadness.

This book is intended to liberate us all as human beings having a human experience. Those who search for freedom for themselves and others are an inspiration. This book is for those who haven't the strength to fight for their freedom right now at this point in their journey.

This hope trans folk provide feeds into our hope for the space we all need to live full, happy lives.

Racial Bias in Medicine

We know that there isn't contraception that is 100 percent effective, so unplanned pregnancies can occur for anyone. Unplanned pregnancies happen to about one in every two women who get pregnant. However, unplanned pregnancy rates are higher for Black folk than for other racial groups.

The difference in these unplanned pregnancy rates, experts think, is down to contraception use. The Black community aged 15 to 49 are less likely than other racial communities to use birth control regularly. Those between 18 and 24 prefer condoms. And condoms on their own have among the lowest rates of effectiveness.

When we discuss long-acting reversible contraceptives (LARCs), we are referring to copper intrauterine devices (IUDs), progestin-only IUDs and birth control arm implants. Those in the Black community are less likely to use prescription contraception, which includes the pill and LARCs.

There's a racial difference in birth control use, which makes perfect sense. Experts mainly blame centuries of inequality and racial discrimination. It's simple: people face social and structural hurdles to reproductive health care.

---

[v]   'TERF' stands for 'trans-exclusionary radical feminism.'

There is so much medical mistrust due to how the Black community has been treated and is continually treated. Loretta J. Ross is an African American activist who advocates for reproductive justice. Loretta used the Dalkon Shield (a contraceptive intrauterine device developed by the Dalkon Corporation) and kept asking her doctor for support post-insertion. Her doctor ignored the IUD and treated her for everything else. Loretta ended up with pelvic inflammatory disease (PID) caused by the Dalkon Shield, which led to a hysterectomy at twenty-three years old.

Millions of these Dalkon Shield IUDs were sold for years before the parent company went bankrupt due to patients organising class-action settlements. The 1960s and 1970s Dalkon Shield had a design flaw that caused miscarriages, infections, fertility loss and, in some cases, death. There were over three hundred thousand lawsuits brought by patients. Did Dalkon, the PR company, A.H. Robins or medical professionals listen to the patients? Absolutely not. They said it was down to poor hygiene or even riskayyyy sexual behaviour. Another example of a contraception pushed onto a marginalised group while their side effects were ignored.

Medical mistrust must also be discussed in how the line between medical advice and coercion is easily blurred. Starting in the twentieth century, the US government institutionalised policies to sterilise Black, Latina, and Native American folk without their informed consent.

Targeting Black folk with long-term birth control has its roots in white supremacy and the desire of white people to have control over Black bodies, which dates back to the era of chattel slavery.

Then there's the early 1990s trend in the US to financially incentivise or even require people to get the long-acting contraceptive Norplant to receive public benefits. Of course, this kind of prevention pressure backfired and resulted in people using less effective, less reliable or no contraception.

The cost of birth control can exacerbate racial disparities. Structural racism means people of colour are less likely to be able to access the medical care and insurance they need to purchase expensive birth control, if they so wish to.

Another reason for these stats showing the racial differences in contraception use could be a desire to avoid hormones. Many may not feel comfortable using hormonal forms of birth control. And we only have to look at the history to understand why.[27]

This implicit bias among some health practitioners and in healthcare continues to be problematic. In the UK, Black folk are five times more likely to die in childbirth than white folk. In the US, a 2016 study shared that Black patients are less likely to be prescribed painkillers than white patients. These stats show that Black patients aren't being prescribed painkillers for the same pain being endured by white patients.[28] The legacy of racism continues to affect Black health outcomes negatively.

We must acknowledge and amplify Black folks' voices in advocating for their health.[29]

Porn: One-Third of All Internet Traffic

Choosing a film with my husband that we can both agree on is hard work.

When we decide on a film together, it has to have a couple of elements for us both to be happy. I like a romcom where there's a final kiss. My husband, however, is into what he would deem 'good films'. How he places *Bridget Jones*, *Bridget Jones: The Edge of Reason* and, of course, not forgetting *Bridget Jones's Baby* in the 'not good films' bracket, I don't know.

But here we are, the battle of finding a romantic thriller to sit down and watch together.

Porn is no different; not everyone will enjoy the same types of porn films.

Free online porn, the one nine-year-olds are getting their hands on through the phone given to them for texting home, isn't going to be great for several reasons. But we can't place all porn in the same bracket because some producers are making ethically produced porn. (We will discuss what the term 'ethically produced' porn means later in this chapter. Bear with.)

This porn industry is one of the fastest-growing web-based industries, with a report showing that a third of internet traffic is porn.[30] So what do people do if they haven't received excellent sex education and are watching poor TV shows or films with sex scenes, or poorly made porn? They then learn nothing about their or others' needs when engaging in sex in real life. Absolutely not a scooby, babe.

This means that when it comes to voicing our needs, we don't actually know what they are. We are all scrabbling around, sometimes quite literally, trying to work out what consent looks like. What it means to meet our needs. What our vulvas need to open to the experience. What safety looks like in any given sexual scenario, whether on a one-night stand or in a long-term relationship.

We try to explain that we need more time to open into the sexual experience. Partners are often confused, because when they watched sex in a movie, on a TV show, or in a porn film, it showed people ripping each others' clothes off and engaging in penetrative sex, complete with an over-egged climax in one minute flat. What do you mean I need to honour your needs, comes a confused retort when you've avoided touching your partner for three months. Meanwhile, we don't know what honouring our needs looks like either.

In this scenario, we all feel shut down, lost and confused, pushing away the one person we want to bring closer.

A study reviewed the fifty most viewed Pornhub videos of all time to find how focused they were on showing sexual stimulation before orgasm. About 18 percent of these videos showed visual or verbal cues to show the woman had actually orgasmed, while it showed visual or verbal orgasm cues for men in 78 percent of the videos. The videos, on the whole, showed that it was the male orgasm that signalled when sex was completed and showed that most women were orgasming from penetration.[31]

Overall, this kind of porn continues to show us nothing of use, and we continue on as lost souls navigating what joy and pleasure look like when engaging in sex. The honouring of the pussy is ignored altogether, leaving relationships in disarray. It often causes conflict and confusion.

Not forgetting, there can be challenges that arise in relationships where porn is being watched without the other partner's knowledge.

To understand what ethically produced porn actually is, I hopped onto a zoom chat with Avril Louise Clarke of Erika Lust Films.

Erika Lust Films is a production company creating sex-positive content, adult cinema made via an ethical production process. Avril is one of Erika Lust's clinical sexologists; she's also their intimacy coordinator and the brand manager for their non-profit project, the Porn Conversation, which can be found at thepornconversation.org. The Porn Conversation provides free and accessible tools to support teaching and talking about all things porn. Helping us to have the #thepornconversation.

Having *this* conversation with Avril was a gift.

A Porn Conversation with Avril

When describing porn produced ethically, I like to use the exact phrase 'ethically produced porn'. It allows us to define it a little more, and it can lead to some really great discussions. Other terms you can google when looking for ethically produced porn include 'feminist porn' or 'ethical porn'.

A lot of what makes porn ethically produced is happening behind the scenes. Behind-the-scenes elements include editing, how actors are treated, post-production, and how the content is distributed. We can see that there are layers to this. Such layers are not visible on your screen.

Personally, I don't use the term 'mainstream porn'. This is because we are moving towards more ethically produced everything, from the products we use on our faces to the food we eat. This has become more mainstream. OK, granted, ethically produced porn may not sell as much as, say, oat milk. But we are finding a way to make ethically produced porn the trend rather than giving any power to what would be deemed mainstream porn.

Using the term 'free online porn' defines it for people and makes it a more transparent term. This is especially useful for the porn conversation, where we focus on opening up these conversations with children and teenagers. One in ten children have watched pornography by the time they are nine, according to the children's commissioner for England. However, this age group are typically not going to have access to ethically produced porn. Simply because other kinds of porn are so readily and easily available, and of course, they don't have access to credit cards to buy ethically produced porn.

It's not bad that they come across free online porn; we don't need to be adding to the shame that already plagues our society around sex and pornography. We don't need to add to the fear-mongering. Instead, we must have conversations around the fact that this may happen. Let's discuss this before it does happen—this being the potential pop-up on their screen and easy access to free online porn.

Society does shame porn, and labelling all porn as evil with such extreme language doesn't lead anywhere and doesn't allow for nuances, discussion or conversations. It brings up this shaming language we already receive from people in our lives and society. It doesn't matter how you feel about porn, whether you detest it entirely or have other beliefs about it. We should welcome these discussions. It doesn't get us anywhere if we cannot have these conversations.

Society is exceptionally polarising; we can't even have political conversations anymore. It all feels very icky. I think it's a very harsh position to take when you don't allow for the porn conversation, wherever your views land. Especially when we talk to young people, adults in pain, or those with sexual challenges. Giving people time to talk, critique and question something is always necessary.

Ethically produced porn typically exists behind a paywall or is subscription based. This is because of the money that goes into production. There are so many people involved in ethically produced porn vs other kinds, from what I have garnered from talking to actors, for example. There can sometimes be as many as fifty people on set for ethically produced porn vs two or three with other kinds of porn. And this number doesn't take into account the editors, the costumers, the makeup artists—everyone that's involved. It's vast; there's so much that goes into it. So it is improbable to find ethically produced porn on, say, Pornhub.

We have high protection at this stage for all involved; we protect the sex workers. If they choose to work with a particular director, we must be clear on where the film will be placed. We can't say that every single video available on Pornhub is unethically produced or that sex workers were harmed during the making of the film. We must remember that we cannot see how the film is made and what goes on behind the scenes. From our end, we will only be distributing our videos in a way that meets our standards. Others will have different standards.

When we watch ethically produced porn, we don't see what goes on behind the scenes with boundaries and consent. I'm an intimacy coordinator on set. The process begins when I read the script, meet the cast, consider the power dynamics and who they are as human beings. We begin to explore consent and boundaries at the very beginning of the whole process. We discuss what they would be comfortable doing and not OK doing, while leaving room for nuances as and when they arise. You'll then find that we have pre-production sex talks, with the most amazing questions and conversations we should all be having before sex. I think it would be a completely different world if we had these actors' discussions.

We check in again on the day of the shoot to see if anything has shifted since we last spoke. There are talks throughout the day and before the performance. What we are doing is ensuring everyone is safe, secure and comfortable. There's also a plan if we need to support further. Power dynamics will always be at play, just like in any job we do. My role as the intimacy coordinator since the #metoo movement is essential. We ensure no one is saying yes when they feel it's a no, just to make someone else happy. We often do this in jobs, say yes to things to make the manager happy, for example. You'll find I am simply standing still, taking in the whole scenario and monitoring all that is unfolding. Everyone understands that they have full body autonomy. That they can stop, change it up, or adjust at any time. We encourage this level of communication.

What I am sharing here is that even if you don't see 'it'—it being all these nuances, needs, safety points and conversations on the final cut—there will have been this level of support within the sex. I'm there with my headphones on, thinking, 'Wow, this is the most consensual sex I have ever seen, way more consensual than the sex I was having in college'. Some final scenes show audible consent for us to see its practice. This is important, and you'll see this in all our films. Body autonomy and consent are at the forefront of our messaging. We are media, and just like all other media, we are producing messages too. We always need to consider in every aspect of the films what our messages are for our viewers.

How porn is distributed also impacts the messages we send out. There's so much sexualisation in the queer community. For example, on free online porn sites, lesbian porn is made and constructed very much for a male audience. Therefore, it's not relatable for the LGBTQIA+ community, where they are often seen as simply props. For example, giving leading roles to queer performers and creating a narrative that feels relatable for the queer community will land very differently for many. But what we have to remember when it comes to porn literacy is that people will relate differently to different messages.

When we look at the messages on free online porn sites, the messages start with the categories. Why is there a Latino or Asian category, for example? Where is the white category? This sends a clear statement of white supremacy. It's something that should be fetishized, right? Then we dive further in and find the titles of the videos.

An example may be 'tight Asian pussy gets pounded by big black cock'. This immediately perpetuates the idea and stereotype based solely on race. It does a huge, huge disservice to the Black and indigenous community because of the—quite honestly—disgusting messages it sends out. So again, when we discuss ethically produced porn, it's about creating realistic narratives. These communities, just like white cis heteronormative communities, are deserving of pleasure.

The messaging and distribution within ethically produced porn is clear: we all deserve pleasure through safe, held, loving environments.

During the call with Avril, I was keen to ask about her thoughts on labiaplasty and porn. As we have seen, the rising labiaplasty stats are blamed on porn, but the discussions are rife with opposing views. For example, top plastic surgeons warn that it's misleading and dangerous to blame porn. Avril explained that when she grew up, neat labia was something to be aware of, and one day you may be ashamed of yours. She grew up in Miami, where billboards advertised labiaplasty and the radio shared regular adverts. She knew about labiaplasty before she'd even gone through puberty. This quite frankly blew my mind. I didn't hear about it until I was past puberty. 'The messages are everywhere', she said, 'not just in porn, but yes, porn is part of the issue'.

Avril discussed that porn literacy is about critiquing and breaking down the messages porn sends. Exploring and creating your own meanings and interpretations from the videos. There are many messages porn sends, from the fetishization of BIPOC communities to the sexualisation of teens and young girls to misogyny and violence. One of these messages includes body image. Avril explained that we see some common body types in porn, including huge penises, bleached anuses, and particular breast sizes.

Circling back to the labia, Avril dived into messages around this.

Certain labia are seen as cleaner, tighter, and prettier', she confirmed. 'You only need to search the free porn sites using search terms such as 'tight pussy'. These will perpetuate this feeling that there's a sure way to be sexual and attractive. There's a certain way you are supposed to look, and there will be rewards for that. We get these messages from society through social media to the red carpet; for example', Avril continued. 'Porn does the same thing with messages. We must step away from that and choose how we want to relate to this media.'

When discussing the enjoyment of porn, Avril explained how porn can feel challenging to navigate when it often sends out particular messages.

> Enjoy porn but be aware that these messages don't need to affect you. If they do, you must choose how you interact with it or choose a different type of porn. Perhaps you could begin to critique the video by exploring what it is called, how it is categorised and what its messages are. Realise that perhaps the messages don't align with you anymore. Consider if what you are watching actually makes you feel bad about your body. Be aware of the editing and what goes on behind the scenes. We aren't here shaming the sex workers in these films but are simply aware that this media is constructed to make you feel a certain way.

Some final words then from Avril around ethically produced porn and body types.

> How we feel about certain films will change from person to person, depending on identity. In some, not all, of the ethically produced porn, there will be a more diverse representation of body types. Some people love this. But, of course, this range includes those with the 'typical' free online porn body types we see. What ethically produced porn does is challenge the narrative of having to look or be a certain way to feel pleasure. Look, it's very layered; I feel very opinionated about it. It's not even about looking a certain way; it's about taste and smell. You only have to go to the grocery stores to see, in the US at least, these freshening wipes. It's like something is wrong with us; we are dirty. Essentially, something that is natural is not good enough.

And these final words around allowing ourselves to bask in all our natural beauty land perfectly within the pages of this book.

Gaslit

I was at university post a traumatic car accident.

One morning I was the passenger while one of the girls I was on a teaching placement with drove the hire car to the school like a formula one driver who'd meandered off course and onto a dual carriageway. I clung to the door handle, hoping we'd arrive in one piece, as I saw the mph reach 100. She continued to bomb it down this country road. In front of us was a junction with cars waiting to leave. I didn't feel her brake at all, so I suddenly shouted, 'Brake'.

It was too late, and at around 60 mph, she hit the stationary car at the junction, sending it up in the air to land facing the other way on the opposite side of the road. I went into survival mode and was the first to anyone injured; my phone went off as I became the primary contact for all emergency services. It was, quite frankly, horrific.

But that was nothing compared to what then occurred. The driver kept saying the brakes failed on this brand-new Corsa; she wanted me to say the same. I would not. I marched into university and demanded that I never set foot in a car with her again. Nothing happened from within my university; there were no check-ins for my health or well-being and seemingly no repercussions for her wild Michael Schumacher driving.

She was hell-bent on making my life miserable because I refused to be in a car with her and follow her story. Instead, I said one day at the petrol station (we were riding together for the few days before I demanded otherwise), 'You didn't brake in time'. She declared that she was being bullied by me to the teachers in our placement school.

One morning the placement school teachers sat me down in their staff room, and I was told I would fail my whole university course and never become a primary teacher if I didn't shut up and get my head down. I was labelled rude or petulant by the teachers when I tried to share my perspective on how I was being treated and simply wanted to be heard for the trauma I was enduring.

Meanwhile, someone handed me a newspaper that had published news of the crash under a headline that read, 'Girls Lucky to Be Alive As They Walk Away Unscathed'.

A few months later, this same driver did actually get kicked off the course for a range of behaviours. However, I was left with a beautiful soup of complex PTSD, panic attacks, and depression. My gut health got so bad that I was actually hospitalised a few months after the car accident, and they suspected I might have appendicitis.

The consultants decided to check in with keyhole surgery when the pain became uncontrollable. Imagine my disbelief once I became conscious; they declared they had found nothing. Nothing at all.

The next day, post explorative surgery, I was confused, upset and feeling isolated. I was on antidepressants and having regular panic attacks—ya know, it was quite the vibe. And now, I had no idea why I was in so much pain with my gut.

Just to hammer home that they'd found nothing, while I was lying in the hospital bed waiting to be discharged, a male doctor swung open my curtain, surrounded by several junior doctors with clipboards, pens and eager looks in their eyes.

He went through my admission symptoms and what they had done. He proclaimed to them all that there was fuck-all wrong with me. I asked where the pain was coming from, as it was very real to me. 'You know', he said, 'it just stems from the head', while he tapped the side of his own head, just in case I needed more clarity on his diagnosis. 'You can go home', he smiled. His students lowered their pens. There wasn't much to learn from the 'it's all in ya head' case.

He closed the curtains, waltzing off to share his love, knowledge, kindness and support for his next patient in need. I closed the curtain on this issue, hiding it just like he'd closed the curtain on me in front of his students. Years later, when I started working in the pelvic health field, I did a range of trainings. In my early thirties, during my womb massage training, the teacher, Clare, was sharing about the ileocecal valve (ICV). The ICV is found between the small and large intestines and controls the flow of digested food when it is time for it to leave the small intestine and go into the large intestine to start its journey to become faeces. 'We are going to be massaging it, as it often holds onto tension', Clare explained. My whole body began to tingle, and I almost wanted to cry. I couldn't look at the sheet of paper. We were on day two, and I hadn't had such a physical reaction to her notes until that point. I went into the massage, and my partner started elsewhere before reaching my ICV. As soon as she began to go deeper over my ICV, my whole body began to shake. I could not stop shaking and crying uncontrollably; my head felt hot, my body went cold, my palms were sweating, and I started shouting out. My throat suddenly felt like someone was gripping it, and there in front of me was my father.

I spent my childhood in absolute fear of him. Over the dinner table, he would sit me down opposite him to rage at me. He would shout, hiss and tell me what a waste of space I was, while spit would fly. I learnt to shut down my emotions because if I cried, he fed off this, and I could see he felt like he was achieving his goal.

That day in my training, it felt like he was in the room, and as I hadn't seen or spoken to him for about twelve years, this was the last thing I imagined unfolding. Everyone else had to stop, and Clare came over, soothing me with her words while everyone else held my body and kept the space. She drummed over me, asking me to scream, release or move it through, and I simply couldn't at the time. Eventually, it passed. My training partner, Victoria, had continued to touch my valve.

From this day on, if I feel stressed, busy, or out of touch with my pelvis, I know because my valve tells me so. My IBS may flare a little. I continue to work with my food, being careful of my triggers, but the triggers are a lot less to non-existent since then.

Now I know why I was sent to the hospital at university with suspected appendicitis. The pain was in my ileocecal valve, which held trauma from my childhood. The ileocecal valve sits near the appendix, hence the diagnosis of suspected appendicitis.

It wasn't in my head when I was lying there in agony in hospital at university. It was pain trapped in my body.

Gaslighting is where someone tries to control someone else by twisting their sense of reality. We are made to feel as though we are making it all up. We must be wrong, and the gaslighter is correct.

Except no one knows your body like you know your body.

I find that you can walk into a vet with your unwell cat, explaining you think Mr Tiggywinkles is under the weather, but you can't be sure as to exactly how or why, and the vet will absolutely take you seriously.

'Let me check Mr T's levels. Aw, poor Mr Tiggywinkles, are you feeling a little poorly? We will take good care of you here. Let's see if we can get to the bottom of it'. Mr T may go home with a prescription for something to try and strict instructions for extra cuddles on the sofa. You may even have taken the day off for your pussy cat, to ensure you have all the time it takes.

If you and your pussy wander into the doctor and something is making you feel below par, the care can often be entirely different. Your pussy may be ignored or have a speculum shoved up it with a 'meh' response, or you might be told it must be in you and your pussy's head. You leave and rush back to work, feeling as confused, if not more so, than when you plucked up the courage to talk about whatever is going on.

As it's apparently all made up, you may feel absolutely ridiculous to push forwards without further support, so you shut yourself down and crack on like you never even brought it up. The disconnect between you and your pelvis increases.

I suffered from IBS for a further thirteen years, which sometimes floored me before my womb massage training, but I told no one except my husband. I also suffered from period pains sometimes all at the same time and just lay on the floor sobbing.

I am sure you can think of a time when you have been gaslit. It's a horrendous experience, and I am wrapping you in a hug as you feel into memory or emotion that may arise while reading this section.

While we are here chatting about all things shutdown and gaslighting, I thought I would take a quick pause to share some of the words that landed on my socials when I asked people to share their experiences with medical professionals when they've asked about their periods. Here are some of the words my community shared. I am sharing some words from doctors anonymously here:

> "Your options are to either have a referral to a fertility clinic or go back on the pill."

> 'I got given the coil when I went to the GP with heavy periods. "Many women experience period pain. It is normal."

> "Still, while spotting at the appointment, go back on the pill."

> "This is your third C-section, yes? We can sterilise you during the procedure, OK?"

Take a Breath

Pause.

Tune in to your breath at this moment.

No, seriously, pause. Here are some questions to consider. How fast is your breath right now? How deep . . . is your love? (Couldn't resist.) What is the depth of your breath? Is it into the belly or simply in the upper part of your chest? Is it in through the nose or into the belly?

Since working with my own breath, mainly through circular breathwork, I have learnt a fair few things about the power of breath.

Here's the thing I am not sure I considered before: we can live without water or food for a while. But breath. Well, we are pretty fucked if we are unable to breathe. And yet, we hardly hear anything about the importance of breathing. How to breathe. How to adjust our breath.

So how is your breath right now?

We will explore breath here so you can actively tune in to your breath at all times. So when you return to your pelvic bowl, you continue to be aware of your breath. Essentially, we want to ensure that we are utilising our breath to better support the functions that occur within the body. So that oxygen is moved to all the major organs more easily—think vagina and womb.

Breath by James Nestor is one of my favourite books on breathing and one I always recommend to clients. It will change your life. The book is accessible and mainly shares the story of James undergoing some research on his own breath while sharing the importance of said research.

Within the book, he discusses how our breathing has become so poor over the years that we have literally changed our own skull shapes; we now have crooked teeth and snore. All a result of being pretty crap at breathing. And I can hear you thinking, 'Breathing just happens—it's involuntary'. Yes, but the more we consciously connect to our breathing to adjust it, the more it will change when we are unaware.

Once you tune in, you'll be hooked on how you breathe.

Tune in again right now and count how many seconds you breathe in and how many seconds you breathe out. According to Nestor's research, the perfect breath is 5.5 seconds in and 5.5 seconds out.

I want to share some breath practices for you to work with daily. Tune in when you have a moment.

We spend our time distracted by . . .

'Squirrel'.

Social media, emails, pings and dings and dongs from notifications.

We really don't spend that much time focused on a particular task. And when we are erratic, our breathing also becomes more . . . erratic. It becomes shallow and just a little all over the place. This has a huge impact. Research is looking into how this has affected our overall health. I am not here sharing all things breath for you to skip on to the following parts without mentioning how critical your breath is overall. Ya gotta start tuning in.

Breathing like the above even has a name. It's called email apnoea, where we unconsciously (and that's an important part to note here) pause breathing up to half a minute or longer while doing something on the screen. What does this do? It limits our oxygen intake, thus sending us into a consistent cycle of being in fight or flight; it impacts our emotions, physiology and overall attention. It can affect our sleep and memory and exacerbate depressive and anxious feelings.[32] Essentially, we aren't meeting our basic needs, which isn't going to support our goal of finding happiness.

We could go through all the steps in the book without bringing in breath awareness, but we'd be missing something key in the overall process. Now that would be just plain silly.

Extending the exhale

Extending the exhale is a common practice, and there's a reason for it. A Ukrainian doctor, Konstantin Buteyko, spent his life researching all things human and found people in hospitals, those in the worst kind of states, were breathing too much. He developed the Buteyko breathing technique in the 1950s. Buteyko encouraged people to breathe slower, so people were breathing calmly and effectively.

Key practice:

A conscious breathwork technique to try:

- Begin by sitting comfortably, shoulders relaxed, spine straight, crown lifted, chin lifted.
- Tune in to your natural breath.
- Slowly introduce a deeper exhale. Almost as if you are gently pushing out any 'leftover' air as you reach into a deeper exhale.
- As you breathe slowly, consciously and smoothly, think of a 2:1 ratio. Inhale for 2 and exhale for 4 counts, for example.
- You can slowly move on, inhaling for 3 and exhaling for 6.
- Be aware of your capacity here, as you want this to be easy-going to soothe the parasympathetic nervous system (the rest and restore system) and not the sympathetic nervous system (the fight or flight response)
- Ensure the transition between the inhale and the exhale remains smooth.

You can continue to do this for as long as feels comfortable. Even just five minutes a day will have an impact. Here you are encouraging the body to be more comfortable with higher levels of carbon dioxide, so during unconscious breathing you will breathe less and more effectively at rest or even when you engage in a spin class, for example. Good for you, babe. We will release more oxygen, support our bodily functions and increase our endurance. I personally can tackle a hill here in Margate on my one-geared bike with four-year-old twins in the back in a child bike trailer like an absolute boss. Meanwhile my husband, who snores when lying on his back, is out of breath way quicker.

Key practice:

- Begin by sitting comfortably, shoulders relaxed, spine straight, crown lifted, chin lifted.
- Scan the room for a few moments, finding safety through any sighs or yawns. Rest on lovely objects or objects that aren't as nice. Just be aware of every corner of the room, above you, behind and in front of you.
- Bring your eyes to a close when you feel safe enough to do so.
- Tune in to your natural breath through your nose.
- Nothing to change or do. Just be aware of the in breath and the out breath.
- In breath. Out breath. Without naming it as 'in and out'.
- Be here for as long as you need, checking into your body for any sensations as you do so. You don't need to tend to these sensations. Be aware. Then come back to the breath.

Try this key:

Nadi shodhana

One of my fave ways to breathe is with alternate nostril breathing. This is a yoga practice and one you can find easily on YouTube. If you go thisisnaomigale. co.uk/books, I have a nadi shodhana practice that connects to the ovaries. But for the purposes of this book, let's focus on the inhales and exhales, and in your own time you could explore breathing into the ovaries through the practice on the book's website.

When we see a poorly or distressed animal, we notice they begin breathing through their mouth. Panting even. They stand still, mouth open, looking like they are knocking on death's door. Some humans have landed into the habit of breathing through their mouths too.

When we breathe in through the nose, we allow ourselves to take deeper breaths, which then travel to the lower part of the lungs, where there lies an abundance of parasympathetic nerve receptors.

I like talking about breath because it reminds me of cervical canal chat. The nose is lined with cilia, just like the cervical canal. They filter the air and protect us against foreign bodies; the air then passes through a mucus-lined trachea (windpipe). The mucus keeps out dust, debris and particles from the lungs. Sound familiar?[33]

Essentially when we breathe through the nose, we filter the air and allow the air to trigger the parasympathetic response. Breathing through the nose is where it's at.

A practice for alternate nostril breathing:

- Find a quiet, undisturbed place where you will be able to concentrate fully.
- With your spine straight, crown and chin lifted, begin to tune in to your breath.
- Using your right hand, place your forefinger and middle finger on the third eye (the bit between the eyebrows).
- Place your thumb over your right nostril and close it.
- Inhale through your left nostril deeply and slowly.
- Open the right nostril while closing the left.
- Exhale through the right nostril.
- Inhale through the right side slowly.
- Open your left nostril and close your right.
- Exhale left through the left side.
- Continue in this cycle for as long as feels comfortable. Closing the eyes at a point that feels safe to do so.

Vaginas That Run, Fight or Freeze

Unravelling your nervous system and armouring

There was a sudden banging in my room in the middle of the night. The banging continued. I threw my body entirely underneath the cover. I was around nine years old, and it sounded like someone was knocking around my room. I remember thinking, 'Why would someone be THIS loud if they were a burglar' but nonetheless, I absolutely froze. I was still, hardly able to breathe as the banging carried on.

After a while, I wondered why it was only localised to my dollhouse. A lot of inward self-talk later, I felt I could begin to move after the initial shock of waking to this kind of noise. I began to slowly peel back the covers and turn on the light.

There standing on its hind legs was my Harry, the hamster. All this time when I was frozen to the bed underneath the cover thinking Burglar Bill was in my room stealing all my prized Polly Pockets, it was actually Houdini the hamster exploring his new pad for the night.

Trauma, in the world of psychology, is something we experience that is 'outside the range of a usual human experience and would cause distress'. This includes a serious threat to our lives or seeing something horrific unfold for others. As Peter Levine explains,[34] using this definition doesn't consider that we are all different and all experience life differently. We can't define what would be traumatic for one person vs another. But essentially, we either instantly realise that we have just experienced a traumatic event, or it unfolds that we did experience trauma over time. It may be that we may not realise it was traumatic at the time, especially because our reactions vary at the time of the event.

This topic is vast, but it is crucial to know how trauma impacts us daily and with root work. Often clients ask me if their trauma can be healed. 'Will I feel like this forever?' 'Will sex always be this painful?' 'Will I ever be able to get a smear test?' One thing I see in my space is the importance of understanding that we can't change what happened, the choices we made, and the situations we landed in. We can allow ourselves to work with being in the here and now, moving through the current feelings and memories that arise somatically. We can then land deeper into the body, becoming more present. We would be working with tools that allow us to build resilience and more awareness of what may be threatening situations.

Over time, we see how trauma impacts the body due to not being on any healing path, and due to not supporting our nervous system and how our nervous system is now wired. We often spend our time being, well, super fucking stressed. Dysregulated.

Even when we think we have an excellent grip on life (while doing nothing to support our bodies and nervous systems), we may suddenly lose the house keys for five minutes. We start to lose all grip on life as we know it over the keys. The world ends, and it takes you hours or even days to find some kind of calm once again.

We may live perpetually in either the fight, flight, freeze or fawn mode. These are all innate responses we use to survive. When we go into a fight response, we respond aggressively, assertively, and/or quickly to something threatening. A flight response is when we feel the need to flee. A freeze or fawn response is when someone feels there's no point in fighting or running, so they numb out, disassociate or collapse.

Our life experiences land us in one of these responses often or all the time.

I often slept in bed with all my cuddly toys for safety, and I flicked around repeatedly between the above responses as a child and into adulthood. I suffered from CPTSD (complex post-traumatic stress disorder). Someone else may have realised Harry had escaped and was having an absolute ball, knocking over every item in the dollhouse. But I was shit-scared and went into the freeze response because I had no tools or resilience to deal with my perceived traumatic scenario. I was chronically stressed into my mid-twenties.

We get stuck in the sympathetic nervous system (the 4Fs above) rather than being able to drop into our rest and restore—the parasympathetic nervous system. Pete Walker has an excellent list of examples of what we may see in someone who is experiencing detrimental somatic changes:

· Shallow/incomplete breathing
· Feeling always rushed and exhausted from said rushing
· Unable to properly sleep from being overly alert
· Constantly feeling that rush of adrenaline
· Having challenges with digestion from tightening in the digestive tract
· Excessively self-medicating with food, alcohol or drugs, in a way that leads to physiological damage[35]

Armouring

If there has been a situation involving our body and/or specifically our vulva or vagina, then we can find our pelvis armours itself.

We can think of armouring like knights who get on all the gear, ready to go into combat. Once done, they remove their armour and likely celebrate the fact they are still alive with a beer in hand. While writing this, I was thinking about Heath Ledger, who remains in my top three celebrity crushes of all time. I could watch 10 Things I Hate about You on repeat. But Heath's personal story ended in tragedy; he was self-medicating excessively through prescription drugs and died.

I digress slightly. Armouring. So we see armouring in the root, in the yoni. Think about muscle tightness in general. I use the example of our shoulders; they can often lift when we are stressed, be up around our ears even. We massage them or ask someone else to so they begin to release back down. This doesn't happen in the vagina. Stress, trauma, and wounding can cause it to tighten and remain tight.

If you were about to enter another situation that felt like a threat, it might armour even more or remain armoured, unable to soften and relax into the scenario as it unfolds. It's simply the vagina protecting itself from any further 'attack'. Armour on, ready to go into combat at all times or at those specific times when it feels there's a lack of safety.

The steps this book follows will be life-changing for those who have experienced trauma because the trauma we experience will often show up in our pelvis. Root work is the key to moving through the experiences that have bound us.

If we have been made to feel unsafe, our bodies respond physiologically. The emotional turmoil we have been through has jeopardised our ability to feel safe in our body, to root down and find any level of contentment, let alone joy or happiness for ourselves, or joy or happiness with others.

This chapter could be a trigger for you. Our triggers keep us safe, essentially. Our protectors often speak up. Our inner child wounds ensure we remain in safety. Being 'triggered' shouldn't be seen as a bad thing. It's all part of who we are. Through this book we will never reject any parts of you. Simply welcome all of you in. We are never 'getting rid' of anything, simply bringing in awareness.

We are now going to explore some examples of experiences we may have gone through that can impact our pelvis and our overall well-being.

Post reading this chapter, take time to tend to your nervous system with something that feels nourishing for you. For some of us, that would be a snuggle on the sofa; for others, a session at the gym. Feel your feet on the earth, perhaps to feel grounded and held by the earth below. You do what you need to do. This chapter may feel like there is a lot moving, rising, coming to the surface for you.

Maybe we're born with it

According to research, every year, around thirty thousand people experience some kind of birth trauma in the UK.[36] The elation that we often see post-birth of finally holding the baby just doesn't reflect reality for many people. The whole experience may have been frightening; someone's heart rate may dip, or they may lose too much blood, experience and injury or have an emergency C-section.

I am not here writing this to scaremonger anyone out of birthing a babe. I personally went through a lot of challenges in my births, but I still found it to be one of the most life-changing experiences in so many wonderful ways. We have to remember that two people could experience the exact same birth and process it completely differently. The point here is to acknowledge that there can be trauma in birth.

The issue we have, especially in the way things are post-birth, is that we haven't the time to process what we have just endured. We are given an actual human to look after and sent on our way, often within hours of the experience. Once home, we simply go into survival mode.

What I see is how mothers then often have to rediscover who they are and reconnect with their needs after giving birth. What should be this gentle maiden-to-mother voyage can often be harrowing. In that time, we do what we can to survive. We all do the very best we can. Your mother and your mother's mother did the absolute best with the resources they had within and around them. We also do not often have the support network other cultures or other eras had either.

A traumatic birth can, of course, impact the child. A sudden forceps yank into the world can create a very different landing than floating into a pool in the comfort of the living room surrounded by candles. This birthing can continue to impact on the child. It can impact the way they feed, bond and process their emotions.[37] This can continue to impact the child, depending on what unfolds for them as they transition through life. How the mother unravels into the experience also then impacts how the child copes. And so this kind of cycle continues.

You may be reading this as a child who has been told all about their traumatic birth and how your mother's pussy was never the same again. Your birth story matters and has a huge impact on how your soul entered this world.

Childhood abuse

No parent is perfect. As a parent, I can see how we can easily place unrealistic expectations on ourselves. You can be healing as much as possible on your journey, but there will always be something. Some legacy. My husband and I joke about a separate fund for our children's therapy. I believe everyone should be in some kind of therapy regularly—we joke, but we are being serious.

We can literally give birth to a whole human being and be responsible for said human for the rest of our lives with very little—any—prep or training.

Nowadays, as parents, we have Google. How did parents cope before Google?

Some of us grow up in abusive households. And before you skip on thinking, 'My parents were fine', don't. Just read this section to yourself, so you can be super sure of what unfolded in your childhood. As I said, no parent is perfect.

Some of us will have grown up with dysfunctional parents who react to the baby, toddler or child's call-out for connection and attachment in detrimental ways. Verbal or emotional abuse in the form of rage or disgust, or frustration. When, as children, we experience this kind of reaction, we feel shame. The feels of 'I am too much' and 'I make my parents sad'. What then happens is the child gives up asking for help or connection as often or even at all. The feeling of being abandoned will then unfold.

Some parents can add a layer onto this by bringing in punishment of some kind, adding to the feelings of being unworthy, powerless or helpless. The child may often be confused about where they stand in their parents' life.

And, of course, there could have been experiences of divorces, deaths or adoptions.

Then there's emotional neglect. Emotional neglect can show up in several ways. Some of us may have grown up in households where we had everything we needed: great toys, clothes and food. But cuddles, probs not. Or we had parents who worked all the hours god sends and thus had no time to be with their child. Some parents send their children off to boarding school full-time under the guise of 'providing a better education'. There are so many ways neglect can show up, and they may not be that obvious. Or you may feel your trauma isn't as significant or worthy. As I keep reminding you here, your experiences are yours only.

Parents who often turn their backs on children's need for connection, attention, support and help lead to the child feeling helpless.

Such rejections, as listed above, add to children's layers of fear, which leads to feelings of shame. We hold onto an inner critic or consistent thoughts of being unworthy, unlovable or too needy. The list goes on. The child may have disassociated or numbed out and often lands in scenarios unconsciously searching for love and connection.

Everything we experience has an underlying foundation. None of it was your fault. None of it is here to create a long-lasting impact on you into your adult years. That's why you are here reading this book. You are a chain breaker. The work you do here through these pages impacts you and all those around you.

What we often see is how these childhood experiences feed into our relationships and experiences, how we process them and how we sense our truest, deepest needs. We won't feel like we can trust that we can voice our needs. An example of this may be in voicing our needs in sex. If we have been through verbal or emotional abuse, we may find no or minimal comfort in eye contact or voice support. Maybe we cannot receive or give eye contact, verbalise our needs or receive verbal love in any way. It will manifest (show up) differently for different people, again based on their experiences, their network and the support they go on to receive (the tools they have in their journey toolbox).

Rape

Rape is sexual violence and a crime. It isn't 'forced sex' or 'sex without consent'. Sex only occurs when everyone involved has consented.[38] It is sometimes exceptionally challenging for someone to conclude that they were, in fact, raped. We can often come up with reasons why it probably wasn't rape, or maybe it 'wasn't as bad as you think'. But if you said you didn't want to have penetration, you didn't give them consent—glaringly obvious consent—then it was rape.

Sexual violence is a general term that describes an unwanted sexual act or activity. Sexual violence includes:

·   **Rape:** the penetration of the vagina, anus or mouth with a penis without consent
·   **Sexual assault/abuse:** any act of unwanted sexual contact, including rape, online grooming, domestic abuse and sexual exploitation
·   **Sexual harassment:** any unwanted behaviour of a sexual nature, e.g. sexual comments or jokes that make you feel uncomfortable, distressed or humiliated.
·   And, of course, there is **female genital mutilation** (FGM)[39]

The Sexual Offences Act 2003 explains that someone commits rape if all of the following happens:

·   They intentionally penetrate another person's vagina, anus or mouth with their penis.
·   The other person does not consent to the penetration.
·   They do not reasonably believe that the other person consented.
·   Someone removes a condom or lies about whether they are wearing one in the

first place (stealthing).
- There was consent to oral sex or vaginal sex, for example, but anal sex occurred as well/instead.

What often happens is that a victim finds it hard to express what happened, downplays what happened or is questioned, finding it difficult to articulate the scenario that unfolded.

Sometimes what occurs doesn't fit the legal definition above, which is OK. Your experience is just that—it's yours. All sexual assault and sexual abuse is a crime. Full stop.

Statistics show that in 86 percent of cases of rape against women, the victim or survivor knows the abuser. In 1 in 2 cases of rape against women, the abuser is a partner or ex-partner of the victim or survivor.[40]

It's also not just about whether there has been force. There can be many ways these kinds of events unfold, from bribery, manipulation, threats, drugs and alcohol and other tactics for raping someone.

The long-lasting impacts of rape on someone are huge. And as we know, everyone's experience is entirely different. Everyone's experience after will also be completely different.

Armouring can then occur with the pelvis. This makes sense, right? If there has been entry without consent, then the pelvis will close. For many people, this can manifest physically with vaginismus (the inability to experience penetration without pain), or vulvodynia (a broad term for pain around the vulva/vagina at any time or constantly). What can be frustrating is that this kind of physical manifestation can take years to show up.

Sometimes it shows up after someone has been through one hella of a journey to find a loving partner, and then the pain begins. This can happen as a result of the body finally leaning into safety; it almost gives a big sigh and allows for this level of holding and love. As it does so, it realises it no longer needs to be in fawn mode, so it may move into fight mode, almost like an 'absolutely fucking no way is that coming anywhere near me' vibe.

Rape can also have a long-lasting impact on our ability to find happiness, joy, and pleasure in life because we always feel as though something terrible could happen to us at any moment. We constantly brace ourselves, often unknowingly. We live in fear. We live in the freeze, fight, flight or fawn mode, never feeling as though anything is shiny or sparkly to us.

It can also leave us confused about what it would feel like to be in a healthy relationship, or confused about how to let love in once again. We can also struggle to receive holding, love and support from loved ones. We may give off a vibe of 'It's just me vs the world'.

Sexual violence can leave a lot of damage. Know you deserve all the support you need. There are fantastic resources to support you if you are yet to seek further help. Perusing rapecrisis.org.uk would be a great starting point for additional support.

Consent

Getting clear on what consent means is essential. Consent is where you give full permission to engage with whatever is happening at any given time, moment to moment.. You have the right to remove your consent at any time. In rape cases, the term 'consent' is discussed at length because investigators want to establish whether the perpetrator had established explicit consent from the victim.

When looking at the situation, there needs to be an exploration of whether there was capacity to consent, freedom to consent, steps taken to obtain consent and reasonable belief in consent.[41]

Capacity to consent relates to whether there was drink, drugs, or any medical condition limiting the ability to communicate consent, if they were asleep, or someone has learning difficulties.

Freedom to consent explores just this—whether there was the freedom to consent. Examples of when this may be in question include instances of domestic violence, or when the perpetrator is in a position of power, such as a teacher, employer, or carer, and abusing their status or position. Then there's the question of whether the victim was significantly younger than the perpetrator and whether they were old enough to consent. We should also steps were taken to obtain consent. Was there explicit permission? Or was the victim exploited or targeted due to vulnerability? Also, there should be reasonable belief in consent, whether someone was ignoring signs that the victim did not want sexual activity. Was consent given to all the sex that unfolded?

We must teach our children about consent and bring consent into our everyday language. With our children, this looks like ensuring they are aware that they have to give consent for, say, granny to give them a kiss or for mummy to change their nappy or for daddy to take off their clothes to get ready for bedtime. Suppose we teach our children about consent in everyday life, model not slapping each other on the bottom randomly and share what boundaries look like. In that case, we will be more transparent about what consent looks like in a relationship and thus during sex.

We have a warped view of consent because we do not know what it looks or sounds like. We aren't aware that we actually have to give consent and can, in fact, not give our consent. If it starts with 'Well, I must kiss Grandma because she's my grandma' from the very beginning, then where do we draw lines? Why has the line not already been drawn? Grandma may be confused, but it's time to teach Grandma about consent too.

Another reason we are confused AF around consent? Society's messages. Remember, if you were drunk, you were in a vulnerable position and absolutely not 'asking for it'. If you wore that cute miniskirt from Mango that covers your butt cheeks only but makes you feel like Britney circa 2003, you were not going out asking to be raped. Because you froze and didn't know what to do, you were not accepting anything—you were trying to survive. If you began to befriend the person because you felt your life depended on it, you weren't asking them to sexually assault you. If you reported the incident late because you were shit-scared to do anything else, you feared it all. It doesn't make the situation any less traumatising or necessary to be explored by police.

The list could go on.

We also have to get used to consent in our current relationships to feel safe enough to unravel into the spaces created during intimate moments. We have to get accustomed to phrases like 'I would love to be held by you tonight, but I don't want any penetration; just external touch on the vulva would be great'. Or 'I would love to have sex with you tonight but only with your fingers and not with a penis, pleasure wand or dildo'. Our body surrenders a little more as we practice speaking up for our pelvis and needs in these spaces. A voice in your pelvic bowl cheers whenever you speak up and clarify your needs. Only then will we begin to find safety.

Giving birth

I stood up and pissed myself all over the floor. Not a little bit, not just a lot, a hella of a lot. It was a river, hun.

The midwife stood agog as there was very little I could do to stop it. I had been in agony after giving birth to the second twin, and no one could tell me why. She then explained that as I stood there with the final drips moving down my leg towards the puddle still spreading over the floor, they'd removed my catheter. So the pain was my bladder far too full after bags and bags of drip. I had zero feeling in my legs due to the epidural. I hadn't a clue that this had been removed. This is why gravity supported me with what was needed. A massive pee. The relief, hun.

Her response was, 'You need to work on your pelvic floor'. Ya know, I'll repeat this in this book: do not underestimate what these flippant comments do. They create fire, frustration, rage, sadness and more, sometimes all at once. Babe, you have removed my catheter without telling me, pumped me full of drugs and liquid, taken away my bodily autonomy for the last forty-eight hours. I've pushed out two children and you are telling me that my pelvic floor 'needs work'.

I went through a lot during my singleton birth and my twin birth. Both labours were induced, lasting past forty-eight hours, with tears, stitches, cuts, bruises, threats of C-sections and forceps. If I could go back, I would speak up for my rights again. But quite frankly, three children are plenty for us, and we feel blessed with the gifts we already have.

Births require us to speak up for our needs and the needs of our unborn souls. This is a challenge for some of us, and for others, this comes with ease. But either way, pushing something the size of a watermelon through your yoni or removing it from your belly is quite the journey.

Sometimes, as with all these things, we land in the space of incredible consultants, midwives and before/aftercare. Other times, we do not.

Giving birth changes us physically and emotionally in ways we would never have imagined. We transition from maiden to mother. Our life is changed.

Giving birth can be traumatic, and we also underestimate the impact miscarriage and premature birth have on someone. Every birthed soul, however that birthing takes place, leaves a footprint on our hearts. A memory that moves with us on our life's path.

Sometimes, there's not enough love, time and support for those giving birth. The rise of hypnobirthing and doulas is truly a gift for us all. Hypnobirthing teaches us exactly what we need to know to speak up for our needs. Doulas are there to hold us through the experience, supporting us emotionally, physically and practically.

Those who have given birth need to be given more time to process the delivery. We don't need to go through the ordeal again to rake through the memories, but we must go back to the birthing space to empower ourselves.

I have often given clients a rebirthing session where we celebrate where they are on their path, celebrate the soul and close the birthing field. As we open and give birth, we open a birthing portal. We open the root. What we need to do is close the birthing portal. Such closure and transitioning allow us to heal and bring new energy into our relationship with ourselves and the souls who have passed on or are with us.

At the very least, it takes a minimum of six weeks for the vagina to heal after birth. Stitches from tears take much longer than they say to feel OK, and episiotomy healing takes even longer. I know because I have had both and have heard plenty of experiences from others in my spaces. Everyone who has given birth deserves more time, honour and love.

There are many reasons why people may feel their birth was a difficult or traumatic experience. There may be challenges before or after, such as tears and births that end in emergency care. Others may feel a massive wave of distress or disappointment due to not being heard and losing complete control over what unfolded. As we already have discussed, your birth experience is yours, and your experience will feel very different to your friend Sandra's birth experience, even if you compare notes and it's a 'Omigosh, same. We are basically birthing twinsssss'. Meanwhile, you may have PTSD, post-traumatic stress disorder (birth trauma), or be feeling depressed and have postnatal depression.

PTSD from birth differs from person to person. Symptoms may include repetitive/distressing sensations or images. There may be nightmares and physical phenomena such as pain, sickness, trembling and shaking. You may feel numb to the whole experience, so try to never think about it or avoid people/things that remind you of the birthing event. Tommy's website (Tommy's supports people with pregnancy complications, miscarriage, stillbirth and premature birth) has a great page on PTSD after birth if you feel you need further support.[42] And know you could still feel like this years on from any birthing event you experienced. You are not alone, lovely soul.

For those who care about someone who has recently had a baby: Don't prioritise asking after the baby. Ask after the mother and person who has given birth. We should offer to clean, cook, dust and cuddle the mother and birther before presuming taking the baby is what they need.

Pap smear tests/rummaging from professionals in general

We dream of wandering into a space filled with love. The gentlest of smiles, hands and speculums. Except, this doesn't always happen.

Either way, we must all attend our smear tests and appointments; it's just that sometimes we need further support before this feels feasible. You are not alone. Going through the steps in this book will empower you further. Many clients who follow the metamorphosis process feel they can finally book in for that smear test or appointment.

What often happens at these appointments on all things ya vulva is further pain, distress or fear due to a lack of holding from doctors, nurses, gynos or consultants. For example, when you are in pain, you go into their rooms asking for advice, support and understanding. You get a speculum (likely bigger than necessary) shoved inside your vagina. You know, the place that feels incredibly painful even to the lightest of touch.

Smear tests can be challenging for many. Later in the book, I will share more about dealing with smear tests and how to get yours from a stance of feeling in control. You can also refer to the Dear Vagina section.

I have been at the hands of several people with a lack of love; I get it. During my fertility treatment, the kindest and gentlest place I experienced speculum life was in Athens. Was this Greek life, or is this a reflection of the bedside manners of some professionals there? I couldn't confirm either way.

I know that people often land on my social media account relieved to find someone talking openly about all things pelvic health after feeling ignored, gaslit or put through further pain/trauma in medical scenarios. Some people feel like they've no hope of finding relief from whatever is manifesting for them. Or they don't know how they will ever be able to step back into a medical scenario. Essentially, they go into hiding with the issue.

You're held here in this space, on these pages. I know this book has landed as it needs to if you have experienced any challenges in the rooms you hoped to find love, holding and understanding. I've got you here, babe.

Contraceptives in general

Coils tend to cause the most challenges for people. Most people who stop using them do so because of vaginal pain or bleeding.[43]

'Shit, is it there? Has it gone?'

'Is it supposed to be unravelling from here to Timbuktu?'

'My body simply rejects it'.

'Are you sure paracetamol is enough for, ya know, inserting THAT?'

If you are adamant you don't want to get pregnant, then there can be a lot of fear around contraceptives. Nothing is 100 percent, but finding the one that works for you at a given time in your life can be challenging, to say the least.

Often people feel backed into a corner when it comes to their options.

There's essentially often a lack of consent. 'You're not helping yourself' flippant remarks can push someone into accepting a prescription for the pill when all they wanted was some more answers as to why they have erratic periods. You see, the authority 'they' have makes you believe their offers are your only option.

It's your body, your rules, and your needs. These professionals aren't the ones living with the side effects of a contraception option that doesn't agree with your needs.

If you are experiencing anything that feels wrong, off, like it shouldn't be that way, go back. Say no. You can change your options. You can speak up for your needs. Take someone with you who can support you as you speak up for what you need.

You deserve the very best. And only the best. Your little vaginal cheerleader will thank you for returning to this connection with your body and your root as you speak up for your needs.

Your Vaginal Portal

Anodea Judith, author of *Eastern Body, Western Mind* shares that all foundations rest on earth. Anodea describes how to connect with the body is to connect with the earth, and how our bodies are the homes of our spirits.

The pelvis is powerful. We must take it back to our roots to find stability, love, joy, happiness, and pleasure again. But at a sustainable level. The root space is where we can find a greater depth of healing.

And so, we enter your portal to all that is.

We begin to enter the part of the book where you cocoon to undergo your transformational process. The part of the book where we hold you tight, wrap you in a cuddle while you explore the above and other pelvis-related topics in more detail.

Every day you are birthing something into the world. You plant seeds for new ideas, new relationships, new starts, new jobs, new businesses and creative adventures. You are always planting these seeds, then growing them on, ready to birth them into the world.

Your vagina is a portal. It literally links the outside world to your inside your world. This inside world is your creative centre/hub where you grow, clear and then cleanse, ready to create space for new ideas. Then the cycle continues, this holding, growing, building and cleansing.

As you read this book, I advise you to allow time to cocoon. Give yourself the space you need for the keys. Treat yourself to the things that make you feel good as you process the words on these pages.

As you cocoon, you'll know when you are ready to emerge. Birthing into all that you are. Emerging, never the same again.

You are retreating inside your womb/hara to be rocked, held and loved. Finding true healing from within.

You deserve infinite happiness. You deserve everything that you feel you want and need in life. You deserve the very best of the best from life. You no longer deserve slightly less than. You will allow for it all as you root down and mother yourself through this book. Whatever 'it all' is. Because you don't need to settle for less than sparkly, full-body tingly fuck yeses. You deserve happiness. That happiness really does lie in your vagina.

I'm going to show you the way. Torches out as we explore this unknown terrain. Head torches with Duracell batteries.

Let's do this together. I'm holding your hand as you go through this transformation.

I wake up to him inside me
I didn't know how wrong this was

-2022

Annamaria's Love Story with Her Womb

I've been sitting with this question, 'Where were you before we started this work? What's your story?' and I've realised that I was angry. I came off the pill at the end of 2018 because I wanted my body to return to its natural rhythm (I had been on it for sixteen years!!!) and spent 2019 in survival mode as my pituitary gland and hormones went bonkers. It was a wild ride—trying to figure out what was 'wrong' with me (of course, the blame) while navigating amid dismissive doctors and a lack of holistic support. It was fucking hard!

I was angry at myself, my body, my womb and the system that clearly had no interest in exploring root causes, only in covering up symptoms with surface-level 'solutions'. The endocrinologist I had back then told me off for leaving the pill behind. They literally told me it was a stupid move.

Increasingly, I became desperate to find someone open and willing to listen. Someone who had other tricks up their sleeve other than sending me home with paracetamol or telling me that it was all in my head.

It was a book I found in a second-hand bookstore in early 2020 called Wild Power by Alexandra Pope and Sjanie Hugo Wurlitzer that brought the first big breakthrough. I couldn't put it down. I was entirely mesmerised by it. That was the first time I'd heard about menstrual cycle awareness and the concepts of finding power in my cycle and body. Loving my period was both ridiculous and mind-blowingly exciting to me. I come from a culture where the period is considered disgusting, a burden and taboo. Where the female body has only one power source—its looks. The younger, slimmer and sexier a woman is, the more 'power' she has. At least, that's the lie I was sold growing up.

It became apparent that I wanted to learn more about my body, tap into my feminine power and cultivate more connection with myself.

After I was on Naomi's podcast, I became more curious about FAM (fertility awareness method). FAM sounded like something everyone should understand in order to feel empowered. I also wanted to be in charge of my energy levels and ditch condoms during sex without the fear of getting pregnant.

I was over the moon that I'd finally found someone who understood me and my experiences of struggle.

Reading Wild Power and learning FAM was like opening Pandora's box in a life-changing way. Once I started to experience positive shifts and see things differently, I couldn't unsee them or go back to my old habits and patterns. While my initial 'pain points' were hormonal madness, disappointment in the system and simply the desire to enjoy sex without worries, I was also super curious and wanted to dive in deeper.

FAM training, a workshop with sound healing, a womb connection/creativity challenge and a wonderful womb ceremony with Naomi have contributed to my healing. The connection I felt was just something I had not really experienced before. It wasn't 'just' a pelvic bowl exploration; it was also unlearning the sister wound, letting myself be held by another woman, surrendering to wisdom while nourishing myself through it.

I'm not going to lie; it was not always a delight going into the layers of the shadow (and it's still a process as I go through life). It was a journey that involved all the feelings on the spectrum and demanded commitment but cultivated love and compassion.

There's been so much to work through. I've had to unlearn conditionings about my body, period, womb and sexuality. Release trauma caused by unconsented gynaecological treatments as a child. Release blame and shame around my first sexual encounter with a man. I've moved into learning how to use my body's wisdom to maintain my energy levels and cultivate a more loving self-care routine. There are also the 'basic' things I learnt, like when I'm ovulating—if I'm ovulating, the nuances of my body have given me so much confidence and self-awareness.

When I started using the FAM method, I intended to know when I could have sex without a condom. By the time we decided to have a baby, I had become so attuned to my body's rhythm and messages that I was sure about being pregnant even before taking a test.

Since starting this journey, I have self-awareness, acceptance, more creativity, the tools for tapping into and embracing my body's wisdom—and a baby growing in my beautiful womb.

To my younger self: you are more than what you are allowed to believe. Trust your body, your voice and your intuition. You are allowed to say NO. You are a cyclical being. There's nothing wrong with you being unable to keep up with the linear demands. You've got this, girl! And when you move to the UK, make sure to find Naomi Gale!

Step Two
You Deserve More Mothering, Babe

A Lack of Mothering

To be mothered is to receive. Being able to receive is one of the most complex journeys we can go on. If we cannot truly understand what it means to receive, we will likely find challenge with what it means to experience joy, pleasure and happiness. We need to be able to receive care, affection and love. What would your inner child need to receive to be truly nourished?

We must remind ourselves of the importance of being mothered as adults. We must continue to mother ourselves every day, every week.

Here I am using the term 'mothering' to encompass many different elements. But as you read, you can replace this word with any term that feels best for you.

You likely didn't receive enough mothering. None of us does.

The Western world challenges us when it comes to mothering. We no longer live in tribes, sharing the load. The motherload is real.[1] If you haven't heard of the term, 'motherload', it's essentially a term to describe how mothers hold everything in their minds—having to think about it all. Keeping up with all the needs of their children, the house, the present for little John's birthday next week at preschool (the mother didn't even know a John existed until the invitation landed), the logistics for the Saturday day out. It's exhausting and stressful. At times the motherload tips, tipping mothers over the edge. Mothers need space and time even if that space and time comes from hiding in the cleaning cupboard with a bar of chocolate.

Mothers can only work from where they are on their journey. There will always be times when you, as a child, miss out on mothering.

'Not now. I'm working', one of my daughters insisted on her sister during their imaginative play. I often listen to them playing as it teaches me so much about where they are emotionally and what their household feels like overall. This line took my breath for a moment. 'Not now. Not now I am working'. I will likely never know what she wanted and what I missed out on. However, working brings me joy too. It gives me an identity away from being a mother. It pays towards our essential means. But at that point, despite being with me full-time without a single day of childcare with anyone else until age three, she missed out on mothering and has absorbed that sometimes I have to sacrifice some level of mothering to work.

We all deserve more mothering, love, care and affection. But we have to give this to ourselves. We must mother ourselves into our adult years and understand what it feels like to receive or what we want to receive in our lives. 'Cause even if you are reading this proclaiming your mothering was perfection and you received the perfect amount, you still need to work with tools to sincerely mother yourself. To tend to all your parts and flow with receiving.

Step two is about understanding how to mother yourself by leaning into the great mother. What lessons can we learn from Gaia? How the great mother supports us with receiving and helps us to understand the cyclical nature of our nervous systems. We flow from dysregulated to regulated, and the paramount need of this cycle.

Welcome to the Four Seasons Hotel: It's Time to Check In

There are so many seasons interacting with you simultaneously, which we will go through in stages. There are layerrrsss of seasons.

We start with the apparent seasons:
· The season of goodwill
· The season of chocolate eggs
· The season of cute swimsuits
· The season of buying yet another coat

Winter arrives, and we lean into the cold; there's no other option. The darker and shorter days with colder months stick around. Mother earth's trees are bare, the ground cooler, and there's generally less of a buzz in nature. The great mother rests, knowing exactly how long to lie dormant to have fully restored in time for the next season.

We get towards the end of winter and generally are very much ready for spring. The shops fill with pastels; the supermarket has some spring flowers grown under cover, making us long for daffodils and blossoms. Except winter continues to go on and on and on. We often begin to wonder if spring will ever arrive. 'Perhaps it will now just be winter forever', we question.

Mother earth holds tight, not done resting just yet. Then one day, you realise on one of your usual walks that earth is alive with energy. Buds are forming on the trees, snowdrops everywhere, and that tree is about to burst with blossom. Spring eventually merges into summer, and we move from tulips to roses to dahlias alive with bumblebees. The great mother is buzzing. We crack into our swimwear department and drape ourselves over rugs in parks, on beaches and next to lakes. Summer lands; we make the most of long evenings, warmer days and happy-go-lucky vibes. Eventually, we realise we are making our way through crisp leaves underfoot. We've switched from our Tevas to our Dr Martens once again. We start to layer, and Mother Earth slows. The great mother begins to let go, cleanse and find expansion in the 'making less' approach. There's less activity, and the last of the flowers go over. Mother Earth prepares for the shorter days, slower pace of life and hibernation that comes with winter.

Fluffy pencil cases back out, hunz. It's your first journaling task. Don't skip them. You'll be surprised by what flows.

Unlock your answers

· What season is your favourite season?
· What do you love about this season?
· Which season is your least favourite season?
· What is it that you find hard about this season?
· Which season would you like to love more and why?
· Which season do you feel you receive more from and why?
· How do you pay attention to the changes in the seasons?

Try this key:

When you are on a walk next time, really take in the current season. Consider how the season is presenting itself. What fruits are on the trees? What blooms are blooming? What trees are sharing their seeds? How bare are the trees, or how full are they? What is the grass like underfoot? What does the landscape look like against the backdrop of the coastline? Take in the idiosyncrasies of the season you are meandering through and plant yourself into the season of Mother Earth. Take in these subtle shifts. It will indeed allow you to appreciate the world a little more. You'll deepen your understanding of where the great mother sits while everything else around you feels like it is constantly moving at the same speed. How can you receive the gifts of the great mother as you move through the earth's seasons?

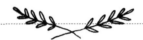

A Bloody Mess

'And where are you on your cycle?'

'My cycle?'

'Yeah, like, what day are you on'.

'I'm not great at keeping track; hmmm, I bled like a week ago, or was it. You know what, I am not sure'.

This is often the response I get when I ask this question. Thankfully, now phone health apps are keeping us on track, or cute period apps are tying in the moon with your cycle. But thanks to the shutdown of our cycles, many of us don't know much about our cycles, especially if we are on contraceptives.

Sometimes we look down and realise we are bleeding and had absolutely no idea we were anywhere near our bleeds. Oftentimes this creates a bloody mess in our fave jeans.

One person DM'd me randomly, and their message stuck with me:

Fun fact. Obvs I've been following you forever, but thanks to you, I can now track my period down to the hour when I'm due on, just

by listening to my body, feeling all the feels, and really leaning into her. It's changing my life. Thank you so much for the work you are doing.
—Jazmin

This person has never worked with me. Not in any container. But just from being a long-term follower and listening to my teachings, they've changed their experience of being a keeper of their cycle. They've become *the* cycle keeper.

One of the reasons we have tuned out of our cycles is that we have avoided confronting the blood. We have either shut it down or ignored it. Shame is the lowest theme (we will discuss the themes later on), so if we feel menstrual shame, then we aren't going to tune in to our menstrual cycle. We are gonna run in the opposite direction. Your period is dirty and shameful, remember?

Not anymore. Dear keeper of your cycle, it's time to tune in with YOURS.

As you do, you put your fingers up at the control others have over your body.

I love seasonal cycle work. It's being shared more and more. It's eye-opening and gives us something tangible to work with, but I was hoping you could learn how to deepen your knowledge. Could you take it to a new level?

Your inner season work will allow you to explore your energy, work with your nervous system and learn what space you need and when. It's your inner compass. When you connect to your seasons, you also connect to the earth. It's magic.

Just like the seasons of the great mother, you too have four seasons. But your seasons may feel very different to someone else's seasons.

For example, you may be someone who can't get enough of summer, but winter feels like a drag. Or you may be someone who adores autumn but cannot get on board with summer. Your energy may vary from your friend Sarah's. Sarah may be a hub of activity in their summer, but you may feel you need to pull back drastically from all social events as soon as you have ovulated.

We will explore the seasons briefly, and then there's an explorative task for each season.

Winter

Day one of your bleed marks the beginning of your winter season. Mother Earth teaches us the importance of rest and restore in winter. You are literally bleeding from your uterus. You are shedding your lining, leaving a trail of bloody goodness as you go. This is an incredibly nourishing time. Your blood is powerful. How can you stand back in awe of the fact that you are a bleeding hero? Clearing and cleansing the previous month for a new cycle to begin. This is the purpose of the bleed. It's a cleanse and a clear chance to start afresh from what was. To rest and then pick yourself up again for a new cycle. A fresh start with whatever it is that's alive for you.

Day one of your cycle is marked by a full bleed, not spotting, but a beautiful flow of red leaving your body. The relief that comes with that can be huge for many of us.

Some of us feel energised during our bleed, which can encourage us out into the world on day two, pushing ourselves hard in a spin class. I get it. But you've got to consider where you could place this energy. Is a HIIT class gonna to make you feel good when bleeding afterwards? At the time, it may make you feel like you are untouchable. Then you go home and wonder why you've less energy for the hours or days to come. Or why your summer is a struggle later on (more on this later). You want to harness that energy, placing it into something less athletic. You may have a vision board you still need to start or a gentle home DIY task such as painting a wall in a new colour. Indeed, use the energy but plunge it into something nourishing, something you'd define as nourishing.

Some of us crawl from our beds to the hot water bottle to the sofa and back again. No, you have started a Netflix series you told yourself you wouldn't start because . . . time. Sometimes we feel all the cramps, twinges and tweaks. For some of us, we are heavy—the weight of the womb physically and the bleed is just constant. There's a general 'meh' vibe so that WhatsApp group message inviting you out wouldn't ever be entertained. Absolutely not, hun.

What I see from clients is a build-up of their uterine lining. If you aren't allowing yourself to bleed with ease, you will find a build-up from one month to another. If you aren't acknowledging the bleeding in some way, you will find that your womb isn't able to fully let go. If you are using tampons that act like a plug, then the blood isn't flowing out with ease. If you are stressed and working all the hours, scrolling the phone late at night and getting less sleep, then the womb isn't able to relax, clear and cleanse. This build-up can cause the womb to contract more during the next cycle. If you're someone who experiences cramping, looking at how you allow the womb to do what it needs to do, so you are working as a team, is paramount for decreasing period pains.

Your winter is yours; just like Mother Earth, you know what you need. There are some ways you can make your bleed even easier.

Unlock your answers

- What do you need for your bleed practically, physically and emotionally?
- What's one thing you could do to make your bleed even easier?
- What do you like about your season of winter?
- What's one thing you find more challenging about your winter season?
- Describe your winter season. Your emotions, your physical experience, your needs?
- How is your actual bleed? What colour, amount and experience do you have with the blood leaving your body?
- Write a list of things you could do in your winter to mother yourself more.

Try these keys:

Make yourself a period box. Everyone needs a period box. I have one on the top shelf of my open wardrobe, complete with everything I need for my next bleed. Organic pads, pants, face masks, hot water bottle, a gift voucher for a massage, rose essential oil, dark chocolate. Think about what would make you feel like the bleeding wonder you are, and grab yourself a box. Any excuse to buy a new basket, hey? You can organise this during the other parts of your cycle and pre-pare it for your first day. Imagine the joy of grabbing this and finding these kinds of goodies inside.

Another key: consider how you connect with your period blood. How do you connect with the blood that passes out of your vulva?

Here are some ideas for you to explore in order of progression. So you'll likely wanna start at the beginning and make your way through the list over time (months, years).

- Allow yourself to bleed into something where you will see the blood. A cup, pads or knickers will help with this, or you can look into the toilet and see the kind of blood leaving. (Putacupinit.com is a free online cup quiz to help you find the right cup for you.[2])
- Allow yourself to free bleed at times into a towel on the floor while connecting to the womb space.
- Collect your blood in a cup, for example, to fertilise your houseplants. Dilute it down with water and pour. Your monstera will be ever so grateful. (Visitors be like, 'Your cheese plant looks incredible'. Maybe it's born with it; maybe it's your fertiliser of choice.)
- Paint with your blood. Use your blood to paint a picture, anything at all. Just the process of seeing your blood glide over the paper will give you a whole new perspective on it.
- Use your blood to anoint your third eye, marking yourself as a sacred bleeding soul. 'I think clearly. I see clearly. I trust in my intuition'.
- Pop outside and bleed onto the ground. Find a remote area in woodland, a space in your back garden, wherever feels private, and allow yourself to bleed onto Mother Earth, feeling this energetic connection. It's primal and a gift.

As you explore ways to connect with your blood, you will come home to your body a little more and realise how incredible it is. You will rewrite the previous narrative of your blood being dirty or shameful. As you come into union with your bleed, you come into union with your womb, your root, all you are. You break the chains that bind us all and begin to pave a new path for us all.

This process takes time. You may feel uncomfortable doing any of the above immediately or telling friends about the work you are doing here just yet. This is big ground-breaking work.

Thanks for doing it for us all. Thank YOU for carving out a new path for generations to come.

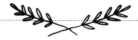

Spring

Springtime, lollipops and rainbows. I'm not joking; I thought it was springtime for a minute in the song, then realised it's actually sunshine, lollipops and rainbows. But you get the intro idea. Sorry, Lesley. It's the fact that you have bled, and springtime arrives. It's like the veil lifts for some of us; we are well into the springlike vibes. When the daffs come out, Mother Earth is in full bloom. If you are British, you are on the beach 'sunbathing' in a coat.

What we find is that we blur when winter ends and spring begins. We often rush out of winter and into our spring before winter is even finished. Mother earth does no such thing. The great mother will only bloom when there has been enough rest. Mother earth wouldn't make it to autumn with ease if all the plants bloomed too early in each season.

You do this when you sack off your winter after three days, or after your bleeding slows or stops. Ideally, give yourself around seven days to be in your winter. Using that vibrant energy for creative endeavours, pulling back to bleed and simply being in your winter vibe. You'll know when you've explored that complete metamorphosis. When ready, you will come out of your winter chrysalis and gently land into your spring.

Spring is when you build up to the biggest event of the month: ovulation. During your spring, you want to be in that springlike energy. For some of us, it will be doing all the things. For others, we find that we limp out of our winter into spring with the pull of oestrogen. Some of us vibe with the oestrogen rise, and some of us find it challenging to navigate this new energy.

Your spring is yours. Just be aware of how you use the energy arising at any time in your cycle.

Unlock your answers

- What do you feel when you move from your winter into your spring? Can you pinpoint that moment?
- What do you do in your spring that always makes you feel good?
- Is there something you need more of in your spring?
- Can you describe the way you feel and think in your spring?
- How can you mother yourself a little more in your spring?

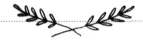

Summer

Around ovulation, you transition into your summer. When we think of summer, we think of full bloom, faces to the sun, short-short skirts and holidayzzz.

For some of us, this is precisely how our summer feels in our cycles. We feel vibrant, like nothing can stop us. Oestrogen has peaked, and we have PEAKED. Progesterone starts to rise, and we get shit done. You'll be saying yes to all social engagements and making the most of this sun on your face.

Others of us find summer more of an inward season. There's this push-pull when it comes to ovulation. As progesterone is about pulling you back into your body, it can feel like a rise in progesterone almost creates this 'off' energy. In our minds, we are told that our summer season should feel good, but we feel inward. There may be anger, frustration or just a general gentler mood. Know that this is also OK. Your seasons look different from everyone else's.

Lean into what is alive for you. If socialising is where you want to be, then socialise. If pulling back and having more solo time feels necessary, then do that. We do not need to feed into another system telling us how we should feel at certain times.

I say this because clients often share how frustrating they find the push-pull of their summer. Your extroverted time may peak in your autumn when you've got used to the rising progesterone. Your output may be better in your autumn than in your summer.

Your challenges may also arise for a short while in your summer, just around ovulation for a couple of days.

The only way you can pin down how you feel daily on your cycle is by journaling daily. When you get a complete picture of your cycle over three months minimum, you will see the patterns and be able to better mother yourself. You'll be able to predict where you will need more support and where you can plan your social engagements. Navigating those yes and no answers that honour you as a whole.

Unlock your answers

· Do you notice any shifts when Mother Earth moves from spring to summer?
· What do you do in your summer that always makes you feel good?
· Is there something you need more of in your summer?
· Can you describe the way you feel in your summer?
· What do you need to receive in your summer?

Try this key:

Journal daily across your whole cycle, considering:

· Energy levels
· Highs of the day
· Lows of the day
· Desire (sexual)
· Appetite/cravings
· Triggers in the day

Set an alarm to remind you to check in, and keep your journal with you to make notes as you go, or round it all up at the end of your day.

You can use this acronym from clinical professor of psychiatry Daniel Siegel—SIFT—to support you further with feeling where you are. It stands for Sensing, Images, Feelings, Thoughts. Pause with the alarm, feel your feet on the ground, and perhaps your back supported straight but relaxed.

· Sensing: What are you sensing in your body? This could be your heart beating or the temperature, for example.
· Images: What comes up for you in your mind's eye? No need to put words to the images.
· Feelings: What feelings are arising? Being aware of the emotions, you could label these.
· Thoughts: Are there thoughts flowing through your mind?

SIFT will enable you to come into communication with your body at any given time.

Once you have journaled for three months, in a journal or diary, on a cycle tracking sheet or a mood tracking pad—whatever sticks over time—look back over the three months and see what patterns arise.

Are there any particular days that seem to mirror each other every month?

Once you have this pattern, what can you do to support yourself on those more challenging days?

You will find your cycle and certain seasons easier to navigate when you soothe yourself through tricky sections. This kind of work is a true gift.

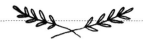

Autumn

Mother earth prepares to sink deep within when the leaves begin falling from the trees.

What's your autumn like for you?

Once you tune in to the idiosyncrasies of your seasons, you will feel the moment you transition from summer to autumn. Like that day you wake up and go on the same walk you took yesterday, only suddenly you now feel autumn in the air.

You may begin to feel frustration, anger, tiredness and more in your autumn. PMS stands for premenstrual syndrome.

I would challenge my autumn regularly. My relationship with my husband was a struggle. I often felt like I was going to land in a panic attack. I have been known to get all the contents of a cupboard out in despair. I've shouted, cried, screamed and lost my mind in my pre-bleed feelings. But I knew I wasn't allowing myself to feel into what it was I really needed at this time.

A note on PMS Vs PMDD

In *Sexy but Psycho* by Dr Jessica Taylor,[3] she writes about how someone contacted her asking why the Western world had spread the term PMDD (Premenstrual Dysphoric Disorder) to her non-Western country and culture. How this will now be another tactic for men to control the women in her country. She was raging. And rightly so.

I have always disliked some of these terms bandied around, the labels. Sometimes we need labels in life. And sometimes, they are used against us. As cyclical beings, sometimes labels are used to coerce, manipulate or micromanage us.

At least five of the following eleven symptoms (including at least one of the first four listed) should be present to diagnose PMDD:

· Markedly depressed mood, feelings of hopelessness or self-deprecating thoughts
· Marked anxiety, tension, feelings of being 'keyed up' or 'on edge'
· Marked affective lability (experiencing strong and variable emotions)
· Persistent and marked anger or irritability or increased interpersonal conflicts
· Decreased interest in usual activities (e.g., work, school, friends and hobbies)
· Subjective sense of difficulty in concentrating
· Lethargy, easy fatiguability or marked lack of energy
· Marked change in appetite, overeating or specific food cravings
· Hypersomnia or insomnia
· A subjective sense of being overwhelmed or out of control
· Other physical symptoms, such as breast tenderness or swelling, headaches, joint or muscle pain, a sensation of bloating or weight gain[4]

Hunz. If you asked me whether I felt 'on edge' alongside feeling bloated, tired, craving dark chocolate and feeling as though work or parenting feels overwhelming, it would be an absolute yes.

What happens here is that when someone is struggling with PMS and feels like they have nowhere to go, they get increasingly frustrated. They then lean into the idea that they may even have PMDD. They read the criteria and agree to this psychiatric diagnosis.

Pharmaceutical companies make pretty antidepressants nowadays, especially for PMDD. Essentially, they rebrand their pills in pink and purple avec a sunflower for extra cute points. Sarafem is a standard antidepressant, and with FDA approval, it is now given out with a smile for all things PMDD.

I am not here shitting on people who suffer from challenges before their period. FAR from it. It's debilitating. You genuinely would lean into a pretty pink drug to help you if it felt like there was nowhere else to turn.

Losing yourself to the latest message from *that* friend is OK. You realise you are done with this shit—this being anyone and everything. I get it. I hear you.

But we have to be careful with the language we use. I am finding people flippantly saying, 'It's probs PMDD', which further shut downs our needs.

Unlock your answers
- What does your Mother Earth autumn feel like for you?
- During Mother Earth's autumn, what do you do that makes you feel good?
- How could you mirror what makes you feel good during Mother Earth's autumn to your inner autumn?
- Is there something or someone who always 'triggers' you during your inner autumn?
- Do you feel energised or tired in your autumn?
- How could you honour those feelings unconditionally?
- What do you need from others and from yourself to be able to honour the feelings that arise?

Try these keys:
See if you notice when you shift from your summer to your autumn.

There is sometimes an exact hour when this occurs, and you may suddenly feel a wave of something, like a general feeling of wanting to be more inwards or more sociable before your winter. It could be any feeling.

As you feel into this shift, mother yourself. What would our inner child need and deserve at this time?

What are those triggers, and how can you write them down into a list to be dealt with at another point in your cycle when you feel less challenged by the progesterone rise? What needs to slowly but surely happen with those things or people?

Mark the days (or weeks) when you feel most challenged on your calendar and that of any partners, mothers, or friends. Hey, hunz, I am less emotionally and physically available on those days.

You will then need to dive into the why of those triggers. Why do you feel resentful, angry, and frustrated? Where does this stem from? Any particular events or scenarios you can pinpoint? Grab someone who can be a sounding board at these times, a therapist or a really bloody good friend where there is a give-and-a-receive scenario, i.e., you listen to them, and they listen to you.

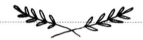

A note on perimenopause

Your perimenopause is when your periods start to shift before you enter menopause. Your menopause is when you have not had a period for a full twelve months. This can only be assessed retrospectively. It's also important to note that periods can go AWOL during perimenopause. This is when some of us have significant life shifts, such as children leaving home, new careers, relocation and retirement. Any level of change can bring about a change with our cycles.

Your perimenopause can feel very autumnal, like a thin veil drops, and you suddenly realise who YOU are and what YOU need. Fewer shits are given. It's a gift; your autumn is a gift. The more you learn to lean in and notice the importance of prioritising yourself, the easier it will be for you to navigate your perimenopause. The time is now to practice working on mothering yourself and putting yourself first. No one else will do it for you.

The Seasonal Mirrors

Your seasons mirror each other. There are seasonal opposites. So how you support yourself in one season will reflect how you can navigate the opposite season.

Winter/Summer

Your winter mirrors your summer. If you find that you haven't honoured your winter in the way you needed to honour your bleed, then you may notice your summer being more of a challenge. Someone who adores the earth's summer, is super sociable, and loves getting through a list but finds themselves slumping on the sofa scrolling their phone, whinging that they have no energy, needs to consider their mothering levels. Ask yourself, did you pause and honour your uterus shedding and bleeding out of your vagina? Because if you didn't, you might likely feel the impact in your summer.

If you go all-out in your summer through work or socialising, you may need to rest more when your winter arrives. Your winter may need to go on a little longer than usual. You may need to mother yourself for longer. Or at least pull in a little deeper.

Likewise, if you didn't honour your bleed as much as you required in your winter, you can't chastise yourself for slumping in your summer.

Spring/Autumn

Your spring mirrors your autumn. You can't be rushing out of the gates in your spring like Noble Yeats in 2022 at the Grand National. You know, out of the blocks, like Usain Bolt singing, 'Don't stop me now', when you usually need more time to get up to speed. With this rushing, you may land in your autumn with a heavier kind of land. More Babs from *Chicken Run* off the top of the chicken coop than Ginger. A louder thud with wide eyes, continuing to click your knitting needles at 100 mph and wondering why you're ready to do time after spending three hours with your mother-in-law.

It's OK to fall off the mothering wagon, but know that it may impact elsewhere. And when it does, you can be with your autumn with more compassion. Rather than damning yourself for the anger you feel in your autumn, you can give yourself a hug and remind yourself you were super busy in your spring: 'I just need more love here in my autumn'.

When you speak to yourself with kindness and understanding, it's revolutionary.

Try this key:

You can work with these mirrors by simply tuning into your cycle through journaling. Keep track and check through each season to give yourself more respect and love when you don't feel like going out. You're not letting down friends. You're honouring your needs so you can be the best kind of friend and showing your friends what boundaries look like for better self-care. When you cancel that date night with your partner, they will thank you for it later. Utilise the language of your cycle. Model it. You are changing the world one WhatsApp text at a time, explaining your cyclical needs.

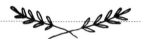

It's SO This Season

We don't just go through the seasons of Mother Earth or our inner seasons; we go through the seasons of life. How we manage our life's seasons is shown through how we manage our inner seasons, i.e., how we are mothering ourselves.

Sometimes we go through incredible life seasons where it feels like we are riding high on the gift of life, and other times we go through more challenging seasons.

Your life seasons are basically the different points in your life that become a priority. Some examples may include university, new jobs, new homes, new pets, new relationships, babies, career changes, courses, traumatic scenarios, relationship breakdowns and awakenings to new perspectives.

We have to prioritise certain things when we go through a particular season. For example, if you are embarking on a new relationship, you will prioritise how you feel unravelling into the space created by this partnership. This is the current season of your life. And that's OK. You can't be everyone to everyone, ya get me. You have to spend time navigating the season you are in. And this season will vibrate with the season Mother Earth is in, alongside vibrating with your inner season. And I have yet to mention astrology . . . OK, I won't be diving into astrology, as this isn't something I have expert knowledge on, but know that the moon cycles will impact you. And if you don't bleed, you can use the moon to guide you instead.

There's a lot of layyerrrsss.

Whatever is alive for you will be around all the layers interacting with you anytime. I share this because we don't give ourselves enough credit for everything we are navigating simultaneously.

Seasonal affective disorder, where you can feel pretty low during the winter months, affects two million people in the UK and around twelve million across northern Europe. We know it's a blip. It's us just feeling all the feels. Even those ring lights can be helpful while ensuring we are including more vitamin D. But if we are feeling SAD and then we go through a breakup while landing in our inner winter—well, fuck. You are going to be feeling all the feels. You deserve more mothering.

If you are in your inner summer and need to pull back a little more because you usually love navigating the summer through being more solo, except it's also Mother Earth's season of summer, when everyone else is going to all the festivals. Oh, but you've also just started a new job. That's a lot. When you can, you will want to find more alone time.

You've had a baby, and they begin to reach crawling age, so you know you need to go out more to entertain the crawling babe, except it's winter, and you like to be less sociable, plus you have just finished your bleed. Those days will likely be more challenging. You're a mother, and you also need more mothering yourself.

There are endless examples, but know that you are cyclical, trying to manage a lot at once.

You have to prioritise.

For example, I am writing this book, so I decided to support myself by hiring a cleaner and asking my husband if he can put away the washing. This is a luxury; only some have a partner or the ability to pay for a cleaner. But I asked myself: 'What do I need right now?' As I write this chapter, it's also the summer holidays. Technically the priority would be my son, who is on his holibobs. I'd park this and be with him, except that's not the reality. My outer season is this book, and I verbalise this to those around me.

I up my self-love, talk to myself with more compassion and take my son out for shorter, more manageable trips.

Despite chastising myself for feeling less than a tip-top mother this holiday, I asked my son what he enjoyed the most about his break. 'Being with you', was his reply. This took my breath away because it made me realise how much pressure I was placing on myself to be perfect for all.

Your nervous system can only cope with so much at any given time. We must honour the space our nervous system needs to feel held in life. We also cannot trust in the universe fully unless we can soothe our nervous systems into any given season that we are in.

Overwhelm is feeling challenged in our body/mind to flourish, cope, and deal with life.

Feeling like:

· We aren't getting enough.
· There's too much.
· There's too much too soon.
· We aren't in control, and others seem to be instead.
· There's not enough time or space to heal from a life event.
· We aren't able to resource ourselves enough, given the current stress factors that exist.

When we feel overwhelmed, we generally risk not coping with everything life throws us. It can, in some cases, lead to experiencing trauma.

You deserve more. You always have, and you always will. Whatever that 'more' is depends on you slowly feeling into your needs.

Feeling into the dysregulation, what's coming up for you? What are the current rising emotions? What can you feel in your body? Refer back to SIFT as you notice a shift in your energy.

Try this key:
Make a timeline.

Sit on the ground, grounding into Mother Earth, and begin to soothe your nervous system by holding opposite arms. Squeeze each arm with the opposite hand (right hand squeezing left upper arm, left hand squeezing right upper arm), move all the way up to the shoulder and then squeeze back down. Touch each side of your face and cover your eyes. Hold one hand on your forehead and with the other gently squeeze the back of your head. Breathe into the womb space and exhale out of the mouth to land deeper into this space.

On a large piece of paper or across two pages of a journal, mark your current age at one end, zero at the other and then the middle of your lifespan in the middle of the line. Write out the seasons of your life. Explore the more significant outward seasons you have been through. Stand back and contemplate how much you are managing at any given time.

Unlock your answers

- What is the current season you are in? What do you need to prioritise? What do you need right now?
- Always ask yourself at any point in the day: What do I need?

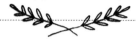

Mama Earth

On a Friday, I was attending a weekly silent disco. It was lovely spinning and moving into my body as the sun rose on the beach. At one of the sessions, someone had popped along with their mum. They were dancing around, and at one point, I turned around to see them having a cuddle. I felt this pang. I have always felt as though I lacked mothering from my own mother. It's been a long process of realising how little there was. It wasn't her fault. She could only do the best she could, given her own circumstances.

I have always craved more holding, hugs and love. But I have also been poor at verbalising this from those around me. I feel abandonment and rejection at such a deep level. I am a recovering CHRONIC people pleaser.

Suddenly I felt tears in my eyes. One tear trickled down my cheek, and I swung away towards the sea. I walked closer to the shore. The clouds covered any blue sky on this day, while the wind prevailed.

I held myself in an embrace as the tears continued to pour, and the wind blew around my being. I paused, breathing into it all. Breathing into that moment. Right there, even though I didn't have my mother by my side giving me a cuddle, I had Mother Earth wrapping me in an embrace.

I stood, rooting down through a grounding cord, being nourished by her; the wind moved around me, holding me, the sea with its constant gifts of being able to hold and cleanse me at any point I needed.

Mother Earth is mothering me always.

The great mother is always mothering you. Guiding you. Holding you. Teaching you. You can work with Mother Earth in so many ways. I've listed some below.

Key practice:

- Breathe into your heart space, and imagine a rose in your heart space, slowly unfurling, petal by petal.
- As the rose unfurls completely, there will be a golden light in the middle from the fertile, golden, pollen-filled centre.
- Allow the centre of the rose to become brighter with every breath.
- Suddenly, the centre is alive with a golden light that can no longer be contained in the centre of the rose. It begins to travel down into the womb.

- Breathe into your womb with the golden light touching the edges of the womb.
- The light fills your womb with every breath.
- This light extends down through the womb, out of the cervix, down the vagina, out of the labia.
- It begins to pour into Mother Earth below, penetrating the ground.
- You are now plugging yourself energetically into Mother Earth.
- Wherever you are, the grounding cord finds its way into Mother Earth.
- You are now plugged in until you feel restored.
- When you are ready, you can allow the light to fade, knowing you can plug yourself back into Mother Earth's placenta whenever you need.

Try these keys:

Floating in the sea

I'll be honest. I have always loved the sea, but I have not been able to go into the sea. Swimming was never my strong point, due to mostly freezing my tits off in an outdoor secondary school, plus wearing a swimsuit at school with body dysmorphia . . . need I say more?

Whenever I went on holiday, I wandered in the waves, never wading further than my knees.

I have never watched *Jaws* for a reason, hun.

However, I've snorkelled a few times because I could look under the sea and see any sharks approaching.

But my determination to live by the sea meant I needed to change my relationship with how I worked with this body of water. My husband is a keen swimmer. He likes to do breaststroke across the sea and frolic in the waves. One day I announced in October that I'd like to join him in the sea; what gear did I need? Starting your sea swimming hobby off as the sea temperatures drop here in the UK wasn't the best idea I'd had. Doing so involves boots, gloves, a woolly hat and a dry robe, and a costume if you wish.

The first time I did it, I got why everyone was buying ice baths during lockdown. I was ALIVE. I dipped in slowly and just stood there breathing.

I did this for months, come rain, shine or hail. I adored surrendering into the arms of Mother Earth while putting down my grounding cord. I floated while using my affirmations. Sea bathing helped me endlessly during the winter.

Around April, when the sea was warming up, I began to engage in light breaststroke. I extended the length of time I was in Walpole Bay, the largest tidal pool in the UK, spanning four acres. Then, I began dipping in the wild sea, not just in the tidal pool.

One day I went in without a bikini top on.

On another date night, I took my husband skinny dipping with the full moon.

I'm a sea swimmer now, hunz.

Many clients who come to me also begin their sea swimming journey post-sessions. I have been sent pictures of naked bodies running towards the sea and photos of post-sea swims galore. It's a calling, for sure. It's changed my life and clients' lives, being held by the great mother in this way. Do you feel the calling right now? Perhaps in the future. This may never align for you.

Begin dipping into the water, feet, calves, and entire body progressing to swimming if this is attainable. Where could you go to be held in water? The sea? A river? A local lake? A pool? Your bathtub? Begin to cleanse and clear. Use the mantra while you surrender to the water: 'I am safe and held'.

Nature's gifts

Work with herbs/nuts/vegetables/fruits. Herbal teas from your own herb patch or just beautiful organic teas. Honour the food you get from Mother Earth. Thank you, thank you, thank you, Mother Earth, for these gifts. Start your own vegetable patch (it's easier than you think), and/or start a flower patch. Watch them bloom into all they are as a result of simply rooting down into Mother Earth.

Houseplants

Apparently, houseplants are now classed as pets. I get it. I've cried at a fallen houseplant. You too could own houseplants or more plants. Do you need an excuse? Mother your houseplants. Watch them thrive in response. See how this works in tandem. Meet their individual needs, knowing how different they all are. Split them and create multiple houseplants. Money plants, for example, are great for this. Or take cuttings and allow them to root down in a vase of water before transplanting them to the soil. (Feed them ya period blood.) You get the point.

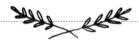

Your Menarche Exploration

Our first bleed is truly a beautiful time, but it can be a turbulent time for many of us. For example, it may not have been truly honoured. Or our bleed may have been completely ignored. Others of us may not remember our first bleed at all.

Unlock your answers

- Free-write: How do you find your periods now?
- Free-write: How do you find your connection to your womb space now?

Once you have begun exploring your current feelings around your period and womb space, you are ready to explore your menarche.

In society, we have long ignored the fact that we bleed red blood from the vagina, which is filled with magic. Instead, we hide the red blood in the toilets and comfortably watch the actors in the adverts poor blue liquid onto menstrual pads. Wtf? 'Oh, she's on the blob'. 'Oh, shark time'. 'Oh, the time of the month'.

Let's first acknowledge what is happening: we are shedding our endometrium lining from our wombs out into the world through our magical gateways. Through our vaginas.

When we can describe what is happening, that will be the first step towards society overcoming this weird relationship with period blood.

Let's share what is happening with young menstruators everywhere.

There is so much to share about menstrual blood, and we have already begun this exploration. But there's more. (There's always more, hunz.)

This is my understanding of menstrual blood. Take and leave what you will, babe.

Menstrual blood has, in fact, been revered through ancient societies before we concealed it to avoid offending the patriarchy's eyes. Healing properties, history, birth and renewal are all held within menstrual blood.

In fact, it is said that the blood caught at the bottom of Jesus's cross represents birth and renewal from the birth/renewal of menstrual bleeds. The red wine drunk every Sunday is representative of this. The Bible even calls menstrual blood 'the flower' in Leviticus. And what is meant by this? Menstrual flow.

Menstrual blood is our feminine wisdom when considering its association with Mary Magdalene. The fact that Magdalene went on to teach through love and womb renewal only guides us further with the understanding that menstruation is the gateway to God. And when we refer to God, we mean however you refer to God: your guides, your lightworkers, your higher self even. We've discussed the importance of opening our hearts and minds to the term God previously. (Cue reviews on Amazon all about how the book was far too 'godly'. Soz.)

To really tap into the energy of our blood, we must take the time to consider a womb space as a portal of renewal. We come from the dark and into the light renewed. An *ahem* resurrection, if you will. We talk about going into the belly of the earth and coming out changed. Whole perhaps. The list is endless when it comes to comparisons.

We know witches have been persecuted due to menstrual blood, as mentioned at the beginning of this book.

Stem cells held within the womb were believed to only be activated with pure love, which gave rise to love from courtly love. Ya know, the kind of love from knights, troubadours. A gentlemanly sort of love.

Those bleeding should be honoured and cherished; instead, the power has been misused over the years. 'Virgins' sought after with perfect womb spaces or their first menstruation. Power was ripped from young menstruators. Periods were seen as a portal to the higher realms, like an actual path to heaven. People wanted a piece of this.

It all makes sense when you consider how lucid we are during our periods. We can birth creativity and love in ways we can't do the rest of the cycle. Progesterone and oestrogen are at their lowest before oestrogen begins to rise once again. We are the closest we ever are with spirit during menstruation.

And if you think all the above sounds far too wild for you right now, just consider that menstrual blood is only now being looked into for its ability to heal with menstrual-blood stem cells. Stem cells do respond to love, desire and intention.

Unlock your answers
- What feelings do you get when you start to bleed?
- How do you feel each time your bleed arrives with you?
- What language do you use to describe your bleed?

Try these keys:
On your next bleed, consider this wonderful ceremony:

Write down how you wish you were honoured when you bled as a younger girl.

What would you celebrate? What would you gift yourself? What would you buy yourself to make it more nourishing? What promises would you make yourself?

The overarching question here: How would you mother yourself, and how could Mother Earth mother you each time you bleed?

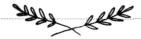

Awakening our wombs
We are going to explore what it means to awaken our wombs.

Our wombs are being awakened. You are here to awaken your womb, and as you do so, you support awakening others' wombs.

Though you may have heard of womb awakening, we need to start back at the beginning. Where did this even come from? Then we can dive into what it means to awaken your womb.

These teachings come from way back when. They were shared by Jesus and Mary Magdalene, in fact.

When Christ was on the cross, Magdalene was depicted wearing a red cloak, symbolic of a female shaman or womb priestess. She was there catching his blood, weeping for her lover, Jesus. Magdalene was the first prophet. The apostle of apostles. Jesus shared things with Mary he didn't share with others.

The apostles were all like, 'We know that the saviour, AKA Jesus, loved you more than any other woman, so tell us the things you know that we don't'.

Mary responded, saying she would teach them about what was hidden from them, the gospel of Mary Magdalene.[5]

Except Mary Magdalene has been written out of the Bible as much as possible (it's the patriarchy, hun). Her teachings have been hidden—quite literally buried. It was only in the 1950s that Magdalene's gospel was published. But actually, Magdalene teaches us much about the feminine. There are different stories about what happened to Jesus after being nailed to the cross. For some, it would be too much to consider the idea that Jesus lived on with Magdalene afterwards, but some stories say they went on to have a family. Other legends and folk tales share how they lived near Rennes-le-Château in the South of France, where they continued their work. Their work was all things sharing their teachings of love. The 'Fountain of the Lovers' now exists, where they are said to have baptised people.

In her book *Mary Magdalene Revealed*, feminist theologian Meggan Watterson writes over and over how this isn't the Christianity we know; this is the Christianity we haven't tried.

Why Magdalene in this part of the book? Well, this is where the education about the wonders of menstrual blood really began in the western world. Such education has been kept alive where possible, taught in feminine mystery schools around the globe. Here we are today, sharing the same messages.

Magdalene likely came from a line of feminine prophets known for their spiritual and sexual ecstasy. We must shift our usual views of prophets as all-knowing, wondrous, non-purple-parsnip-hiding men. What? A female prophet. I shit you not. These female prophets taught the importance of sexual desires, menstruation and love. But their stories have been suppressed by the patriarchy, which would hate for us to know the extent of our spiritual and sexual powers.

Really, we are just here to open up the conversation between your mind, your heart and your pelvic bowl.

To begin this conversation, we must awaken your womb (your hara) and allow it to finally come alive. It's the inner knowing, the knowledge you've always had. Your internal energy is being awakened. Imagine a plant blooming and growing. The petals unfold and spread through your pelvic bowl. The energetic awareness enlivens, and you receive guidance, support, messages, ideas, dreams, and knowledge.

This work is profound. It uncovers truths and suppressed feelings. Don't be fooled into thinking you are on an easy path. But know it is the RIGHT path, for you have found yourself here for a reason. You are ready.

Currently, most of us are plugged into an artificial placenta rather than the placenta of Mother Earth (Gaia).

We are plugged into social media, the news, fast culture, poor diets, electronics lights, money, and jobs which don't provide what we need. The list is endless. Take what you will from the list, loves. We spend our time grappling with it all and looking outside of ourselves. In fact, we should stop, look inwards and closer to home.

Womb awakening is taking time to pause and tune in to our pussies, when we sit with our wombs, our pelvic bowls, our yonis. When we tune in to the energy in our centre, we awaken our womb. We just need to be with our wombs in this way. Nowhere to be, no goals set, just be. You will quite literally ask what your womb needs. Your womb doesn't need to be physically there. The energy will always be held in this place and can be awakened.

Think Adele. You could imagine Adele singing to her womb: 'Hello, has it been me all along that you've been looking for?' Your womb, in time, will eventually respond with 'Fuck yeah; I have been waiting for you, and here you are listening'. When you are ready, when they are ready. When your feminine energy is genuinely ready. This is years of neglect from the world around us. This is you breaking the chain and paving a new path.

Many believe this kind of relationship is outside the realm of possibility. I am here to tell you it isn't.

Making the most of the exploration

What is our menarche? Menarche, pronounced 'men-ar-ki', means your first period.

There's a tantric festival where those experiencing their menarche are respected and honoured. There's a ceremony, and they are worshipped as goddesses. Uma Dinsmore-Tuli writes about visiting and meeting those involved, how they radiate great beauty and confidence.[6] We should prepare our young people to enter this season of their life, conscious of their strengths and powers.

Try this key:

You will want to give yourself around eleven days to journey with your menarche. You can do this at any time and, of course, can continue to read this book and go about your everyday.

Working with goddesses (especially dark goddesses, I find) gives us the support we need when going through challenging seasons. Dark goddesses are deities from various traditions who support us on darker paths. They are often called on by witches or practitioners like myself to guide and support us through our shadows.

Shadow work is essentially the subconscious: The thoughts/feelings/experiences hidden in the shadow for safekeeping, or for supporting with sex or dark magical work. These dark goddesses have darker sides, the kinda energy we all need to lean into. But the 'darker' sides, our shadow selves, are demonised as 'bad', when they're far from it.

I often work with Mary Magdalene or Persephone (goddess/queen of the underworld), for example.

With your own menarche exploration, you could call on support from Sodasi (one of ten Hindu Tantric goddesses, as mentioned in the beginning of the book).

Research Sodasi. Give Sodasi a google. Then print out a picture of Sodasi to place on an altar or somewhere you will see it.

Creating an altar means finding a space to place things that matter a lot to you. This can be anything from crystals to candles to shells you've recently found, to photos or cut flowers. It can be a small table or corner somewhere in your home.

Light a candle for Mahavidya Shodashi (Sodasi).

Recite this mantra: Hreem Ka Ae Ee La Mahaasiddhim Om Phat.

Use it/print it/YouTube this mantra or a version of this mantra. (There are a fair few!)

This mantra is said to be the most important mantra created by Lord Shiva, bringing you closer to shiva and shakti life-force energy (divine masculine and divine feminine energy).

You will begin to feel it vibrating through your body as you work with it. No one needs to hear you or know that you are reciting any daily mantra. Just explore how it lands and how it moves through your body. How does it feel? Does it feel like it resonates with you over time or not at all? Recite the mantra until you feel a vibration on your lips, perhaps. The vibration may be felt elsewhere in your body.

Repeat this process of lighting the candle and reciting the mantra. Do this once or twice a day. Each day you do it represents one year. If your menarche arrived when you were, say, eleven, do this for eleven days. If your menarche came when you were seventeen, do this for seventeen days.

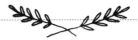

Continuing the exploration

The shaming of periods continues to cause havoc on our experience of menstruation, from severe period pains, avoiding periods altogether through hormonal contraception, endo, a 'plough ahead even though I am bleeding' approach. I could go on.

We don't celebrate, acknowledge or even take the time to rest during our periods in general. But that's why you're here reading this, right?! Any work we do to heal for ourselves heals for the collective. Heals for the next generation.

As a society, we are holding onto energetic blocks, traumas that aren't even our own and emotional holding patterns. This list also goes on.

When young menstruators first experience their periods, what are we doing if we aren't acknowledging, guiding, supporting and holding them?

Perhaps just shoving pads in their knicker drawer and speaking no more of the blood they found? Taking them to the doctors to mask the pains with contraceptives from as young as nine?

Seriously, what are we doing as a nation? What could we be doing for the next generation?

If menarche is surrounded by secrecy, shame, embarrassment, negativity and lack of education, this undermines someone's confidence. This disempowerment can have a long-lasting impact on someone's general experience of periods and femininity. Even the language we use around periods creates long-lasting impact: 'woman's troubles', etc. Anything negative will have a negative impact.

When people are first introduced to the idea that young people often have a dramatic fall from self-confidence around their menarche, they remember their own silencing. They reflect back to the strong, vibrant person they had been before the lights went out and may feel grief at first, but then . . . something more. They feel empowered. Like a wave of determination passes over them. A determination to break the silencing cycle. They meet themselves, the parts of themselves they'd left behind.[7]

As we have our first period, our body has started this clever, delicate conversation between the HPO axis, the hypothalamus, pituitary and ovaries. Our cycles are a gift. They help us tap into our creative potential. From the very beginning, our sexual hormones have been rising and falling. As they do, they provide us with sexual energy. Our sexual energy is our life-force energy, the flow of shakti (divine energy) through our bodies. Our cycles provide us with pure and abundant magic if only we listen and take the time to tune in.

As we bleed, we have clarity and a sense of awareness that only comes from the ebbs and flows of a cycle. The hormonal dance which occurs in our bodies is an emotional, physical and neurological dance. This conversation provides us with changes we haven't experienced before, giving us time to travel into the underworld to have conversation and support from the spirits. We open ourselves up to sexual love. We find ourselves navigating our true feminine gifts.

Research shows that our brains grow and develop in vast ways during puberty. The prefrontal cortex, amygdala and hypothalamus are all areas where growth occurs. Neural connections grow too; thus, our smell, spirituality, dreamtime and sexuality all develop and provide us with a new perspective.

As we aren't accustomed to being celebrated, honoured and understood when we hit our menarche, we cannot feel these positive shifts with ease. Instead, we are taught to not trust our bodies. That our bodies are 'out to get us' in some way. Such distrust from the start severs the relationship we have with our bodies. We are unable to build trust from such broken foundations. We end up plugging our umbilical cords not into mother nature but into false placentas, trusting elsewhere and accessing our 'wisdom' from anywhere else but within.

When we explore our first period, we also experience our first sexual experiences. Taking time to explore both to uncover wounds, traumas and imprinting, which have continued to impact our cycles moving forward, is where we are going with these lessons.

We are now approaching your menarche again, looking back to look forward, allowing those who felt 'meh' or unsupported with their menarche to feel that support and love, rewiring the neural pathways formed way back when. So when you feel into your bleed, you feel into a new narrative that's no longer negative but filled with more positive emotions, though this is a process, of course.

What are we exploring?

Our exploration of our first period takes us back to the moment. Ideally, you will explore this moment, the experience, the smells, and the sensations. To move with the initiation you experienced, we need to go back and explore how your menarche felt.

Some were lucky enough to experience their first period with joy and reverence. Others felt shame. There may have been pain, embarrassment, discomfort and loss. It may have arrived too early for you to fully navigate or too late, when the damage to your sexual, feminine being had already been done.

To heal whatever occurred, we must explore the experiences with the respect they deserve. Your first experiences have left an imprint. We are referring to your periods and sexual encounters with yourself and others. If we find that there was difficulty at the beginning, then these experiences leave wounds. Those neuron connections are made through suffering and hardship. It's kinda like the wiring is left like that of an old house. To rewire, we must consider our first experiences to understand what we are working with. Imagine your neurons forming where there was stress, violation, dysfunction or pain. Every cycle remembers. Sexual experiences can open old wounds.

Such wounds and traumas are not just yours. They are your culture's, your parents', your grandparents' and so forth. Though you will be unlikely to ask your ninety-year-old nan about her experience of being a sexually feminine being, after a while, you will tune in to these imprints and navigate them as yours or your ancestors'.

We must consider the blueprint of our sexual energy. We must look at what we have been left to navigate since our menarche. Poor relationships, lost sexual desires, embarrassment around periods/sex. So much understanding can be gained from such an essential exploration, one you may not have ever considered.

Key practice:

The exploration

Below you will find a list of prompts to guide you in exploring your menarche after listening to the meditation you can find at www.thisisnaomigale.co.uk/books.

You will need the following:

- Journal/pen or pencil
- Candle
- Sage or palo santo (if ethically sourced, obvs) to clear the energy
- The menarche visualisation
- A photo of you around the time of menarche if you wish

Read all the way through before you get started:
- Find a quiet and comfy place where you won't be disturbed for 30 to 60 minutes.
- Clear the energy.
- Take time to sit with your womb space. Resting your root on the ground, tune in to the energies, especially around your perineum area, as this is what really rests on the ground.
- Place the photo in front of you
- Take time to clear your thoughts, and when you are ready, play the visualisation.
- Once you have finished the visualisation, take time to feel the body. What sensations, thoughts and feelings arise at this time?
- Light the candle to represent your first bleed.
- Take time to use the below prompts to explore your menarche.
- Once you have finished, thank your womb and your pelvic bowl for this time.

Blow out the candle, and as you do so, allow yourself to clear whatever feels ready to be cleared.

Journaling prompts:
- How old were you when you had your first bleed?
- Where were you when you first bled?
- Was it a surprise, or did you feel it was time?
- What support did you receive from your parents?
- Were there any negative remarks around your first period?
- Did you feel celebrated?
- Did you feel held?
- Did you feel guided?
- Did you understand what was happening?
- How did you feel when you first saw the blood? What thoughts ran through your mind?
- How did you feel about your first period?
- Did you experience any pain with your first bleed?
- Did you give yourself time around your bleeding days?
- Did you tell any friends? If so, how did they react?
- What happened immediately after your first period? For example, were you offered more (any) supplies/support for next time or put on hormonal birth control?

Those who recall very little about the experience can take time to be with the meditation. Perhaps tune in to your feelings about your periods growing up.

Key practice:

Post-exploration, write a letter to your younger self.

Writing a letter to your younger self is not a new practice but a somewhat cathartic one. Take the time to be in stillness after you have been through the previous lesson. Do this directly after the above key practice or do it another time, ensuring you are in a ceremony with yourself.

Write a letter to yourself at menarche.

Mine would begin, for example:

Dear seventeen-year-old me,

I look back and realise we got off on a bad foot. I knew it was wrong to be put on the pill straight after my first bleed. I knew it wasn't about a poor pain threshold. I am sorry . . .

However your letter begins, let it flow, darling one.

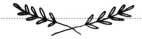

Experiences with your bleeds

Before we completely wrap up, let's explore how your menarche may have impacted your experiences with your periods a little deeper.

As mentioned previously, your first bleed anchors in those neurons. Wonderful neural pathways will be formed if you experience beautiful, orgasmic energy alongside your menarche. If your period wasn't respected, you experienced pain or discomfort, shame or embarrassment. Without rewiring these neural networks over time, you may continue to experience pain, discomfort, shame or embarrassment when you have your period.

We continue to experience our monthly bleed through the traumas experienced with our menarche. You may not have even considered them to have been traumas, but a snide comment from a brother or a lack of feeling held by a mother will have an impact.

We must remember that those around us could only offer support from wherever they were on their journey. No one is to blame here for what happened around your menarche. But know that your experiences were valid and may have shaped your experience of periods.

Our periods provide us with the creative flow we deserve every month. If we cannot embrace this flow, we also limit the energy flowing through our core. With such blockages from the traumas and wounds that have manifested themselves, we cannot access the full range of our creativity.

We unconsciously hide our creativity and creative desires, which lay deep under unresolved wounds traced back to adolescence. Every unfinished project or creative dream that's not been carried out stems from blocked roots. We don't move with this creativity to protect ourselves from previous discomforts unfolding again.

All we need to do to move forwards is rewire our neuro-chemistry so we can experience more bliss and love around our monthly cycles.

This takes time and is very much doable. Suppose we can experience our periods through ecstatic joy, sensual power and love. In that case, we can re-establish our connection with our roots and tune in to our centres, thus rewiring our experience of the monthly cycle. Tapping into such sexual energy only then supports us with opening up our creative energies, as these are intertwined.

Sexual experiences

Once we start having periods, we start exploring our sexual energy too. This energy comes from many forms: pleasure in day-to-day life, our femininity, our own touch or the touch of another. How open or closed we are energetically, emotionally and physically could stem from our first experiences.

After looking back at our first sexual experience, we can look into how this has affected our future relationships.

When engaging in new relationships where previous wounds and traumas are yet to be worked through, issues can arise, such as giving yourself or others the respect needed. Your sexual desires and needs may continue to be unmet. There may be embarrassment around requesting what you need. The list could go on.

Do you often give away your sexual energy without wanting to, for example?

To heal our sexual shadow into wholeness, we must explore these firsts. When we feel we can energetically and emotionally open up to them, of course. Don't rush into moving through painful experiences if your menarche was a challenge to explore. Give yourself time. Soothe your nervous system by coming back to the tools in this book. Immerse yourself in mother nature.

Once we explore these firsts and empower ourselves to move into a new frame of mind, we can allow our sexual energy to bloom into being. We can tap into our full creative potential.

Again, this is to be explored delicately; it may be weaved through healing your womb in time, or it may be when you feel ready to explore this experience independently. For some, their first sexual experience was empowering; for others, traumatic. Some may have found that it occurred too soon or that their first sexual experience was taken away from them due to assault or rape.

Try this key:
Explore your first sexual experience with yourself and/or others in the same way you did with the menarche exploration, in a ceremony, marking this with a ceremonial vibe.
- Send down your grounding cord.
- Journal through what unfolded or write a letter to yourself again.
- Write a letter to the other person and burn it safely in a fireproof

bowl outside.
- · Remember, this experience doesn't mean when you first had 'penetrative sex'. This is your first sexual experience.
- · If you can't remember this first, be with your general sexual experiences as you moved through your teens and twenties.

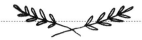

Plugging into Mother Earth

Plugging back into Mother Earth's cycles will only be of benefit for healing your wounds. As you plug your energetic umbilical cord into the centre of Gaia, you will feel the healing elixir of the great mother's womb centre. As you release, release into Mother Earth. Let the great mother carry away your wounds and replace them with love and support. Make time to look at the way Mother Earth expresses her sensual energy, how earth acknowledges birth and rebirth.

It's time for you to move forwards with a new narrative. It's time for you to rewire those connections, feeling the love and joy that comes with your sexual pleasure. It's time for you to reclaim that first bleed. To claim the firsts.

Look at how we are gifted with the flow of a cycle, allowing us to birth and rebirth each month, giving us the gift of hormones. Hormones which dance. Notice how they ebb and flow, allowing your sensual pleasures to come alive and wane as you move through your cycle. Enabling you to renew, rest and restore your sexual energy monthly. This is a true gift worth celebrating and acknowledging fully.

Integrating this experience

Exploring such firsts can surface many emotions, such as loss, sadness, isolation, grief, happiness or joy. These emotions will vary for everyone. Everyone's experiences are so unique to them. Moving forwards from this experience in a way that aligns with you is essential. You may need to go back to the place where you first bled. You may need to speak to your parents about your experience, or to friends or loved ones now in your life. Perhaps you experienced a feeling of grief. In this case, grief needs to be explored more, given more time.

You may need to bleed after the exploration to navigate the feelings that arise during your period. This will allow you to consider whether this exploration impacted your monthly bleed.

As ever, it is crucial for you to honour yourself. To feel your emotions and know they are valid.

You may need to journal further as the days or weeks unfold. Know that any exploration this deep is to be honoured and revered.

We see you. Honour yourself and give yourself the respect you deserve.

Lessons from Peony Season

I bought my first peony bunch of the year and placed them in the vase on my kitchen table. Peony season is one of my favourite seasons. It's June, and you know that the warmer weather has already hit or is about to. It feels like there is so much energy around this time.

These peonies began to open, petal by petal; they unfurled in the vase on the table while the sun beamed in. Every evening I smiled and was in awe of how huge the flowers were getting as they danced under the light of the disco ball's reflections.

HUGE. They were the largest peonies I have ever had. They revealed their golden centres and reminded me of the beauty of my own fertile nectar in my centre. Even my husband kept commenting on how incredible they were.

Best six pounds I had spent in a while.

Except there were two that hadn't quite fully opened. Three of them stole the show, so you hardly noticed the two that hadn't quite opened fully until the other three began to gently fade. I tried spinning the vase around so they too could face the same sunshine the other three had received. Except they never entirely made it to the same level of vibrancy. They weren't made aware that the sun was available.

I contemplated this for a long while after. How those three peonies bloomed into their full potential and there were two that just ... didn't.

They were all in the same water, cut at the same angles and in the same space.

They'd missed out on the sun. They didn't manage to bloom into all that they were because I didn't turn them to face the sun.

You are here, unfurling petal by petal, to truly bloom into all that you are. These pages are the sun. You're finally facing the sunshine fully.

You cannot dance fully under the reflections of the disco ball until you allow yourself to take all the time you need to receive everything you desire. All the rays of the sunshine.

Every day you have the chance to explore your needs to unfurl another petal.

There will be keys in this book that you don't feel you are ready to use just yet, and there will be answers you wished you had unlocked years ago.

Take your time. There's no rush. It can take a long time to reach full-bloom status, and that's OK.

Just continue to mother yourself every step of the way so you can finally unlock it all, whatever 'it all' is for you. Be gentle with yourself as you continue to explore the next step. The mother wound is real.

She sobs

What would it feel like to be safe again? I ask

Tears continue

Her vagina softens

*What would safety feel like, to know you are safe
and loved? I repeat, gently*

My finger remains still in the middle

*The walls ease both in her root and around her
as a feminine soul*

—Sexual Assault

L's Love Story with Her Vulva

I was in a loving relationship. A very safe, caring, loving, adoring relationship. But my body and vagina would not allow me to have sex with my partner. Absolutely no penetrative sex. Over time it obviously became a bit of an issue in our relationship.

For me, it didn't actually harm the relationship. Still, it became an issue for me, thinking I was broken and my body wasn't working the way it should. I became extremely frustrated at myself, my vagina and my body. That's the start of this journey into this kind of work.

I kept putting off doing anything about it. I really thought, 'It'll go, it'll go, it'll figure itself out'. And after just over a year of this intense pain, every time I tried penetration, I realised I needed some help.

Having a vaginal massage with Naomi was the obvious choice for me. Because firstly, I hadn't really heard about this work before I found her. I was ready to give it a go and trusted that it would help no matter what happened. I felt it would still be a liberating process.

Growing up and into my early twenties, I wanted nothing to do with my vulva. After working on this a lot, I had intense feelings of disappointment and sadness that I had spent so much of my life hating my vulva. Then, in the last few years, I came to embrace and accept her exactly the way she is. My vulva and I were the closest we'd ever been. And then this pain happened. I was angry and frustrated initially: 'We're meant to be good right now. For the first time, I thought we were friends. Why are you doing this to me now?'

So, when I had the experience of working with Naomi, the thing that stood out most was an intense release of emotion that I didn't know I was even holding or carrying. It just burst out with me. Whether it was just the endless trickle of tears coming out of my eyes or full breakdown mode, that's one thing I didn't particularly expect.

I thought I'd worked on my childhood traumas and many things about who I am. Many things came up for me that I wasn't expecting. Though sometimes, I didn't have particular thoughts when I was crying. It felt like a great release to cry and let it all out, as my body clearly needed to shift the emotions.

Physically, in the beginning, it felt painful, tight and uncomfortable. But by the end of the session, when Naomi was pushing on the same point, it wasn't painful at all, which was amazing.

While attending the sessions we had over three months, my relationship ended as beautifully as it could. And since then, I haven't experienced any pain in my vagina from penetration. Many factors likely contributed to the fact I no longer felt pain. This may have included coming out of a relationship I knew deep down wasn't the one for me at the time.

Since connecting with my vagina this way, I feel I have a much stronger connection with her. Simply taking the time out of work and my busy life to sit with Naomi in her cabin, and giving myself this time to work on healing my vagina and my wounds was so powerful.

I am so much more trusting of my vagina. I'll never not listen to her ever again. She knows what's happening and is looking out for me, yet I was battling it with her. I was furious at her, but now I can see she was looking out for me and had my best interest at heart. I feel that now. It's brought us closer together. I have finally listened to what she was trying to tell me all along.

Step Three
Look Your Vulva in the Eye

They spread their legs. Their vulva winks at them. A knowing wink. Like a welcome home.

After much exploration of what it means to look at your vulva in the mirror, I came up with the term 'mirrovulva work'. This term incorporates using the mirror, looking at your vulva and, in time, using a camera. It's also more than just looking at your vulva. It's about working on the relationship with your whole body, using the mirror as a tool.

You may have heard of the terms 'yoni puja', 'pussy worship' or 'pussy gazing'. None of these are new. The idea dates back to likely around the Dravidian period of India. So like, thousands of years ago. Nothing is unique in this work; really, it has been suppressed.[1]

In this book, I want to share the importance of doing this kind of work where you feel held and where any trauma is acknowledged.

You may have already felt a physical reaction when reading the words 'look at your vulva' because it is not as simple as whipping it all off to gaze adoringly at your vulva. That kind of approach can feel overwhelming and unattainable for many.

So in step two, we will be journeying to the point of looking at your vulva in the mirror—a slow, beautiful, integrative process. At the end of the chapter, you may still not be ready after exploring the tools. And that is as it needs to be. You are unfurling slowly.

There's a reason you've been taught to fear your vulva for so long. You have to go to the places you've been disillusioned into fearing.

What is the subconscious mind?

We must be aware of the subconscious mind when working through this section, as it plays a critical part.

When present in the here and now, we are consciously aware of what we feel, see, touch, do and experience. We don't store anything when conscious, as we are just here and now. We utilise our conscious minds to make choices.

Our subconscious mind drives us 97 percent of the time. You may have also heard it called the unconscious mind. It's always working in the background, but you are not necessarily aware of it.

Your subconscious mind contains all the stored information of everything you have ever experienced. Think of it like the hard drive of your mind.

Your subconscious impacts how you react to scenarios and influences your personality traits. For example, there may have been some abandonment in your past. And now your subconscious reminds you of this abandonment again; as a result, you people please with everybody. Exhausting, hun.

Struggle to form a positive relationship with food? There may have been challenging mealtimes or a flippant 'You can't leave this table until you have finished'. Subconsciously this may have impacted or continue to affect how much you eat, whether you feel comfortable eating out with others or whether you control what you eat to control how your body looks.

Find that you numb out of relationships? You never felt safe in your relationships with your parents, so trusting in someone doesn't feel accessible. You subconsciously numb out if there are any challenges in order to protect yourself, just like you did when you were growing up.

This chapter explores the subconscious and how we can consciously, positively influence what is happening subconsciously.

What is the ego?

It's the ego that can, at times, keep us stuck. We can work through our limiting beliefs, but our ego suddenly appears, wagging a finger. 'Are you sure, babe?' It will find a story to prove the point. 'You won't find Mr Perfect because Mr Perfect doesn't exist; do you remember the last date you went on with Mr Snorter? Well, that proves that Mr Perfect ain't out there, so you might as well give up now and imagine yourself lonely and alone, being eaten by Alsatians after all'.

The mind will always happily remind you of failures to keep you bound to where you are. You have to be able to recognise the ego and talk to it.

Spiritual teacher of Australian Indigenous heritage Isira Sananda explains how the ego is a veil between what you think you are and what you are, how we live under the illusion of the mind, unaware that a load of stories guides us.

The ego will also remind you of good narratives. What's important is that you learn to recognise the ego and separate yourself from it. To hear it, acknowledge it, but not attach yourself to it. True freedom occurs when we allow ourselves not to be attached to anything, when we execute non-attachment and live in the here and now.

The ego is made up of a story and personality. The story is made up of beliefs, ideas and sensations about:

· what you have experienced before
· who you are at your core,
· what you are excellent at
· what you are not so great at

For example, I love knitting. When I was younger, I was taught by a neighbour, and I created the worst scarf that was inconsistent in width and filled with many holes. I decided to try crochet in my twenties and found it challenging. So I hung up any form of needle in favour of telling anyone who brings up this kind of craft that I am shit at crochet and knitting.

In my late twenties, I stumbled upon a chunky knitter and longed to knit her patterns. But of course, my ego would say, 'Ding dong, remember that when you knitted a home for mice rather than an actual scarf? You'd never be able to take those cool selfies in the mirror with hand-knitted clouds of joy draped around your shoulders'.

All the ego wants for you is for you to be kept safe.

I recognised that the ego was protecting me from further disappointment and financial ruin (from buying expensive wool). So I got my husband to buy a kit (I didn't pay for it, hun), and then I tried a chunky knitted scarf. I remained present with the pattern; I'd heard the ego and sometimes agreed I was rubbish at knitting. Then the next day, I would crack on again.

Eventually, I had a ridiculously long scarf I wore for years. When I began looking at other patterns over time, the ego would pipe up: 'Oooo lovely, remember how you knitted an actual cardigan? You'd be able to knit a narwhal for your son'. And so I did. He was welcome.

The ego involves using 'I'. The ego encourages beliefs the subconscious has already formed from past experiences through stories and then voices them. 'I can knit'. 'I will succeed at knitting'. 'I know I will try my best with that knitting pattern'. It will simply exaggerate what you already believe about yourself. It expresses what it considers to be accurate based on the stories we have.

Tune in to your ego and what it is saying, become aware of the stories, and you will be able to remove the safety armbands to throw yourself into the deep end a little more. At the same time, you'll be soothing your nervous system every step through your favourite tools, of course.

But first, we must find further safety in our bodies to stand on solid ground so we can stand up to the more challenging stories.

Look at YOU

Working on finding safety in the places you find yourself in is essential. This kind of tool, the tool of bringing in felt sense wherever you are, will give your body the space to root down, unravel a little, expand and feel safe.

Key practice:

Find yourself seated or lying down in the space. Begin to look around you, taking in your surroundings. Find yourself looking at tiny and larger details of the room as you gaze around above, behind, in front and below you. Set your gaze on something nourishing, pause for a moment and allow the feelings to land. As you look at this detail, ask yourself what the colour is. Consider labelling the colour as if it were for a paint colour chart: 'Whisper White' or 'Glorious Yellow'. You'll notice how your breath's speed or depth may adjust as you gaze around you. You may find yourself exhaling deeply, sighing or yawning. Lean into this unravelling. Continue to look around you for as long as you need while noticing your body adjusting in the space, noticing a surrender. When you feel this adjustment, you can gently close your eyes and breathe into the body. Place one hand on the heart and one hand on the womb to breathe deeply.

You can utilise this key before going into any activities shared in this book, but you could now consider where else it would be helpful. For example, when you are landing in a consultant's room, before you lie down in bed, before a smear test, before a one-night stand, give yourself time to check in with your body and ensure this is where you want to be and what needs adjusting to help you land in the space more gently.

You could then move straight onto the following key.

Key practice:

Find yourself in a seated or lying down position. Place one hand on the womb and one hand on the heart. Breathe through the heart into the womb. Feel the rise and fall of the belly as you do so. You could also bring in a count of breathing in for four and exhaling for six.

Imagine a peony or other flower of choice in your heart. Breathe into that flower, allowing the petals to unfurl one by one. After a while, you will find that the centre reveals itself in your heart space. Breathe into the golden nectar there until it turns into a golden light. Allow the light to fill the heart space until it can no longer be contained and begins to flow down into the womb. The light swirls and whirls around the womb, touching the womb's edges and flowing to each fallopian tube. The right fallopian tube and then the left. It glows in the right ovary and the left ovary. As you breathe into the womb, the light continues to shine. When you feel the heart-womb connection has been fully formed, you can allow the light to fade and the flower to close petal by petal. You know that this bloom with its golden glow lies within your heart space. You have access to this whenever you need it.

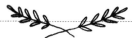

Mirror work

Using the mirror as a tool is work. Sitting with the mirror can be a lot for so many of us. Essentially mirror work is life-changing magic work. It combines using affirmations and looking in the mirror. The term 'work' in mirror work is there because it can take a lot to sit facing the mirror, telling ourselves something we have conditioned ourselves not to believe or to not feel for so long. There's no escaping it all when you sit looking in the mirror.

Affirmations are messages you are giving your subconscious. Your subconscious feeds messages to your conscious without you realising it daily. As I mentioned earlier, you are actually impacted by your subconscious 97 percent of the time. If your subconscious is feeding your conscious restraining thoughts like 'You never deserve love' as a result of being told this when you were a child, this will play out consciously. If you tell yourself consciously, 'I deserve love', this feeds into the subconscious.

Positive affirmations allow you to plant seeds of positivity so you can grow them.

If you then say these positive affirmations aloud in the mirror, the mirror will reflect your feelings. You'll be able to see the body and how it reacts; you'll be right there looking yourself in the eyes, telling yourself what you need to hear.

Now before you slam the book shut with 'Sounds a load of bollocks', remember that the most straightforward methods are usually the most powerful and the ones we resist the most. Your ego (your subconscious) will rise up with all the negativity to keep you safe. Safety can also mean keeping you bound. You can clearly feel where you have the most resistance as you share these affirmations with yourself in the mirror. Which words give you the most 'meh' or 'eurgh' feels. How illuminating this is.

It's easy for us to rely on others for affirmations. To rely on them coming from work, friends, and partners. But when an affirmation comes from within, that's where true transformation and self-belief unfold.

The art of healing comes from deep within.

Try this key:

Grab a piece of paper and a pencil/pen/colours. This paper could be a large A3 or A4, or this could simply be in a notebook. Take a moment to breathe into the body. Feel how the body feels. You will draw your body on your piece of paper based on how your body feels. You'll be doing this without a mirror, just simply drawing based on how your feet feel, legs feel, bottom feels, tummy feels and so on. Once done, you will have explored your whole body based on how you feel. Allow yourself to take all the time you need with this. Pause, breathe and reflect. You are exploring the edges of your body and any thoughts that arise as you do so.

Once done, you will find a mirror with your piece of paper. You will stand in front of the mirror with your drawing. You should really give yourself time to explore how you have drawn your body based on your feelings about what you are looking at in the mirror.

There can be resistance to these kinds of activities. The more we explore the keys, the more resistance may come through. We want to dance on the fine line between resistance and something being overwhelming. Something that would overwhelm the nervous system—a 'too much too soon' kinda vibe. We are stretching the nervous system gently. It's a challenging dance, but tune in to the challenge presented. Come into union with your body; what arises for you? Does this feel like there's too much coming up at once? In this case, you need more time before this key practice. Or are there sensations that wane, and it feels like the practice could be engaged with?

When standing in front of the mirror with your drawing, allow yourself to feel the emotions that arise. If there are tears, welcome them. Come back to the breath. Hold yourself in a hug. You can do this by placing one hand on either elbow and squeezing the arms to the shoulders.

At some point, you will feel as though you have explored this enough, and there will be a point where you are ready to come back into your body away from the mirror.[2]

Unlock your answers
- What do you notice around what you have drawn? Were there any areas that stood out to you?
- Did you fill your page, draw yourself small or run out of room? Why do you think that was?
- What emotions rose for you as you drew your body?
- What emotions rose for you when you stood in the mirror with your body?
- How could you bring in more love to one part of your body?

Key affirmation: 'I am here'.

Try this key:
Look yourself in the eyes every time you pass a mirror or catch your reflection in anything. Even if that's the bottom of your mug or in a spoon, repeat the affirmation 'I am here'.

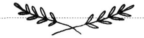

Sadussy to Happussy

One of my viral videos on Tik to the Tok is about the vagina holding onto emotions. Someone duetted with me, sharing a joke on the sadussy, which then hit millions of views. So this chapter is everything sadussy—sad pussy, to happussy—happy pussy.

There are many reasons why you may feel the feels when we discuss all things vulva. If feelings of shame, guilt, judgement, hopelessness, grief, fear, desire or anger arise when thinking about or being with your vagina, it is likely because you have been through experiences that have threatened your survival, which has then impacted your roots.

This is why root healing is so important on a journey. We have to heal from our roots.

Many experiences we go through that may impact our survival, we take with a pinch of salt, snort at or completely downplay. This chapter aims to explore some of those experiences and see how they may continue to feed into the narrative you are in.

The here and now
You won't always have a sadussy. When you are aware of the challenges you have been through, you can turn that frown upside down, finding a happussy once again. There

is light at the end of your tunnel.

Healing your roots means you are working on a sustainable approach to your healing. When your roots are A-OK, you will stand firmly on solid ground. We are exploring the root cause of your limiting beliefs.

We must explore the themes of our vaginas to find the keys to our happiness once and for all. To do so, ya gonna need to surrender a little. You're going to need to sit with the emotions and experiences arising. This takes time but is oh-so-worth it.

What we sit with most of the time is that life is hard. In fact, it has been ingrained in us that life is supposed to be hard. The news and media push negative stories, perpetuating the cycle of 'Well, life is just a constant battle'. But it doesn't need to be this way. There is long-lasting happiness that actually sticks. Turn off those BBC news bulletins pinging on your phone, sharing cherry-picked doom and gloom. It's your time. Your time to explore your feelings and level of consciousness based on your life.

If you want daily joy, pleasure and happiness, then you will need to explore what you have been attaching yourself to. What stories, untruths, emotions and experiences have you been carrying with you every single day? What's been holding you back from it all? Whatever 'it all' is for you.

True happiness comes from letting go of what is and will be. It comes from living right here and now. Nowhere to go, nowhere to be, and nothing to achieve. Just being aware of what is right now.

The challenge of life

Exploring your healing journey isn't going to be all light and love. People will come in to piss you off, your work won't go as planned and you'll get back into the thing that allows you to bypass (ignore) any current feelings, like getting back into the phone-scrolling habit. However, if you can sit with the root cause of sadness, your happiness will be long-lasting. You'll give fewer shits when your neighbour, Barbara, puts the wheelie bins out to save her car space. Or when Dave at work talks over you in a meeting. Or when your bank account drops into the overdraft . . . again.

You'll be able to sit with those things and know that they aren't your narratives to take on. Barbara isn't aware of how annoying it is, and you just park elsewhere, knowing you could mention the old bin chat to her nicely one day. Dave grew up in a home where 'real men speak louder', so he struggles to understand any different. The bank account drop is temporary, but you will ask for that pay raise once and for all. None of those three things on that one day impacted you because you are vibrating in a higher theme of consciousness.

Themes of consciousness

You're on your holibobs, and you pop on some goggles. You dip under the water, and through those goggles, under the water, you see darting zebra fish. Then another day, you see a flushed floating tampon from 1997, now free as a bird in the Mediterranean. You come up from these two snorkelling activities, taking off your goggles, with two very different experiences. One was filled with joy and heart-opening love for the ecosystem underwater, and the other was tainted by seeing a rogue floating tampon.

Themes of consciousness are simply how we view reality. That tampon had been there for years; you didn't see it the first day. The next day you saw it but allowed this to ruin the whole experience. The ocean is still incredible, filled with darting zebrafish; we just need to continue to educate others.

On day one of your holiday, you were living the dream. On day two, you just couldn't let go of how awful humanity can be.

What takes up your being, soul, mind, body, days, and life? The theme you are in and the goggles you wear will dictate how you navigate your days. Where you vibrate on the themes of consciousness scale will inevitably adjust how you experience life.

The Themes[3]

You should also be aware that we move up and down through the themes of consciousness depending on our experiences. We can drop into shame from pride, for example. But you'll rise again like a phoenix from the ashes back into courage or acceptance with more ease as you find more tools to support you on your healing journey.

I see the bottom themes as a surrender into the darkness. When we sit in the lower themes, such as shame or guilt, we allow ourselves to be in the velvety darkness of the womb. Surrendering into the feminine flow of feeling all that needs to be felt. This is your time to just be. Once you are ready, cocooned and given guidance, you will be prepared to transition from the darkness into those higher themes.

Shame is always the more challenging theme to land in or sit with. Some of us live with shame for many years, and others feel it for a fleeting moment. It's the

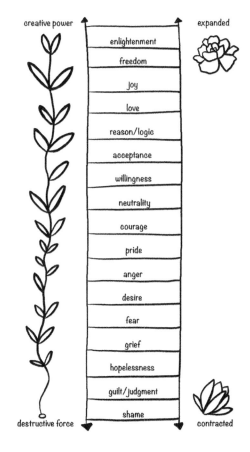

creative power — expanded

enlightenment
freedom
joy
love
reason/logic
acceptance
willingness
neutrality
courage
pride
anger
desire
fear
grief
hopelessness
guilt/judgment
shame

destructive force — contracted

lowest theme. We find ourselves separate from ourselves entirely—often completely numb to life. True freedom and lasting happiness will be where we find things more manageable and pleasurable.

We could look at this as the pleasure scale. It is not pleasurable to be feeling shame or guilt, or hopelessness. There's pleasure when we feel desire or courage, for example. However, every feeling and theme is welcomed, filled with gifts.

Damaged roots impacting your 20/20 vision

Feeling safe in your body is challenging if you have been through experiences that threaten your very existence.

You are not broken; you are not 'damaged goods'; you have all it takes within. We are in the Aquarian Age, no longer in the age of the guru, where we need someone else to heal us. It's all there within your root space, within your womb space. You have what it takes to surrender into the experiences and move into those higher themes. To have the tools to sustain that level of healing. To be aware of why you feel shame, to sit with it and move it through, to be able to dance with it and learn from it rather than dragging it around every damn day for months or years.

The issue is that being disconnected from our bodies is endemic. How can we be expected to navigate the themes of consciousness if we feel completely and utterly separate from our bodies?

'This is me, hi. And meet my body . . .'

'Helloooo'. The body waves in a robotic manner.

This is how we will greet each other in the future if we don't start actively coming home to ourselves.

If we separate ourselves from true existence, we lose ourselves in everyday existence.

Our roots are plugged into the false placenta; we look for happiness outside of ourselves, and we find little sustained joy and pleasure because we rely on the external for such freedom. We glide on through life, believing this is it. Life is simply 'meh'.

I see disassociation in my spaces with clients and their bodies, 'I don't feel much at all' kinda of vibes. Or there's the numbness they feel in their vagina: 'You said you were on the right side, but honestly, I couldn't feel where you were at all'. Or they haven't the understanding they need around their bleeds: 'It came out of nowhere'.

Society has told us that the mind is more powerful. People will hound me when I share videos online about how the body stores our memories and emotions. This is the conditioning we have had. The body is incredible; it knows, guides, and remembers. Science needs to catch up.

In this section, we begin to explore your foundations. Ya know that Bible story of the foolish man who built his home upon the sand? Let's consider your foundations. Oh, how we ridicule that guy. Sand. What an absolute plonker, Rodney.[vi]

What is your home built on, wonderful soul? As you work on your foundations

---

[vi]   Only Fools and Horses (a sitcom from the 80s) joke.

and move through the themes of consciousness, you may feel emotions in a way you have never felt. There may be anger, frustration and tears. It's OK. It's all welcome. You are held.

If our survival has been threatened or regularly threatened, it takes over our whole being. We have already discussed the impact of abuse on our bodies. Now we will discuss experiences that threaten our survival which would have meant our roots were built on a rocky foundation. When our existence is compromised in this way, we can never meet our basic needs fully. We struggle to survive, essentially. Think challenges with our health, money, work and putting down roots somewhere (home).

It's like this. I often hear someone saying, 'Listen, I have done all the healing, and nothing has changed'. Plant medicine and ceremony work have a space for those who feel called to it. However, when someone tells me they've done ten ayahuasca ceremonies and still can't form long-lasting relationships, I gently remind them about the importance of coming IN and DOWN. Literally right down into the roots, gently. Working from the root upwards is the key. This is the whole point of this book. In my spaces, I saw a lot of bypassing of the deepest parts. The most necessary part of a healing path is to provide stable, long-lasting healing work. The trouble is, acknowledging or exploring such deep work can feel overwhelming, too overwhelming. Hence, it's easier to go to experiences that allow you to be doing something, but not necessarily IT.

This is it. This is the work.

In my opinion.

The news and society, in general, can perpetuate this issue, the challenge of damaged roots. This is because the news sometimes forces us back into survival mode, removing our trust in our natural instincts. The news wants you to feel the fear. Fear-based news stories prey on the anxieties we all have and then hold us hostage. Being glued to the television, reading the paper, or surfing the internet increases ratings and market shares—but it also raises the probability of depression.[4] You'll fall back into the arms of the media again and again, removing yourself from this inner work. The trust. The necessary need to come back home to yourself. To plug yourself into the placenta of the earth.

Living in fear is easier, though. We actually find safety in the fear. That's why we go back to the news again and again. Reading about the doom and gloom and pushing us back into those 4 Fs (freeze, fight, flight, fawn). Our focus goes to the threat; we can't find the calm that we need, and we focus our attention back on the mind with the energy moving upwards and out. We almost feel energised by the surge of chemicals like adrenalin.

We have to be able to work through this cycle of fear, but to do so, we have to recognise where the fear comes from in the first place. Then we have to acknowledge what our response to fear looks like. Acknowledging this fear teaches us, guides us and reminds us of our needs.

Triggers are a gift; they keep us safe and remind us of the work yet to be done.

My children love to run and chase each other around the house. Sometimes they run and bang a door behind them. 'Ha, ha, you're not coming in here', they shout while the other child screams. They continue to play this game until I realise and acknowledge that my whole body is tensed, my heart rate is faster and suddenly I jump. Usually, I find myself yelling, 'Stop banging the doors', in a sudden unacknowledged outburst.

Where do I go at this moment? Why the fear-based response? I go back to living in a home with a tricky amount of aggressive behaviour. Where I didn't know what mood my father would come home in. He'd bang around often, shout at me or anything. I'd live in fear of what his mood may be.

The body remembers this when my children, simply playing, bang around with their feet and doors, screaming and making loud noises. Sometimes, I have to work on calming myself in the evening after a response like this. Coming back to my body, home to my roots. I can find safety there once again.

Another example of this was when I was on a vipassana course (a course where you meditate and live in silence for a set number of days) I was eight days into noble silence. In one meditation session, a couple of people on the men's side started to laugh at a bird making noise outside. The teacher bellowed. It echoed around the whole hall. As I was deeply in my own body during this experience, I suddenly completely disassociated and couldn't concentrate on meditating for the rest of the day. I simply had to hold myself in my room. To witness this disassociation was a gift but a stark reminder.

In fact, I have broken the pattern. I know where the fear comes from and have recognised where the original trauma came from. I can express a response to the initial trauma to finish the trauma. I express my response by curling into a ball and crying, running away from the house on a run—things I wanted to do in my childhood but couldn't.

If my nervous system is regulated, it will take big bangs or shouts, but smaller bangs and shouts would also trigger me if I am dysregulated.

So when the threat of loud noises comes back, I need to be built on solid foundations with my basic needs met, such as enough sleep, water and headspace. I struggle with the situation and need further support to manage my reaction if my foundations aren't nourished.

So this work is about:
· Acknowledging your basic needs
· Finding where the fears lie
· Acknowledging the fears
· Repatterning your responses to the threats that come again
· Continuing to work on your basic needs to be in the best space to respond

If you look at a tree, those roots started at the very beginning of the tree's life. The tree may have started in poor soil, so the roots have travelled as far as they needed to find more fertile, hospitable soil. We must acknowledge our past. We don't need to dive into it and dredge it all up, but to have compassion for ourselves, we must be aware of where we have come from.

No longer can we bypass our history in favour of the future. When on a healing path, we must work on our energy supply from our root system. The chakra in the system is called 'Muladhara', which means 'root support' and represents the earth element. If our roots from the beginning, as babies, were not growing in the most nourishing soil, then we have to remember this is what 'nourished' us from the start. We now need to find better ground for those roots.

Let's explore some of the challenges you may have faced during your childhood that potentially still have some kind of hold on you today.

Abandonment

We need to look at abandonment in a whole new way. When people read this, they automatically think of a baby being left in a cardboard box, and that's the level of abandonment we are talking about. One of the most common wounds I see in clients is the abandonment wound. Abandonment can be physical or emotional. Abandonment is linked to survival, as it makes us feel like we are unwanted and thus have no place in this world.

Children who are separated from their parents can feel abandoned. Short periods are manageable, but more prolonged separation through relationship breakdowns like divorce, hospital stays, longer work trips and boarding school can create this abandonment wound.

Adoption also creates an abandonment wound as a child is given up by their birth parent(s), so those who adopt have to make up for this space created.

If there was a lack of love in the home environment through touch, this also is abandonment. We need touch to regulate ourselves. Letting the baby cry it out couldn't be more ludicrous. A baby is crying because it needs something, whether that's support to regulate, touch, food, or nappy changes cause they've done the 456th shit of the day. I remember when my mother-in-law came around, and I was navigating my firstborn's needs in the first few days. She encouraged me to pop him down in the kitchen in his pod, shut the door and sit in the lounge with him screaming. 'Oh, back in the day, we'd put the baby in a pushchair and wheel them to the bottom of the garden'. Don't get me wrong, I can see the allure. More so when I had the twins and was on a constant conveyor belt of cries. But from that moment on, I gripped that little bear harder than ever. It didn't feel right. He has since trotted off to preschool and nursery with absolutely no problems. He hugs me daily, tells me he loves me and gives me impromptu kisses. He walks to me for a cuddle at the end of the school day. I am truly blessed. His foundations were built on the strongest ground I found for him.

With the twins, it's been slightly different. Both of them have struggled a little more with going to school, and I genuinely feel that's because they were twins, and there would have been times, despite my tandem baby-wearing days, when they were left to cry a little longer than my firstborn would have been. And because I cannot split myself three ways, I do my best.

As adults, we can be super responsive to times when the abandonment wound is triggered. For example, if someone says something negative to you, there may be a response that doesn't feel aligned; you may physically respond by going into one of the 4Fs. Or if there is a relationship breakdown, you may feel this more than someone else who never had the abandonment wound activated.

We lose trust in others or ourselves. We often find that we cling to food, others, routine or security (such as crappy jobs rather than committing to the self-employed life you crave). We also find that we abandon ourselves, never feeling good enough or worthy of whatever it may be. The abandonment of self.

Birth trauma

Postnatal care has been a struggle for years. Doulas are becoming more common, postnatal care needs are being assessed a little more, and breastfeeding is back in the spotlight.

As our souls come into our bodies with our first breath, we experience the world for the first time. How we experience the world at this point impacts our survival. So if we are born and taken from our mothers and placed in incubation, for example, we will have a very different experience to a baby birthed into a water pool, placed in their mother's arms, and surrounded by candles in their home environment.

The birth of the baby impacts those initial days. I have seen this firsthand in my twins. The first twin left with ease (albeit after a forty-eight-hour labour), but once she made it into the world, I held her for a moment and then she was skin-to-skin with my husband. The second baby took forty-five minutes to make it out, but this time her heartbeat dropped; they grabbed the forceps and yanked her through but couldn't do delayed cord clamping as they were worried about her heart rate. Twin A went on to have a bit of jaundice but was a feeding queen. Twin B went on to have low blood sugar levels and was forced to have her blood checked while being prodded and poked, shoved with formula and taken into the NICU for all of two hours. Afterwards, she continued to find feeding a challenge, gave up the boob first, at two, and needed much more soothing than Twin A. This is still plain to see at four years old. Birth matters.

Proper foundations at birth and post-birth will likely mean a baby who feels nurtured with ease finds calm in general, accepts positive support with more open arms and experiences a more calming initial few months as the first roots are bedded in.

Food

Our relationship with food can be impacted by how our parents navigated our mealtimes and snacks.

Here are just a few examples: If there wasn't enough food growing up. Poor-quality meals. Mealtimes that were stressful. If food was used in response to behaviours, to cheer you up or as a reward or bribe for being good. If you had to eat when you really weren't hungry. If you had to fight with siblings for food. If you had to wait for other family members to eat before you could eat. If there was shouting at the dinner table. The list goes on.

These kinds of experiences then land us into adult challenges with food. These can include not being aware of when we are full, addiction to food, controlling and manipulating our diets and digestive issues such as IBS.

Other experiences may include being breastfed when the mother felt all the feelings, seeing parents grow up with an unhealthy relationship to their food or being in a challenging environment when eating.

I can really speak to the last challenge. Remember I spoke about my digestive issues. How I was in agony and ended up in A&E and had unnecessary surgery. Then when I did my womb massage training, my ICV was holding onto emotions and the repressed emotions of growing up in an emotionally abusive environment. Well, I had a poor relationship with food growing up. As I got older, I avoided eating with my parents, mainly living off baked beans on toast. I often found myself sitting in a chair being hurled abuse by my dad. It was horrendous to me. I learnt to not flinch and to turn off my emotions to keep myself safer in the scenario. Often my dad was angry or frustrated during mealtimes. I was emotionally 'full'. So when I couldn't eat, my parents would be pretty frustrated, telling me I was fussy. I was really slim in those later teen years. So much so that my period didn't arrive until I was seventeen. And we know we need enough fat to have a period. That's why those who are anorexic or bulimic often lose their period in time.

Now, I have an excellent relationship with food. I understand that I need to eat in a harmonious environment. When my children were younger and being, ya know, children at mealtimes, I found eating challenging. So my husband and I spent a couple of years eating our meals together after the kids' bedtime. This was so much easier on my gut.

Nourishment comes from a plethora of sources, not just food. So the kinds of challenges with food may also come through from other areas of our lives. It makes sense, for example, if you aren't satisfied at work, that you will try and find satisfaction through food.

Physical abuse

Children of the 90s (and of course, kids from the eras before this) grew up with smacked bottoms galore. Hitting children in the 90s seemed to be a given after years of normalising this punishment tool. I witnessed my friend being slapped by their mum, for example. But it doesn't make this OK. As a child who went through physical abuse beyond just a smacked bum, I find it a real challenge when I still hear a parent flippantly say, 'You'll get a smacked bottom'. The Crime Survey for England and Wales (CSEW) estimated 1 in 5 adults aged 18 to 74 years experienced at least one form of child abuse, whether emotional abuse, physical abuse or sexual abuse, or witnessed domestic violence or abuse, before the age of sixteen. This totals 8.5 million people.[5] My husband actually has to remind himself not to cheekily smack me on the bum. It's not OK. He knows that. It's just this is what we grew up seeing. And some of us may enjoy that. This is where we really have to think about these foundations and how they can continue to impact us, so we draw boundaries. And drawing boundaries is hard when boundaries didn't exist when we were growing up.

When we were hit as children, we would disassociate from our bodies, creating a pandemic of people who numb out from their bodies in general. We often find ourselves in potentially dangerous scenarios because we are very good at disassociating. If we grew up in pain, we find pain a source of holding. We appreciate feeling the pain because that is familiar, so we will likely find ourselves back in scenarios causing pain, so the cycle continues.

This kind of strain on the nervous system will ensure we develop some coping strategies. Either we disassociate and numb out to bodily sensations, or we obsess over the body, for example, through dieting. Calorie counting is a way to control something when everything else has been out of control. It's how Slimming World get ya.

We often come back to fear, as that feels safer. We can end up living in constant fear of being physically abused. We relate to walking on eggshells. We will find ourselves in future despair and catastrophic scenarios, as we understand catastrophe. If everything feels quiet and wonderful, that can feel unsafe. Living in dysregulation when you come from dysregulation is hella easier and more familiar.

Boundaries

My first-ever coaching session for my business was a thousand pounds and spanned over a whole day with two weeks holding. It was all around boundaries. Before that, I had spent six months with a therapist every other week, focusing on boundaries. After coming home to my body and feeling safe in my own body, I started to recognise my patterns around allowing people to take the absolute piss. But this was a journey, for sure. And it was showing up like a red flashing light in every part of my life, but I had no idea what a boundary sounded or looked like.

I remember telling my therapist about being on the beach and having a book in my bag. My children began playing with another child, and their parents were there. We ended up chatting to the parents except, quite frankly, I couldn't give a shit. So instead of getting out my novel, lounging back and enjoying this time where my husband could watch the children, I sat talking preschools, schools and obstinate behaviours in four-year-olds. I didn't know the parents or the child and didn't fancy making small talk. She asked me why I didn't just get my book out and say, 'I'm just going to read my book now'.

'What?!' I exclaimed. 'This wasn't an option?' We spent the rest of this session discussing why and what that looks like.

This, hunz, is someone with absolutely no clue about boundaries. What do they look like? What do they sound like? What do they mean for me and others? Not a scooby.

Why? Because when there is a lack of safety or predictability, our understanding of boundaries goes out the window. Your boundaries are vibrations that people pick up on. When they see you lack them, they are subconsciously like moths to flames.

They will know that you can be easily manipulated to meet all of their needs, leaving you feeling like you're constantly lacking. But hey, you're likely used to that, so you don't notice it until you feel like screaming, 'Enough is enough'.

You may likely go through a huge awakening with boundaries, from someone with none to someone who wants to build a wall around them. I remember when this occurred, and my first words of a session with my therapist were, 'I basically just want everyone to fuck off'.

When we know our roots are of deep, nourishing support, we can say enough is enough for whatever it may be. Examples may include your mother insisting you have another slice of her lovingly made apple pie, your friend who puts out her bottom lip to ensure you do another three shots of tequila with her because this is also HER night, the friend who comes around and never leaves when you have work to do, but you can't face telling her because SHE is feeling bored with her own life at home.

That phrase 'stand your ground'? You can't do that if your ground is rocky, made of sand, and your roots aren't penetrating deep enough to allow you to do just that. We need boundaries to feel good to you, and if you are still determining these, then it's a journey you need to take, one that begins by working on your foundations. Your boundaries will likely come later as you awaken to your needs.

What vagina? What womb?

People who land in my spaces often do so because they have ignored their vagina or womb for a long time. Decades. Sometimes people come in their menopausal years, realising that they have never acknowledged their pelvic bowl. It was always seen as an inconvenience.

Except it is intrinsically part of you and your whole system. Your period reminds you of your health. It's your fifth vital sign.

The body then becomes separate from who we are. Except when you realise you are at one with each other and can work as a team, you begin to work with the reflection your pelvis is giving you at any given time. For example, painful periods reflect where you are emotionally and physically.

It ain't yours, hun

At times this damaged root scenario isn't even yours. It's fear of pain that has travelled down the lineage.

Often those parents who have experienced miscarriages place this fear on their child without even realising it; the womb remembers. You were once in your mother's womb, and the fear they had carrying you is then passed onto you. You may feel anxious on the regular but with no real clue as to where this is coming from. Perhaps it comes from the anxiety you felt in the womb from your mother's understandable fear of loss.

If your parents experienced war, racial abuse, loss or physical abuse, then you will feel that too. This may come through in stories or how they behave around certain aspects of life.

It's not yours, and it never was yours, but recognising this is part of the journey. Then, building on your foundations will only ever be supportive.

Often, when we do this work it has ripple effects to those around us. So if you begin to stand firm, this will be felt and only have a positive impact on those around you. (Even if that is challenged by others while working on your boundaries to begin with.)

Try this key:

Take time to sit with yourself in the mirror once, twice or even three times. Build up from five mins to fifteen mins. Work on just being in the mirror with yourself. You could add in being with a playlist. Simply head to www.thisis-naomigale.co.uk/books for the playlist.

Key affirmations:

Choose one or two affirmations to work with when with the mirror. Or write these on a mirror where you will see them daily.

I am allowed to be here

I love my body

I love you

I trust in the wisdom of my body

I am loved and nurtured

The earth below holds me

We can now team up our experiences with the themes to explore the themes of your vagina.

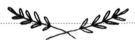

The Theme of Your Vagina

If we are within the negative themes, then it makes sense that we will feel negative thoughts, feelings, desires. If we are within the positive themes, we will feel positive thoughts, feelings and desires.

Each theme is rooted in repeated feelings, actions and thoughts.

As you become more aware of the theme you are in (the goggles you are viewing life through), you will be mindful of the inner dialogue and be able to make the shifts needed. The ego-mind, however, will do all it can to keep you stuck in a theme because it wants to keep you safe. You are challenging this sense of control by awakening to the challenges you have faced and how they have held you where you are.

Let's explore these themes in more detail so you can consider whether you have been wearing these goggles or whether these are currently the goggles you are donning.

Shame

Wound: Rejection

Shame is all around the feelings of being unlovable or unwanted.

This very much can come from the abandonment wound. We may have been rejected, neglected or abused in some way.

We can lean into thoughts of being a waste of space, for example, not needed, feeling as though we are pointless, unworthy of any kind of love and acceptance, ashamed or easily embarrassed.

This is the most challenging theme, as it is the lowest theme we can sit in. The despair can be crippling.

Anytime anyone has made us feel ashamed of who we are by poking fun at us for some reason or leaving us behind somehow, this is shame. It can also come from those of us who experienced a very God-heavy environment: 'You'll be rejected by God; he won't love you for that choice'.

The ego will continuously try and prove how unlovable someone is in order to keep us safe from being unloved. For example, 'Mr Perfect does exist'. Or 'That guy I was on a date with who seemed to be a wonderful man will leave me, so I shan't date him again'.

How many rom-coms are genuinely based around shame? The whole story is around one of the main characters sabotaging the relationship in favour of being kept in perpetual shame. We throw cushions at the TV: 'WHY? Why did you leave her standing there, you absolute prat'. Oh yeah, because later it's revealed that he lost his father and feels as though he would be left again, so feels unworthy of love. The ego keeps him safe by reminding him of this story and any other story that has proved he is unlovable. He feels ashamed to even exist and leaves her standing there because that is the safest option.

Shame may be triggered if there is a traumatic, abusive or humiliating scenario. Thoughts: 'I am disgraceful, I am ridiculous, I am awful, I am unworthy of love, I am ugly, I shouldn't exist'.

Shame is the most challenging to move through because shame stems from deep-seated experiences, buried deep, deep down. It can be a challenge to access the narratives that are keeping you in shame. Living with shame is easier than finding those stories that perpetuate your self-destructive self-talk.

The shame is not yours. It never was yours. It comes from experiences out of your control or words given to you.

It's time to hand back the shame.

New soil for those roots

When you realise that you are worthy of love, always have been and always will be, that's when you can begin to move through the themes. Even when you are most challenged, you are still worthy of love. Those who try and project their shame onto you are only vibrating in the theme of shame themselves. This shame isn't yours. Society works with shame to keep people stuck in old thought patterns to sell you the next product or experience; shame is being used as a weapon and isn't yours. You deserve to be here and always will. You move through previous stories that have kept you stuck and lean into feelings of being worthy of love because you are loved as you are.

Key overall affirmation for shame
I am loved.

Key shame table:

Thought	Feeling	Result	Current rooted belief	New soil for those roots
'I never feel pleasure when I self-pleasure'	Humiliation	You aren't present with a self-pleasure scenario or you don't self-pleasure	I am disgraceful	I claim back my body as mine
'I hate my belly and I look gross'	Sadness	I won't eat out with my friends tonight	I'm unlovable	I am grateful for my body and all that it does for me
'I am unworthy of love'	Rejection	I will find people who reject me to prove being unworthy (e.g., I like 'bad guys')	I don't deserve love	I am worthy of love
'I don't want my period'	Humiliation	I will stick with the pill even if I feel as though it's adding to my depressive feels	I am gross	I deserve to bleed and cleanse each month

'My labia are too big'	Humiliation	I want to get labiaplasty surgery because mine are different to everyone else's	I am ugly	I am loved exactly as I am

Key practice:

The ego can be exceptionally strong-willed here. We want to work not on removing the ego but moving through these thoughts. If it starts to feel overwhelming at any given time, you can work with the ego eradicator to quieten down the ego. The ego eradicator is a kundalini kriya practice. Kundalini is the feminine form of the Sanskrit adjective meaning 'circular' or 'coiled', and in kundalini yoga it refers to this life force coiled like a serpent at the base of the spine that can be moved along to the head through postures and movement. Kriyas in kundalini are where we use a sequence of physical actions, working towards a specific goal. They say that the best way to work with a kriya is to choose one and do it for a full forty days and see the impact it has. But you can use them as and when you choose to, of course. This is your journey and practice.

In this case, it is to quieten the ego. Here's what to do:
·   Sit with legs crossed (easy pose).
·   Lift the arms to a 60-degree angle.
·   Keep the elbows straight, reminding the shoulders to relax and allow the crown to be lifted.
·   Reach up with the thumbs up as if you are pointing to the sky with your thumbs.
·   Your fingers are then folded to the base of the fingers. (Rather than thumbs-up like you normally world, the fingers curl round to sit at the base of your fingers.)
·   Keep your focus above your head. If you feel safe enough in the space at the beginning or over time, you can bring your eyes to a close.
·   You will then begin 'breath of fire'. This is where you breathe from your belly by exhaling only and allowing an automatic snapback with the diaphragm. (Head to thisisnaomigale.co.uk/books for more about this practice). Continue for 1–11 minutes. Start for short periods and build up.
·   Doing this daily for 1-3 minutes will support regulating you when the ego pipes up.
·   At the end, inhale deeply and bring the arms above the head so the thumb tips touch. Open the fingers to point up to the sky. You can then do, if accessible, a mula bandha lock, which is where you do a pelvic floor hold (Kegel), hold in the breath and do this for as long as you need

(though not everyone has access to their pelvic floor).

· Exhale by lowering the arms down to brush the aura around you (your energy field), sit and pause with palms up, for energy to be received, or palms down, to keep the energy contained.

· Take a moment to sit with the sensations in the body.

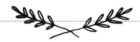

Guilt and Judgement

Wounds: Judgement

Next up, guilt and judgement are trotting closely behind shame in the ring. Oh wait a second, shame is sniffing guilt and judgement's arse. And now we can't tell where shame started and morphed into guilt and judgement.

Guilt and judgement are super close to shame. The way to recognise that you are moving on to guilt and judgement is to take a step back and see that the shame you carried/carry or that is/was projected onto you. It ain't yours and never was.

When we feel judged, we feel guilt.

Shame is around feeling unlovable, while guilt and judgement are about our choices and whether they are wrong or right.

You know when you spent 3,456 days overthinking the conversation you had when you met your friend's friend at that party, and you made a joke? 'It was a funny joke. Or was it funny? Or did it simply piss her off? Maybe she will think I am a right dick. What was it I said after the joke to lighten the mood?' You get the idea.

When it comes to experiencing joy and happiness, we must learn from the feelings of guilt to not repeat patterns. But when we overthink everything, we are hard on ourselves, cruel and just damn right mean. We can never experience the joy of, for example, meeting our friend's friend because we overanalyse and sit in a pool of frustration.

Perfection doesn't exist. In our world, when guilt and judgement are running amok, it is like we are continuously striving for perfection, which is unattainable, so we are in a constant cycle of feeling less than.

When we are children, we make plenty of mistakes. Adults around us should remind us of the importance of those mistakes. They cheer us on as we fall off the bike and get back on. Except over time, errors are lost on us. Some of us cripple ourselves over doing anything we dream of or anything that truly brings us joy, for fear of it being less than the perfection we had sought in our minds.

There will likely be judgement from somewhere and then the rising feelings of guilt from the lack of 'perfection' or 'wrongdoing' that stems from being intimated into those feelings of never making an error.

Make an error, and there will be consequences (punishment). If we grew up in an environment where we were punished for 'wrongdoings', then we find ourselves wading around in fear of being useless, no good, a loser of sorts, stupid. We don't get back on any bike. We feel like shit.

Placing these dizzy heights on a child comes from a place of love (mostly), except we are destined to fall into a pit of suffering. The ego bloody loves clinging to judgement.

To move guilt through, we need to surrender to the reminder that we cannot make the best judgements at all times. We are not perfect. We can tune in to our softer side when we break from this perfection cycle. The side of us that allows in mistakes.

We make choices from a space of knowing. We don't know everything.

We do our best with our experiences, the physical place we are in, the current understanding of the repercussions of said choices, the inner strength we have at the time and the headspace we occupy.

There are so many idiosyncrasies when we make choices. You're doing your bloody best, hunz. You are loved and held as you step from one space to another on your learning journey.

New soil for those roots

Remind yourself regularly that you didn't know any better at the time. You are navigating from a place of understanding that you are only human with your own human experiences, doing the best you can, given the experiences you have had. Everyone else is also working from this space, doing their best. No one judges you with the choices you make. Know that you no longer need to judge yourself through this critical eye. Without your mistakes, you wouldn't be where you are today. They allow you to grow and learn. You knew that, though, didn't you?

Key overall affirmation for guilt and judgement

I forgive myself.

Key guilt and judgement table

Thought	Feeling	Result	Current rooted belief	New soil for those roots
'I am bad at sex'	Embarrassment	I do not feel any joy or pleasure during sex	I don't deserve pleasure	I deserve joy and pleasure
'I can't dance with my body like that'	Humiliation	I will just watch others dance or I'll dance with rigidity to avoid being fully seen	I don't 'look' good when I dance	I deserve to express myself through movement
'I can't be in a long-term relationship'	Unworthiness	I will avoid relationships or find the relationships I know won't last	I am unworthy of love	I deserve respect and a deeper love
'I have too much baggage to be a mother'	Unworthiness	I will put off having children until I have sorted out my 'shit'	I do not deserve to feel unconditional love	I am worthy of unconditional love
'I don't know how to self-pleasure properly'	Embarrassment	I avoid self-pleasuring because everyone is having orgasms and I am not	I am broken	I deserve touch to feel safe and loved

Try this key for guilt and judgement:

Grab a large sheet of paper or stick a few A4 sheets together. Grab a fun pen or lots of pencil crayons. Allow yourself to sit rooted on the ground, sending down the grounding cord. Once you feel safe and held, begin writing down where you still judge yourself or others. Get messy with your writing, your words and your exploration. Feel into the experiences you've had, and the feelings that arise. Where in your body do you feel guilt and judgement? Feel your body's sensations.

Begin to breathe in deeply into your root, into your womb. Allow yourself to scrunch up the paper. You could later burn this in a safe way outdoors.

Breathe into the knowledge that this isn't your judgement.

Repeat the mantra 'I forgive myself'.

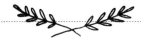

Hopelessness

Wound: Overwhelm

Moving onwards and upwards, we land in hopelessness. Ah, yes, where we become numb to it all. When you have a shitty day at work, and post logging off you lie down for three hours wondering if it is even worth removing yourself from the sofa to eat, pee or drink water. You feel the weight of the world.

But the positive here is that you aren't ripping yourself to shreds. Yay! The issue is that you can block the sad feelings/pain by numbing them out. You're, like, paralysed into doing absolutely nothing. You're unable to help yourself. You realise the weight of whatever it is and feel that everything is pointless, you don't matter, 'it' doesn't matter, you're beyond help. Ah, yes, this.

When we feel any loss, this is where hopelessness is triggered. When we realise how much time we've lost to the lower themes, when someone close to us passes away, when a relationship ends, when we realise how much someone took from us when there was sexual assault. This loss can be felt through the 'what's even the point' vibes.

Those scenes in films when the character loses the love interest and walks for hours and hours across New York City in rain-soaked clothes and lands back at home at 5:00 a.m. placing their keys on the side table, throwing themselves headfirst onto the bed with cheeks smushed into the pillow.

They feel helpless about it all.

The most beautiful way to move through hopelessness is to allow yourself to feel the loss. To feel the grief that washes over us at this stage. We cannot skip GO, collect 200 pounds and bypass this stage. For this stage is vital if and when it lands.

Many clients cry when they book into workshops or 1-on-1 sessions with me. Why? Because they know they are entering into this space of grief. They know they will have to grieve the person who was in order to move into the person they are expanding into. This is the process of being in the cocoon, feeling hopelessness and grief. Surrendering into the darkness that swallows us deeply to be ready to move from the cocoon into the liminal space.

Having support at this stage, where someone can hold you through these feelings, would be advantageous. A 'You've got this, babe' is all anyone needs at these life stages.

New soil for those roots

Many of us who have had a lack of mothering will find it hard to ask for support. But to move from this overwhelming feeling of numbness, you must lean into support. Remember that this won't last, but you must surrender to these feelings to find true transcendence to the higher themes. At this point, as you lie staring at the ceiling feeling all the loss, know that you aren't supposed to have any answers. Your only 'job' on your to-do list is to feel your current feels.

And, of course, numbness doesn't necessarily look like you cannot move; some of us are very good at going about our everyday lives while still feeling numb and hopeless. Either way, you deserve to be held right here.

Key overall affirmation for hopelessness
I am allowed space to feel my emotions.

Key hopelessness table

Thought	Feeling	Result	Current rooted belief	New soil for those roots
'I will never be happy again in a relationship'	Grief	I will avoid dating or just going out in general because there is no one out there for me	I am not compatible with anyone	I deserve to grieve the loss I have experienced in my own time
'The pain in my vulva will never get better'	Helplessness	I will put up with the pain or not ask for any help with it anymore	I have been through too much to ever find relief again	I can ask for as much help as I need to find freedom from my pain
'I will never love my body'	Despair	I will not buy or wear what could make me feel good because I don't know what that looks like anymore	I can't find anything I like or love about my body, and I never will	I allow myself to cry as my feelings arise around my body

'No one can help me with my period pains'.	Helplessness	I will avoid my period by going on contraceptives, which seems to be my only choice	I am a burden to anyone I speak to about my period pains	Others want to support me with this pain
'It is too late now to do anything about my contraceptives'	Despair	I will continue with this contraceptive choice and put up with the side effects.	I cannot ask for help because no one wants to help me	I deserve to be heard.

Try this key for hopelessness:

Aura-building kriya. Your aura is the energy field surrounding your body, also described as the subtle body.

- Kneel on your heels or sit cross-legged.
- Bring your arms up to a sixty-degree angle with elbows straight.
- Keep your palms flat and facing each other overhead.
- Concentrate on the space between the palms.
- You're beginning to feel like you are building energy and light between the hands.
- Bring in your breath of fire.
- Engage with this from one minute to three minutes or longer.
- Bring your arms down, brushing your energy field as you go.
- Place your palms up to receive. Allow your feelings to flow.

This kriya builds strength around your energy field. You can extend this by bringing the palms down, which are parallel to the ground outstretched. Your palms are facing up. Do another one minute to three minutes of breath of fire.

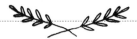

Grief

Wound: Loss

When we are numb and unable to do anything, including asking for support, we know we are still within the walls of hopelessness.

When we allow ourselves to fully feel, lean into help and move through the challenges we have been through, we know we have entered the theme of grief.

Grief clings to what was. It can't deal with this transition with ease. The ego, keeping us safe, resists this kind of change in favour of keeping you safe on the shore of grief. 'You stay there with the loss flowing, see the loss, feel the loss'.

Here, you cannot see how you are simply shedding a layer, expanding and moving into the highest realms. As we grieve in this theme, we are aware of the totality of our life and realise there is a life worth fighting for while feeling abandoned by everything and everyone around us.

Grief attaches itself to whatever is currently being moved through, thus something temporary. Attaching ourselves to something temporary can only lead to further pain.

Grief is triggered by the loss of something temporary in our lives, like an item, a beloved possession, relationships, people, pets, jobs, and circumstances we thought would exist. Allowing ourselves to detach from anything temporary will only allow us freedom from grief.

When we set such high expectations for something to work out, and then it doesn't, we may trigger back into shame and move on through the themes, landing in grief.

Relationships are an excellent example of this impermanence. We may believe that a relationship is the only way to true happiness. That person is our only current way to happiness: 'This person is gonna change my life'. We pin it all on having and maintaining this relationship. We have an incredible first date. We go on twenty more dates, feeling like they are the one. Then they ghost us. 'I can't believe I lost the life I've dreamt of for so long'. 'My life is never going to be happy now'. A tragic end. But we can see how challenging it is to pin so much onto something easily changeable.

New soil for those roots

We must detach ourselves from the impermanence of life. To remove this kind of upset, we will have to remove ourselves from the outcomes of life. Change is necessary, a given; nothing is permanent. As we accept change, we allow ourselves to detach from everything.

When we remind ourselves that the universe, god, our lightworkers or whatever lands here has a plan for us, this can bring about tremendous relief—granted, not a view shared by us all but one I find cathartic, and I know many who do.

There is a wonder in the ever-changing aspects of life.

Continuing the relationship example, you didn't continue in that relationship but found the most fulfilling relationship months later. Or when someone you know ends up dating the same person who ghosted ya, but later you find out they do the same to them and others—the whole 'I want 2.5 children and a white picket fence' spiel they gave to you is bollocks because they got some inner work to do. *Sighs of relief*.

You are constantly thrown into life for you to rise like the phoenix you are.

You, darling soul, live in a cyclical world where the cycle of death is necessary for there to be space for renewal. Allow yourself to accept life as it is at the present moment. It will only ever allow us to reach true, long-lasting happiness.

Let go. Move it through. Dance gently with yourself in the present.

Key overall affirmation for grief
I lean into the flow of life.

Key grief table

Thought	Feeling	Result	Current rooted belief	New soil for those roots
'Life will never be the same without that relationship'	Fearful	Give up on love	Nothing will ever change. It will always end up like this.	I turn to face my fears of what-ifs
'My mother will never be the mother I need'	Woeful	Can only think of the negative experiences with the mother	My mother was my only source of hope	I need to mother myself more
'I will never get the time back they took from me'	Loss	Reflecting back on all friendships, longing for ones that have dissolved because they were so good at the time	It's my fault friendships don't last	I only deserve nourishing friendships
'I never enjoyed my body and lost so many years to dieting'	Loss	Disassociating further from your body to avoid any kind of feelings	I've lost too much time to find joy with my body again	My body changes with me as I journey in this life
'Sex has never been pleasurable, so I have missed years of enjoyable sex'	Woeful	Avoiding sex with a partner	I have never been a worthy partner. They wasted their time with me.	I am worthy of pleasure
'I never understood how my body works, and I've run out of time to understand'	Loss	Disassociating from the cyclical nature of your body	My body and I aren't at one and never have been	My body loves me and provides for me

Try this key for grief:

Sit with yourself by placing your right hand on your left shoulder and your right hand around your waist. Hold yourself in a hug. Feel any rising sensations. Be with these sensations for as long as you need. It's OK to feel this loss, this sadness and this grief. Be with it.

Once done, thank yourself for mothering yourself through this grief in such a gentle way. Choose something that will bring you joy after this short practice by referring back to the mothering section if needed.

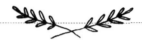

Fear

Wound: Distrust

Of course, the ego is always trying to keep us safe. Once we allow ourselves to feel the flow, lean into all that is, and accept that loss is inevitable, fear can rise. We begin to consider all the 'what-ifs'.

When we have been through challenges, traumas and woundings in life, fear is a theme we can easily find ourselves 'stuck' in. Being safe, happy, loved, held and content is scary when you've lived life in fight or flight.

It can feel pretty energising to be in fear because it means you are thinking about how to survive. That takes a lot. Fear is a higher theme because you now actually fear that you have something to lose.

We get in our armour when we perceive a threat, ready to fight.

There are constant thoughts around what if 'this' (whatever 'this' is) goes wrong.

Often those of us who feel like we have something to fear will make enemies rather than support others to rise with us. We do this because we fear someone is trying to take something from us.

There's fear of loss, rejection, being poorly, dying or social anxiety.

Grief is around what we've lost. Fear is around what we could lose.

Fear can keep us bound to the pill, for example. Fear is instilled in us around the pill too. When someone wants to come off it but they fear the what-ifs, they google it and find statistics to back up their point. The ego clings to stories from friends around a girl at work who got pregnant within two days of coming off the pill 'cause she looked a sperm in the eye. And remember, that's what your geography teacher with squeaky shoes and polystyrene penises said would happen. You can't trust your body. Best to stick with the pill, after all.

All the what-ifs keep us bound by fear—paralysed by fear. Fear is what drives our media outlets.

New soil for those roots

We need to switch from fearing the what-ifs to moving into the desire for the potential of what could be. You will never know what could be.

You ain't got a crystal ball. Not even a tarot reading will ever confirm the future.

It's exhausting leaning into the constant 'what-ifs' and 'what-could-bes' when we need to remain present in the now. Fear keeps us stuck in the 'what if it goes wrong cycle'. But we must consider 'what if it all goes right'.

Fear also perpetually works on keeping us safe; it makes so much sense to feel the fear too and really navigate where it is coming from. Is it actually going to keep us safe, or could we explore the concept of the desire for something better?

There is nothing to fear because when you jump, there will always be a featherbed, as American ethnobotanist Terence McKenna rightly reminds us.

What if there is love? What if it does all work out? What if I learnt about my body? What if I am supported fully?

There is never anything to fear because you are always held. You just have to re-mind yourself that you are guided. You know what you need in any given moment when you lean into your trust in yourself.

Key overall affirmation for fear

I am always protected.

Key fear table

Thought	Feeling	Result	Current rooted belief	New soil for those roots
'I can't try a new period product'	Paranoia	You stick with the period products that work for you, but you know you'd prefer something else	I bleed too heavy and will bleed everywhere	Trying something new is part of my journey
'Sex will hurt with every partner'	Unsafe	You avoid sex with everyone including yourself	Sex is supposed to hurt for me	I can find further safety in my everyday life

'Relationships are meant to hurt me'	Dread	Remaining in hurtful relationships or unable to work with boundaries in relationships so hurt is inevitable	What if everyone is just in relationships that are overall painful	I am worthy of boundaries and trust myself with these
'My mother hurts me, but what if that's how it is supposed to always be?'	Dread	Putting up with hurtful behaviours or comments in case your mother leaves you completely	My mother will never change, so there's no point trying	When I teach boundaries to others, I am showing them how much I love them
'My children will grow up to hate me'	Paranoia	Subconsciously pushing away our children	My children will feel the same as I feel about my parents	Everything and every relationship works out as it needs to
'Exploring my sexuality is dangerous'	Unsafe	You keep yourself stuck in society's 'acceptable' kind of relationships	Only 'typical' relationships are acceptable	When I explore my sexuality, I am honouring my needs

Try this key for fear:

· Extend your arms to the sides, parallel to the ground.
· Make fists with the hands with the thumbs tucked inside, touching the mound at the base of the fourth finger.
· Inhale through the nose, bending the elbows so your fists come to your shoulders.
· Place the mouth into an O as you exhale.
· Exhale through the mouth and straighten the arms out to the sides.
· Do this rapidly and breathe powerfully.
· Continue rhythmically while coordinating the movement with your breath.
· Do this for 3–6 minutes, and then relax your breath.

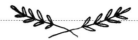

Desire

Wound: Inadequacy

The knowledge that pleasure can and will exist opens up desire. This space has way more energy than the previous spaces. When we feel this excitement around the potential of there being joy vs just fear, this gives us the motivation to create the life we deserve, versus being in hopelessness or paralysed by fear.

Though this theme gives us more space to feel what we want from situations/scenarios and life in general, it is essential to remember the skill of detachment. If we focus on a particular object of desire in a way that becomes an obsession, then we cannot step back and look at the bigger picture.

For example, if you remove free porn from your life and continue to think about the next time you may be able to watch free porn, then free porn has more weight than you want in your life.

What we want to be able to do is remove the object we desire and feel present in our daily life. What will be will be kind of vibes.

This is a sign that you are remaining grounded in your desires. If we feel a loss somehow, we are sliding back into grief.

What we want to avoid is merging our ability to achieve happiness through desire. One more orgasm, the next relationship, the next time we watch free porn, the next skincare product, the next clothing item. If we place our happiness on the next thing to bring us desire, we constantly strive for more when we want to feel pleasure. We need to come home to ourselves in the here and now, feeling loved, held and safe without looking to external scenarios/people/things to feel joy.

The source of long-lasting happiness is within ourselves.

When we attach to the seeking or wanting of more of something, that's when suffering ensues. The feeling of being unsatisfied unless X, Y or Z. Not having enough of something. Wanting more of something.

New soil for those roots

We cannot place our ability to feel happiness through things/others/experiences. We can only find true happiness from within our own bodies.

The most important aspect is to tune in to gratefulness right here and now. We don't often look at our journey and what we currently have to be grateful for.

Some of us write gratitude lists to remind ourselves of what we have to be grateful for right now in the present moment to prevent us from seeking more.

We are looking for something other than a silver bullet. We are looking to the nuances of what exists in front of us as we journey towards goals and new experiences. We cannot attach ourselves to the outcome but merely the here and now of the journey.

That's the magic of desire, the hope, the potential.

You bought this book in search of more happiness. But placing this book on a pedestal as the thing that brings you happiness means you'll always be on the back foot. You bought this book out of a desire for more.

Thus, you are now reading these words on your journey for more happiness. But this book cannot give you happiness, joy and pleasure. You cannot buy it.

It's not about what you want to do with your life but what you want from within your life. Now there's a subtle shift right there in that sentence.

You were whole and complete before you bought this book. You likely knew that anyway, but I am reminding you of this. When you thank life for its rich tapestry and the journey, and release attachment to the outcome, you will genuinely feel what it means to luxuriate in more joy. You have everything you need within. You already house the power you need to find more happiness.

Key overall affirmation for desire

I have everything I need within me.

Key desire table

Thought	Feeling	Result	Current rooted belief	New soil for those roots
'I need to look like X to find love'	Disconnected from self	Repressing desires	I am undesirable unless I change	I am worthy of love exactly as I am
'I have to have that pleasure tool as it will solve my problems'	Frustrated	Bypassing inner needs	Outside tools will relieve my pain	I soothe my nervous system daily
'I want a perfect relationship only'	Tired	The perfect partner exists	Someone has to be perfect before we date further	I meet my own needs first
'I want to orgasm'	Frustrated	Bypassing other forms of pleasure and joy that exist	Orgasms are the be-all and end-all	I deserve pleasure and joy in my day-to-day doings

'If I have their life, everything will be better'	Tired	Aspiring to others' lives (probably via social media), ignoring own desires	Everyone else's life must be filled with pleasure and joy only	I create my own desires for my own life
'I want to be desired as I am'	Longing	Exploring your deepest needs	I am worthy of being wanted as I am	I explore my own desires and needs daily

Try this key for desire:

During this ritual, feel into gratefulness, while moving through everyday processes, like when you are cleaning your teeth. What brings you happiness within this moment? You could write down five things that bring you joy when journaling or before you start your day in your diary or journal. Begin to remind your mind to stay focused. Note this is a challenge, given social media, our phones, the cost of living, advertising and the lure of shop windows.

Or keep a gratitude journal with the same format each day:

Morning:

I am grateful for:

1.

2.

3.

Daily Affirmation:

One thing that will make today great:

Evening:

Three great things happened today:

1.

2.

3.

Tomorrow will be even better because:

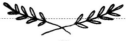

Anger

Wound: Violation

Moving onwards and upwards to one of my favourite themes. Our anger has been chastised. Society ain't into the whole angry women vibe. Isn't it wild that, based on your genitals, society instantly separates how men and women should utilise their anger?

Thus, we struggle with anger, what it means and how to use it. Anger, when used to empower, has way more energy than any of the lower themes. Whenever a client has messaged with, 'This week, I just feel so fucking angry', I celebrate them for feeling this anger. They often explain that they are never angry and enjoy navigating this new emotion. The patriarchy has suppressed your anger, and where would we be without the leverage of well-placed bubbling rage? I'll tell ya, for one, you wouldn't be reading this book. It was not shame, grief or any of the themes we have discussed so far that drew me in front of a laptop to write a whole book in the face of the social media shutdown of 2022.

Desire is about wanting something, whereas anger places expectations on a scenario. We aren't longing; there's an urge instead. We want to make whatever it is happen.

This empowering anger is used for good, making a difference for us and those around us.

What we need to be aware of is anger used in a forceful way, where it can become destructive.

It is essential to note what's beneath the anger because it will come from within and empower you in any given situation. Acknowledge the feelings. Where is the anger felt within the body?

When we set goals and have these expectations, we often cling to achieving them. Anything that prevents us from reaching these goals will instil anger. We need to be aware of how we use our anger. When it comes out as impatience or frustration, or forceful and violent, this isn't energy stirring from within; this is an external force that will lose traction quickly.

Please give yourself a safe space to feel your anger, then work with it to surrender to the present. This approach will allow you to work with your inner power. We know life won't go 'our way'. It will simply flow. Go with that flow, following your needs while you navigate where the anger stems from in the first place.

If we are gentle with anger, if we mother it, hold it, it will shine a light on our needs in return.

New soil for those roots

Anger is married to self-esteem. When we go around stomping our feet on everything and everyone to get out of our way, it leads us nowhere joyful. When we realise we are worthy and deserving of it all, we know there is no need to come from this place of vulnerability. We must remember that only some things will go according to plan. Life unfurls as slowly as it needs. Whatever happens unexpectedly is meant; you can handle this efficiently as you tune in to the needs of your nervous system.

Key overall affirmation for anger
I let go of control, allowing life to flow through me.

Key anger table

Thought	Feeling	Result	Current rooted belief	New soil for those roots
'The system ignores my needs'	Resentment	Ignores all advice to be left lost in the system	No one will ever listen to me anyway	I respect my needs and others in the system
'I'll have sex with whoever I want whenever I want because nothing else has helped with the pain'	Lonely	You don't honour the body as is, and this makes the pain more unbearable	No one wants to help me or hold me in a way I need	I focus on my own needs first
'I hated every part of my childhood'	Bitter	You may begin to isolate yourself from family-orientated scenarios	My childhood will impact me for the rest of my life	I can move through previous challenges
'The pullout method will be my only option now, and I don't care'	Sadness	You put yourself in situations that you don't want to be in	I will never understand what my body needs when it comes to contraception	I put my needs first

'No one will ever be good enough for me'	Resentment	You end up looking for perfection and ignoring the need for growth on both sides	Everybody is out for themselves, and no one will meet my needs	I surrender to the process, growing as I date others
'I won't ask for help with my baby because no one cares about me anymore'	Sadness	You may begin to isolate yourself from others	I need to do it all myself as no one understands	I deserve help and take pride in receiving support

Try these keys for anger:

In a journal, write the history you have with your anger. Is there any aggression? Tune in to the specifics of what you do with anger/aggression.

If anger arises for you, focus on the anger as it arises. In a quiet voice, aloud or internally, speak to this anger by acknowledging it. Say 'Anger' as you feel it. Take deep breaths into your womb space, and exhale deeply from this space. What do you need right now as you feel into this anger? Where is it felt within the body? Are there any other emotions present with the anger?

Explore your answers to the below:
· I feel really angry when . . .
· I try and control my anger when . . .
· My parents dealt/deal with anger by . . .
· I feel scared of anger when . . .
· I notice my anger switches to aggression when . . .
· My anger is reactive when I . . .
· If I express my anger, I worry that . . .
· When I feel angry, I see . . .

If you're unsure why you're angry, you can imagine that anger is an iceberg. Primarily, an iceberg is hidden underwater. Anger protects other feelings that may be arising. It's a quick protector of these, and so there may be plenty of other emotions under the surface. There are plenty of wonderful illustrations on Google if you search 'the Anger Iceberg'. Have it with you, and see if you can detect other emotions and feelings such as embarrassment, fear or loneliness.

Pride

Wound: Insecurity

Pride comes before the fall unless you acknowledge how to work with your pride to transition into the higher themes, starting with courage.

Pride ensures you are truly loved and heard amongst the rest of the noise. At the heart of pride is the voice of speaking up for your worthiness.

Every theme's new roots need tending to. Pride reminds us of this love to keep you back out of those lower themes. Pride is proud. Proud of you and all you have achieved in facing life's challenges. You incredible soul you. Look at you. You're doing wonders; celebrating you. You're worthy of it all.

We have to dance with pride with a little more care when it pushes for this love and worthiness; thus, pride is moved to an 'I am better than you' and 'I am more deserving than you' kinda space. Here pride stems from the validation of always being right or the best. It's a very self-centred form of pride: 'Me, me, me'.

Of course, this will stem from feelings of not being safe, loved and held. Fear of judgement and guilt. Trying to prove yourself. There are no deep roots to this kind of pride.

If you end up feeling like you need to earn respect, or if there's any kind of humiliation or a lack of respect, then pride will do all it can to protect you. You'll approach a scenario or person from a space of needing to be better than anyone else. But underneath, this is someone feeling unloved. Of course, this makes so much sense.

New soil for those roots

Soothing ourselves into the knowledge that no one is better than anyone else, worthier than anyone else or more loved than anyone else allows us to see that we are all equal. There's no need for this strife to prove anything to anyone else.

You are worth unconditional love. Those respected in all their humanness know they've nothing to prove.

Therefore, they approach scenarios and people from a space of love because there is enough love to go around.

We know from the previously discussed themes that allowing emotions to flow comes from this rooted knowledge that we are doing our best. We aren't perfect; we are human and still feel vulnerable sometimes. Allow yourself to feel that vulnerability. This vulnerability can feel scary, but it is the way to finding more love, purpose and meaning on our paths.

You are loved. You do not need to garner anyone's love. You will be celebrated in return when you celebrate others from a rooted space. You are worthy of it all, and it all is available to you. Whatever 'it all' is for you.

Key overall affirmation for pride:

I receive love and give love to others in return.

Key pride table:

Thought	Feeling	Result	Current rooted belief	New soil for those roots
'I will only be loved if I engage in the sexual acts they ask of me'	Vulnerable	You put your needs to the side in favour of not wounding their pride	I deserve to get whatever I need because I do the same for them	Love should not be conditional
'My period product choice is the only option everyone should choose'	Self-absorbed	Others' experiences are ignored	Your choices are better than others' choices	I make informed choices for myself
'I deserve to get whatever I want from a relationship'	Insecure	You ignore that everyone is on a growth path as they enter relationships	My demands outweigh the other person's needs	I am safe in my knowledge around who would be a good match
'I can ask all the personal questions'	Insecure	Probing questions are asked without understanding that there are boundaries	I deserve to know everything about people I interact with	There is no competition
'My sexual needs come first'	Vulnerable	Ignoring the other person in the relationship's needs	I am not safe in sex unless I come first	I exercise boundaries rather than demands

Try these keys for pride:

The vagus nerve (love nerve) is activated with compassion and empathy. This would be for yourself and others. Working with your vagus nerve would be perfect when landing in pride, giving yourself more compassion while also giving compassion to others. We want to be able to feel healthy pride, something some of us find incredibly challenging. Being proud of ourselves ain't that easy for some of us.

Activate the vagus nerve with diaphragmatic breathing

Place a hand on your stomach and another on your chest, between your heart space. As you breathe in, feel your stomach expand and return as you exhale. Notice the breath pass from your belly through the diaphragm as you inhale. This, in turn, supports lowering our heart rate and blood pressure.

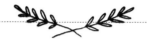

Cut a Cord with Your Root

Energetically, we are connected to the people who interact with our lives. Some connections are fleeting, and others are more binding. When working with the spiritual and energetic body, we can allow ourselves to feel into these energetic ties.

When we feel into rising emotions around a scenario, we can check in around whether these emotions stem from an experience with someone. For example, if it feels unattainable to engage in sex, but there is no pain or anything particularly physically challenging around it, where does this challenge stem from? There may be a past relationship where the narrative of sex changed for you. Once the situation/person is identified, you can begin to look at the bind of this scenario.

A cord-cutting ritual may sound scary, but in fact it can be one of the most liberating experiences. It does, however, mean exploring rising emotions with honesty. This can be exceptionally challenging if the experience feels raw.

I want to remind you that cutting the cord with someone doesn't mean that's it, job done. We are cutting the cord from something very specific, a layer of the overall experience. This gives the experience a new energy in your life, but one cord-cutting session will not necessarily be enough for you to feel completely free from the current bind. It will give you something tangible to move through. You can also cut the cord from people in your life; these people do not need to be out of your life. This process can apply to all relationships, from long-term partners, to best friends, to children. It basically allows you to explore your emotions and feelings around a scenario transcending the energy.

When you work with cord cutting from a rooted space, you can really tune in to what's arising for you around your current safety. Where do you feel unsafe, landing you in one of those lower themes? Repeating the same patterns over and over because you are unable to move through the experience safely?

When engaging in cord cutting, I advise you have a safe person you can speak to around what came through for you. If you have a wonderful friend or partner, you could message or explain that you are doing this cord-cutting thang (no need to go into the ins and outs of it) but you wondered if they could simply be there energetically or maybe physically so you feel as though you have this level of support. If not a friend/partner, then you might seek a professional in the form if a therapist or coach to speak to. It may be that you feel great afterwards and have no need for such support, but it's wise to be clear on the safety net you have to catch you as you surrender into the process.

How to cut the cord from a rooted space

Key affirmation:
I love you.

Try this key practice
You will need:

- a large piece of paper or A4 sheet at the very least (x2)
- a thick pen or pencil
- a rope (or wool or string) around five metres in length
- an object to represent the person or experience
- a safe space to set up the ritual
- space to move the body

1. Ensure you have everything ready and are in a space where you won't be disturbed.
2. Breathe down through the nose into your womb space. Feel your perineum rooting onto the ground. Your perineum lies between your vaginal opening and your anus. Breathe down and imagine roots extending down from this space through the earth.
3. If you feel you know what and who you need to cut the cord from, then skip this section and move to step 4. Draw a vulva outline on one of your sheets of paper. Breathe into the space you have created internally and on the paper. Write down any words that land as you explore your vulva in this way. You can explore all aspects of your pelvic bowl here, as there may be something specific around an ovary or the vagina, for example. Continue to write freely even when you think you may be done. Be as thorough as you can be. Once done, consider what messages are coming through the strongest. What do you feel needs to be worked with?
4. Choose the experience/scenario/aspect and the person involved. Begin to write on a separate sheet. Really dive into all the words that land and come through you into your hands as you write. Sometimes we think just thinking about it will be enough or that we won't have the words, but

really begin to explore the phrases/words/sentences that come through by writing them down.

5. Sit with the paper and really feel into what aspect comes through the strongest. It could be that there is a particular part of the experience/a particular emotion/a particular overall feeling.

6. Sit with an object that represents the person/experience, feeling into the emotions around this. Really allow the emotions to rise through the body while rooting down into safety.

7. Attach one side of the rope/string/wool to the object and leave the other end in your energetic field resting on the floor, or hold it in your hand. How does it feel to be in this energetic space right now? Feel into this specifically.

8. Now tie the other end around your waist, wrist or ankle. Feel how you are connected to this object and emotions. Breathe into them.

9. Once you feel the emotion begin to change, remind yourself how this experience was given to you, this person came into your life, these actions came from someone else's theme of consciousness. It isn't yours to hold onto. When you feel ready to move this through, untie yourself from the object. Move it all out of your energy field.

10. Move your body, shake your body, sigh. It wasn't yours to hold onto, whatever it was.

11. You can now safely get rid of the object. If compostable, it could be given to the sea or placed in the garden. If you're struggling for object ideas, I sometimes advise writing a name on a pebble that could be given to the sea, giving this person freedom in the sea, encouraging them and you to go with the flow of life.

12. You could also go outside and use a safe metal container to burn the piece of paper and give the ashes to the earth, giving the challenges you faced to Mother Earth to hold.

13. Feel into how the experience/person now feels.

You can come back to this as many times as you need after you've integrated the experience over a period of time. The particular experience/person may need to be worked with a few times.

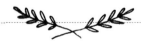

Worship Your Vagina

He should place her on his left and worship her hair-adorned yoni. At the edges of the yoni, the devotee should place sandal and beautiful blossoms.

—The Yoni Tantra

Worshipping the pussy isn't new but will sound wild to the Western world wrapped in a patriarchal system that's shamed the pussy for decades.

How do we transition from feeling our vulvas are dirty to worshipping them?

What a leap to make.

We live in a society where worshipping the cunt couldn't feel further from our reality, but around the sixteenth century, The *Yoni Tantra* text was birthed. We can learn how to make this transition with it. You can easily access it online,[6] but I have cherry-picked aspects of it as, ya know, things were slightly different in the sixteenth century.

Worshipping and working with your pelvis will bring you your desires. I see this in my journey and through those who enter my spaces. It is well-known in all things spiritual-pussy-working spaces. Worshipping the vulva and being rewarded for doing so is described in The *Yoni Tantra* text: 'After performing yoni puja using these methods, the devotee attains whatever is desired—there is no doubt of it. The fruit of doing puja to the great yoni, deliverer from the ocean of misery, is life and enhanced vitality'.[7]

Puja means to worship; thus, yoni puja is to worship the pelvic bowl.

You've made it this far into the book; you're a chain-breaking hero, hun. All ya have to do is keep committing to the steps and the process. Don't let society put you off the idea of worshipping your pussy. You do you, boo. As per the Yoni Tantra, 'Worship a woman or a maiden carefully . . . one should never speak harshly to maidens or women'. (KJN, Patala 23).

This whole book reminds you of your inner strength, inner power that's been shut down by a patriarchal system hell-bent on making you feel broken, so you land in their arms of support. This said support makes them money. A system that is driven by fear.

Kaula, also known as Kula, is a religious tradition in Tantric Shaktism and Shaivism. There are rituals and symbols connected with the worship of Shiva (protector and destroyer) and Shakti (divine feminine energy). It flourished in ancient India primarily in the first millennium CE. In Kaula, every woman is considered a manifestation of the goddess. Again, as per The *Yoni Tantra* text: 'No man may raise his hand toward, strike or threaten a woman. Men must kneel and worship her as the goddess when she is naked. She has equal rights with men on all levels'. (Occult World of a Tantrik Guru, Values Vol. IX)[8]

Essentially pussaaayyyy owners deserve to be bowed down to because we house an inner power that contains so much energy. All we can do is stand at the altar in awe of this magic. But the question is, when was the last time you honoured this power? Have you ever accepted, spoken to, or acknowledged this inner life force energy within you?

Sunshine-loving vulvas

Key affirmations:

I trust in the wisdom of my body.
I am loved and nurtured.
The earth below holds me.

Try this key practice:

Please note that this is something some experts wouldn't agree with doing. I advise exploring this somewhere you'll safe enough to engage with this activity.

Find a safe space to remove your bottom layers. Lie down somewhere in direct sunlight. This could be in a room where the sun streams in, your back garden, or a balcony. Somewhere you know you can do this without any sudden onlookers. Remove the clothes shrouding your vulva. Place the soles of your feet together with knees wide (reclined butterfly position) while lying down on your back or relaxing into pillows or onto a yoga bolster. Make sure you protect your knees with blocks or pillows if you need them, and feel your knees just hanging in mid-air.

Begin to feel the sunshine on your vulva. Breathe into the warmth landing at your root. If you feel safe enough to do so, close your eyes.

Bring breath down into your root while sending your grounding cord into Mother Earth.

Engage with this for around thirty seconds to a minute.

Feel this holding, love and warmth as if it's wrapping you in a cuddle.

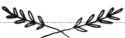

Yoni puja

Science doesn't have all the answers. We are taught that energy is converted from one form to another. The birth of the universe, however . . . Well, cosmologists believe that the origin of the big bang theory stems from quantum uncertainty (where energy comes from, like, nowhere). This cosmic energy persisted long enough to drive the big bang theory in the first place. All life was essentially birthed from the velvety darkness of a womb space. Scientists are none the wiser on where the energy for this said birth comes from.

Hari, Hara, and Brahma—the gods of creation, maintenance, and destruction—all originate in the yoni.

–The Yoni Tantra

All creation is a dance between consciousness (Shiva, the protector and destroyer) and energy (Shakti, the power/cosmic mother). Your womb space houses the creative potential to birth whatever you desire into this world through the vaginal portal, utilising your shakti power. You can literally birth new life. Hunz, is there any wonder your power has been shut down by a society dominated by those scared of it?

We must honour this power, tune in to it and give it the respect it deserves.

I imagine thousands of people reading this book and worshipping this shakti power at home. A quiet protest is rallying us together in union once again. One small step for the pussy, one giant step for humanity.

As I write this, I well up, considering how much difference this will make to the world as we know it, to the next generations, to the previous generations and to you. It's fucking huge.

Tantra is all things ritual, beauty and honour.

Ritual is following a set of steps that focuses the mind, deepens devotion and strengthens our will. They are tools to allow us to move through the themes of consciousness. This gives us space to feel the rising emotions while moving them through simple processes.

Bring in an offering

Key practice:

Consider an offering you could bring for your vulva to represent the love your pussy deserves. You may be on a walk and find some wild grasses, a rock, fallen petals, blossoms or a coin. You may wander past a florist and see a beautiful bunch of flowers. There may be a candle you adore that you could light in honour of this space. On your altar or simply a side table with some space, bring your offering for your pelvic bowl.

Do this in the ceremony. Place your offering near you. Sit by the altar area in a cross-legged position with spine straight, jaw loose and crown lifted.

Breathe into your belly. In time, send down a grounding cord into Mother Earth. Slowly bring your breath into your labia, your vulva, your vagina, your ovaries, your fallopian tubes and your womb. Audibly or internally, whisper your gratitude to this space. Place your offering on the altar once you feel you are ready to do so. Remain in a meditation practice, feeling the emotions that may have risen for as long as you need.

Place one hand on either elbow and bring in a cuddle to your body by squeezing up to your shoulders and back to the elbows again. Be gentle with yourself. Always.

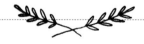

Gaze at your cunt

If a person should gaze at a yoni while ritually bathing, his life becomes fruitful. There is no doubt of this.

—The Yoni Tantra

One of the biggest challenges we navigate with how our vulva looks is with the labia. Most of us will never have looked at our pussy. Nope. Absolutely not. You may have disconnected from the way your vulva looks at the beginning. Even if you have seen your mother's vulva floating around the house or there was an open household growing up, loving yours may still be challenging. This may be a result of society or a previous partner or friends. It only takes one comment or image to throw us.

Our labia are not mirrors of each other. They are not matchy, matchy. Twins Basil.[vii] They are different. One may hang slightly lower or be slightly flappier than the other. While we celebrate our uniqueness as human beings, we must honour our pussies as unique, beautiful souls, changing and adjusting as you do. In one study focusing on all things labia minora and majora, 1 in 10 measured their labia minora to be at least 26.5 mm in width. It is just as common to have visible labia minora as hidden labia minora.[9] The names could be better. Labelling something as 'minora' sounds like it should be smaller, when over half of us have happy, flappy, dangling labia minora below our labia majora.

Many of us as children would have been shamed for our labia because some of us would have hit puberty before others, and those with hidden labia minora would have been interested (which may have been shared in a less than tactful way) in others' labia that didn't present in the same way as theirs.

It's a bit of a mess because society sells us the perfect nipped and tucked vulva. Porn plays a part; the media plays a part. Posters advertising labiaplasty are part of the problem. The fact that we don't feel we can openly discuss our vulvas causes us to internalise our thoughts, thus everything just becomes a solo journey. 'I must be the only one who wants to grab a pair of scissors and cut off my labia'. Except you're not, sweet soul. You're not. And I am so sorry you were made to feel like this was your only option.

What we must be clear on is that if you decide labiaplasty is for you, or perhaps you've already gone through it, then that is absolutely as it needs to be for you. It's your body. What we are discussing here are the underlying challenges we all face.

Consider female genital mutilation (FGM) and female genital cutting (FGC). FGM refers to 'all procedures involving partial or total removal of the female external genitalia or other injury to the female genital organs for non-medical reasons'. Exact numbers of those who have been through FGC are unknown, but it's at least 200 million people across 90 countries. About 4.1 million people are at risk every year. There is an overall decline, but the pace of said decline is uneven across the world.[10]

[vii] Austin Powers reference

You know how real it is when as a classroom-based teacher you go through training to specifically look out for a child who may have been through FGC. According to the Orchid Project, FGC is based on a traditional belief that we need to control a girl's sexuality to ensure her virginity until marriage or to prepare her for marriage. A girl who remains uncut will often be considered unsuitable for marriage. There are also often misconceptions that an uncut girl will be promiscuous, unclean, bad luck or less fertile. There are some communities where there are also misconceptions that it is a religious obligation for mothers to cut their daughters' genitals as theirs were cut.

There's so much that can arise for us emotionally when discussing all things how our vulvas look. It's a lot.

Looking at your own vulva in the mirror can bring up a huge wave of emotions. It's an incredibly powerful tool to work with but one that needs to be done when you feel ready. You cannot rush this process. Your nervous system needs to feel ready for such a practice, and you need to be in a space where you feel completely held. This needs to be approached in a trauma-informed way.

Many of us find forming a relationship with our vulva challenging. Through the practices so far, you may be aware of the roots of this. You are moving through these feelings while creating a safety net around you.

Key practice:

How to gaze at yours:
You will need:
- a hand mirror
- offerings (refer to above bring in an offering section)
- a journal
- a pen

As you read about gazing at your vulva, begin to feel how this lands in your body. Do you instantly feel this is a full-bodied yes by checking in through your centres? Check with your head. Is it a yes? Check at your heart. Is it a yes? Check at your gut. Is it a yes? Check at your root. Is it a yes?

If there is a yes with each centre, then this is a full-bodied yes. You are in complete alignment to move on to the next stage. If a no arises, tune in to where the no is in the body, where that no stems from. You could explore the no through journaling. Work with the no and consider your needs around it. Look back through the themes and feel the emotions. Come back to this tool another day and check in with a full-bodied yes again.

With a yes, begin the ritual:
- Set some time aside to engage in this ritual. Mark it in your calendar, so you know it is coming, and remember to turn off your notifications on your phone.

- Find a safe ceremonial space.
- You could be completely naked or begin fully clothed.
- Put on a playlist. I have an 'empower yourself' playlist you can find by going to www.thisisnaomigale.co.uk/books.
- Begin by moving into your body as feels good by bringing in breath down into your belly. Move gently and into areas that feel good. Perhaps you haven't stretched before this moment, and slower stretches also feel good.
- Place your feet together and stretch into a hip-opening butterfly position, breathing into the vulnerability of opening your root in this way.
- Slowly begin to undress and feel your vulva on the ground below.
- Send down a grounding cord into Mother Earth to feel her safety.
- Bring the mirror towards your root, and in time, hold it to your root without looking in the mirror. Feel the emotions arise while you know there is the reflection of your vulva in the mirror being reflected into the space that you are creating.
- When you feel fully held by your breath, the grounding cord below and the safety of the space you have created, look down into the mirror at your vulva and gaze at your vulva while the emotions wash through your body.
- At some stage, you will feel the emotions change and feel ready to place the mirror back down.
- Once completed, move your body again. Feel the emotions and any tears. Hold yourself in a hug. Squeeze your arms up to your shoulders and then up to your face, to your cheeks. Place one hand on your forehead and one behind the back of your head, squeezing gently. As if you are squeezing your brain a little without the pressure. Breathe in and exhale with force out of your mouth.
- You are held and loved, darling soul.
- You could immediately move into the below journaling questions or get dressed and then do so or journal later once you have integrated the experience.

Unlock your answers

- What emotions rose as you looked at your vulva?
- Where in the body did you feel these emotions?
- Could you look back at the themes of consciousness and consider where those emotions may land?
- Did any previous experiences come to you that would be good to note down here?

- Did your vulva look like you imagined or similar to how it has looked when you've looked at it before?
- What thoughts come to you right now as you think about your vulva?

Try this key practice:

Our partners aren't given the opportunity to view our vulvas in this ceremonial light. You could take this a step further at some point (this could be days, months or years on). Create the same space as above. Ask them to bring an offering to your root space into the ceremony.

Allow them the same experience. The section where we bring in our own hug would be replaced with a hug from your partner.

Share these below questions:

- What emotions arose as you looked at the vulva?
- What emotions arose for you while they looked at your vulva?
- Where in the body did you feel these emotions?
- Where in your body did you feel these emotions as they gazed upon your body?
- Did any previous experiences come through as you engaged in this ceremony?
- Did any previous experiences with this partner or other partners come through?
- What feelings, thoughts, colours and patterns land with you now around the vulva?
- How has this experience left you feeling?

You could verbalise your answers or journal them afterwards. Read them out if this would feel good for you both.

If you are in a same-sex relationship, you could take it in turns within one space or create two separate ceremonies on different days.

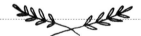

The Legacy of Francesca Woodman

Mirrovulva work

You cannot see me from where I look at myself.

—Francesca Woodman

This book could not be written without a section dedicated to Francesca Woodman. The beginning of this section may be challenging to read, so skip through if you need more time before reading about her life.

She inspires me, and I know her story will inspire you.

Francesca Woodman was a photographer who took photos of herself in nude or partially nude scenarios. She was often hiding behind objects, or she blurred herself through slow exposure.

Who is she? Well, she was born in 1958 in Denver, Colorado. Francesca grew up in a house where art was centre stage with a father who was a photographer, painter and lecturer, while her mother was a ceramicist and sculptor.

Francesca suffered from depression after a move to New York in 1979. A relationship broke down, and in 1981 she took her own life at twenty-two.

When you explore the themes of her images, you can see how she is capturing the ebbs and flows that is being a young woman growing up in the early 80s. She also printed her photos on a tiny scale to emphasise the intimacy and personal stance she was taking with her art.

She was moving with mirrors, objects and the lens, playing with light and movement. Francesca played with the spaces she worked in, creating mystery and atmosphere.

In the 70s, photography wasn't seen as being as necessary as painting and sculpture. In eight years, she worked to create over eight hundred images that explore body image, isolation, alienation, relationships and sexuality.

As she hides behind objects, she represents her vulnerability. The small-scale photos ask us to enquire a little more, noticing her raw vulnerability through being naked or partially clothed.

Francesca was dubbed 'a mirrowoman'.

Taking her art and approach to selfies as inspiration, we can begin to create our own shoots to share our own experiences of self.

People say that there's nowhere to hide when there's a camera or mirror, but Francesca turns this on its head by hiding and yet being incredibly visible for others and herself.

When exploring our own bodies, where the relationship may be fraught with challenges, we can begin to use the tools of mirrors and photography to come into a relationship with parts we love or currently despise.

This practice, where you begin to change the narrative around certain body parts, creates further love, awe and acknowledgement for your body. It is one tool that needs to be worked with repeatedly as your relationship changes with your body.

Key practice:

You will need
- a mirror
- music
- a phone camera or digital camera or 35mm camera (or all three)

Here's what to do:
- Find a safe space and a playlist you love. You could find a room with low light that is dimly lit à la Francesca, such as a hallway.
- Hold your camera, or set up a tripod and have a timer on your phone/camera looking at the mirror or to a part/edge of the mirror.
- Move your body to the music in a way that makes you feel good.
- Send down a grounding cord into the earth to be held.
- Begin to remove layers of clothing and view them in the mirror. Feel into the emotions arising.
- Start by looking at an area of your body you like/love. Place this in the mirror. Create shapes with your body to feel the space you are creating in the mirror. Bring in your camera and take photos of this area. It could be one breast, bum cheek, nose and lips only, or feet, maybe just a little finger. Wherever.
- Your session could focus on the parts (or part) of you of your body you love, or you could choose a part you don't love so much and photograph this.
- Using objects, you could hide parts of your body, such as behind books, fabric, or furniture.
- Spend lots of time playing around. Try different movements. Running past the mirror and taking the photo as you blur on through. Swishing your hair and keeping your body still.
- After a while, begin to look at your vulva in the mirror. Through your pants only or without pants (knickers). If you feel called, take photos of your vulva in the mirror with different angles.
- Once done, you can return to your clothes and peruse your photos.
- Cherry-pick ones you love. Delete others. Keep them for yourself. You could edit them on apps such as A Color Story.
- Further options would be to get them printed (in the UK we have Freeprints, which is an app where you can get photos printed for free once you've paid the postage) or you could post them online (obvs, the ones you know won't get your account flagged). Printing and posting them online changes their energy. What would feel good for you?
- Another option would be to print and frame one for your home or your altar. It could be an image you like of a part of the body you don't love. Looking at this image daily will formulate a different story for this body part. Ensure this feels good.

If Francesca were around today, her work would have been celebrated differently. Incredible selfie-based photographers are doing as above. Sometimes they get banned on socials, but it's worth searching for 35mm selfie photographers on Instagram for inspiration. You could even create a Pinterest board before you begin the selfies. This also can be done outside. You could do this safely outside in safe spaces, hiding in long grass and behind trees, for example. I often find woodlands or do this work on the beach. Grabbing an old 35mm camera and playing with film gives this a different energy. Having photos printed by a company from the film is a thrill I have missed since the 90s.

This is work, it takes time and hard work to create these spaces and to do this work, but it is oh so worth it. Every time feelings arise, you can refer back to the themes of consciousness and explore where these emotions stem from with what you need to move through this theme. I love looking back at my images and seeing the changes I have made for myself.

Celebrating you. Always.

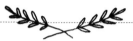

Closing

Gripping

Building its walls again

What is arising for you? I ask as the landscape changes

Anger, she affirms

Let's feel this anger

We can work with anger, I reassure

—The Angry Vagina

Lara's Love Story with Pleasure

I wanted to find my way to sexual pleasure.

Growing up, I often felt deeply unhappy and lonely because there was a lack of deep connection with anyone in my family and a general bitterness every day. Not knowing what happiness or pleasure was as a child affected my sexual development.

Masturbation, for example, was not something that naturally came to me at any age. It was so far from me that up until my early twenties, I could not imagine that that was something that most people regularly did.

When I was about seventeen, I started exploring my sexuality with others, still unsure what sexual arousal felt like or what I enjoyed. For years I had sex with men but never ever enjoyed it . . . at all! Not once did I want to have sex with them in the first place, but I forced myself to continue because I liked the idea of being young and sexually active. I sadly never gave myself the space to think about whether I was into girls because I was afraid of the consequences.

When I was twenty-three, my friendship with my best friend evolved into a romantic relationship after she made the first step.

The first time we ever had sex was amazing and also a truly enlightening experience for me because, for the first time in my life, I was wet and full of sexual excitement, craving her touch and unable to keep my hands off her. I remember thinking, 'THIS is what everyone is talking about!'

I lost those sensations within the first month or so of us dating. Even though I was and am still so in love with her and do not want to ever be with someone else. Two years with that burden on our relationship passed, and I felt hopeless, like I was in a never-ending tunnel.

I worried EVERY SINGLE DAY about whether or not I would ever have an orgasm, let alone feel aroused in any way. I was so afraid of never discovering what sexual pleasure actually was. In my relationship, I put so much pressure on myself to make my girlfriend sexually happy that every time she and I got ready for bed, I started counting how many times we'd had sex in the past week, wondering whether or not she (not me!) was in the mood for sex tonight, and then I felt either relieved or forced to make a move. I was just completely disconnected from myself.

I found out about Naomi's work through her appearance on a podcast. I was already seeing a sex therapist with my girlfriend at this time. The physical and holistic approach to her work contrasted with how talk-sex therapy was working. It seemed fresh, so I knew it was something to try out. I joined one of Naomi's online vaginal massage workshops one week later, and for the first time in a long time, I felt hope because it felt so much like the right thing to do. I was so happy when I found out she was also offering 1-on-1 work because that makes it much more personal and tailored.

It is very wholesome work that requires a lot of commitment, trust and patience, but at the same time, Naomi brings a lightness into it with her very humorous ways that make you feel so much better. What I also love about this work is that it is so empowering. It makes you realise that, once shown, you already have all it takes to heal the wounds behind your symptoms within yourself.

Today our sexual relationship is so much healthier. I take care of myself now—meaning that I learned to accept when I am not in the mood for sex and respect that. This respect allowed me to become wet sometimes when we did have sex, which was a huuuuge milestone for me because it had not happened in two years. It is a long way off from where I'd like to be in my relationship to sex, but I am slowly letting myself lead more and more.

Above all, I was able to let go of all this worrying about the future and how things will or will not change for me, and I came to just trust the process. So far, I still have not had an orgasm yet, nor do I feel I've been close to having one. But still, I know now that that day will come, and I can feel that I am on a path that will lead me there eventually. I am so damn proud of myself for bringing up the patience and strength to actively work with my body, instead of not respecting myself and working against my body.

Be gentle with yourself, darling. There is only you to really take care of yourself.

Step Four
An Orgasmic Cup of Tea

Joyous Pleasure

Joy is a feeling of great pleasure and happiness.

Pleasure is a feeling of happiness, satisfaction and enjoyment.

So they're basically interlinked intrinsically.

Except in society, we focus on the attainment of pleasure through sex. When we find orgasms are aloof, we chastise ourselves for the inability to experience pleasure: 'Well, I must be broken then'.

Except we are missing out on life as a result of chasing what, in actual fact, is far from 'the best bit'. And actually, without the knowledge of what an orgasm really is. You watch films and see people' ooo' and 'ahhh'. We are sold the orgasm packaged in screams of delight and it being absolutely the best bit. I dunno if you've noticed, but the orgasm in these films comes after a long, challenging, joyless chase.

When we experience pleasure, the brain releases endorphins, serotonin, oxytocin and dopamine. These hormones override the shitty feelings, so we feel better/good/incredible/joy. Blood flow increases, and nitric oxide is released, which boosts the production of neurotransmitters like beta-endorphins. Pain is dulled, and we feel euphoric. Stress becomes easier to navigate as a result. We get a dopamine hit when we orgasm, oxytocin and prolactin for satiation. There's also phenylethylamine (PEA), which exists in chocolate. You feel more energised, your mood lifts and you can concentrate better. We know that there are millions of nerve endings around our pelvis. When we orgasm, there are signals sent to our brains. Yep, that was delicious.[1]

I have nothing to give you around any tips or tricks so you can achieve the big O through P in the V . . . and quite frankly, it couldn't be further from what we all deeply need. How you approach your daily life impacts your ability to receive during sex. As you do the inner work and explore your daily doings, your themes of consciousness, where emotions arise for you, how you connect into your root and how you regulate your nervous system, it's these things that truly matter. Great sex is a side effect. A side effect is a term coined by pharmaceutical companies to make 'adverse reactions' sound less scary. I am claiming the term 'side effect' here for positive reasons. Fantastic sex is a by-product, a side effect, a result of exploring your inner needs on a deeper level.

Incredible sex with pleasure, joy and happiness will give you actual chemical shifts only attainable by coming home to your body and your needs. So approaching this differently, then. Therapy is good; chemical shifts feel even better. Wanna be experiencing more pleasure? Well, welcome. There's no getting around it. You're knee-deep into this book and uncovering your needs.

The clitoris houses ten thousand nerve endings (over double that of the penis) and is the only organ that exists solely for pleasure. It makes sense that this organ exists in our root space. It also makes sense that the first comprehensive anatomical study of the clitoris was published in 1998. Hunz, 1998. Can we even let that sink in? Only after this was a study executed in 2005 where they perused its actual shape and size under an MRI scan. What a shocker. It's more than just the little dot we can see. It actually extends beneath the pubic bone and wraps around the vaginal opening. When engorged, it has been compared to an orchid. It's, in fact, a similar size to a small penis.

I haven't finished. Ya know, it was only a cow's clitoris that had been studied until 2022. Yes, in 2022, it was discovered that the clitoris has over ten thousand nerve endings. And who do we have to thank? Seven trans community members going through phalloplasty. [2]

In Greek mythology, the prophet Tiresias irritated a pair of mating snakes. Hera wasn't chuffed, so she transformed him into a woman as 'punishment'. Seven years later, she changed him back. One day, Hera and Zeus argued about which gender has the most pleasure during sex. Hera thought men, while Zeus said women. Tiresias came forwards and said it was women. Definitely women. Livid, Hera struck him blind.

The point is even the Greek gods knew there was a pleasure portal in the pussy, and yet we have had the hood kept over our eyes.

But as we open up to pleasure, the existence of pleasure, the possibility of pleasure, and the knowledge that we can access ten thousand nerve endings solely for pleasure, it changes our standpoint on the point of life.

If life is birthed from our pelvic bowls, and our pelvic bowls house organs solely for pleasure, then it makes sense that life is only for pleasure. We were made in pleasure; we should enter this world with pleasure; we should exist only ever dancing in the pleasures of life.

And yet you are here reading a book on finding more happiness, so chances are you feel like there's more to life yet. More joy and more pleasure to be experienced. Opening our minds, hearts, and souls to this possibility will only allow further joy in your life.

I myself am still on a journey to experiencing life's joys and what that truly looks like for me. One day during a discussion with my husband, I asked him whether he thought I felt joy, as it had been something I'd been exploring for a while. Whether he saw me basking in joy within our lives. This was after I had done so much work on my own journey. He replied with a pretty straightforward, cutthroat no.

Fuck, but yeah, absolutely; I didn't think I did, either.

After this, I worked deeper within my pelvic bowl and worked with my vagina. I'd worked on my pelvic bowl for years, but I'd been missing out on my vagina. It felt too far out of reach, too taboo.

The vagina joins our inner world with our external world. I believe what I have been through is my own vaginal portal. I have had my head up my vagina and am proud to say I have reaped the rewards.

From an outright 'no' back in the day from my husband, to now, where he indeed acknowledges the gifts this journey has given me. And not just because sex keeps getting better.

So yes, the side effect of this deep inner work? More pleasure and orgasms. If you skipped through the book looking for the section on orgasms, I see you. I understand. But orgasms are a side effect of working on your daily connection to your cunt. To your pussy. To your vagina. To your pelvic bowl. To your pleasure portal.

Neuroscience has confirmed the brain-vagina connection. The specific locations linked to the vagina, cervix and nipples on the brain's sensory cortex have been mapped out with actual pictures, thus proving that vaginal stimulation activates different brain regions to that of the clitoris.[3]

And before feminists reach up their hands to argue that neuroscientific data proving a brain-vagina connection would be used against us, or that if we are only going to fully enjoy all aspects of life by feeling pleasure with our pussies, it essentially restricts us to just being cunt-owners, keep in mind that data is always gonna be used against us as women. There are whole books on data biases in a world that spins around four thousand nerve endings instead. We know that. But we should take a moment to bask in these discoveries, as we can use this power for good. We know how to do that nowadays.

When we feel pleasure, we feel more confident and creative. We have a deeper connection with the world and those around us. More pleasure and joy give us more in life. You're more likely to go on a date, wear your favourite piece of clothing, meet up with friends, try for a baby, start your business idea, create art and dance if you're twirling in more sensuality in your daily life.

When we have experienced trauma around the pelvic bowl, we are less likely to feel daily pleasure. This may have been cut off and starved of oxygen by the situation. Only when people return to reclamation with their roots do they bring in the pieces taken from them to experience a little more joy. The more they bring these pieces back in, the more joy they experience, and the more their life expands.

This work is crucial for those who feel less than whole due to others' brutality.

The quickest way to turn off the light from within is to remove our power through our pelvis. Men have known this for years. We have been kept in the dark as to why this was so detrimental. A two-pronged attack on us all. I am sorry that this is the world we have had to experience for so long.

Thank you for being here to explore your joy, your pleasure and the power of your root space. You are turning on the light for us all.

Try this key practice

You may be reading this thinking you already explore joy daily or don't know yet what brings you joy. While you feel into which end of the scale you land on, you can begin to write a list of the things that bring you pleasure and joy. Or a list of things you think may bring you happiness.

As you write this list, next to each task/item/activity, write why you do this. What do you do it for?

Now look back at the whole list and consider whether your list is only for more masculine-leaning gains, i.e., 'Yoga: to keep me fit' or feminine-leaning wins like 'Yoga: to give me more space'.

The feminine and masculine refer to masc/fem energy.

Use the below list to circle masculine-rooted reasons in one colour and feminine-rooted reasons in another. You may not have used the same language, but you can see whether your focus was for masculine or feminine reasons.

Masculine-focused reasons:
· To learn something new
· To feel more proactive
· To keep fit
· For an adrenaline hit
· To follow my curiosity
· To connect with my primal energy
· To make changes in my life

Feminine-focused reasons:
· To surrender into life more
· To enjoy more play
· For more creativity
· To feel more sensuality
· To express myself
· For deeper connections with myself or others
· To experience more energy for daily life
· To experience love
· For more affection
· To learn more about myself

Achieving balance is a challenge, but we're looking for a good mixture of feminine and masculine reasons. This will allow you to explore whether your daily joy and pleasure are still linked primarily to masculine outcomes or to an array of outcomes.

Being able to surrender to joy and pleasure through the feminine should be a focus. Yes, we definitely need masculine-focused pleasurable activities, but we must also explore feminine-based reasons to work closely with our pussaaay-based pleasure.

Orgasmic Pleasure

The lack of P in V orgasm is putting off people in general when it comes to orgasms.

When clients come to me who can orgasm through clitoral stimulation and I exclaim, clapping my hands in a celebration that they can actually have an orgasm, this isn't well-received. They say, 'Yes, but I am not having an orgasm through sex'.

We need to move away from what we see as sex.

We need to understand what we mean by 'having an orgasm'.

Biologists confirm that our moods change when we get a rush of dopamine. This dopamine rush exists as we prepare to orgasm. Once we have orgasmed, we can go on and have another orgasm straightaway. Thus, if we go on to have more orgasmic pleasure, we receive more dopamine hits. This refractory period—the span of time after having an orgasm where the person is not sexually responsive (ya know, snoring on the pillow or just ready for the day ahead)—varies from a few minutes to over twenty-four hours, depending on the person.

Floating through life with more orgasmic pleasure will only ever support our daily lives.

However, let's note that we don't need to 'go over' into this orgasm to experience this dopamine hit. At orgasm, dopamine drops, and prolactin rises. If we work with our breath to soothe our body into a more relaxed state and find what brings us pleasure during sex, we can peak and peak without actually going over and getting that hit of prolactin to then have to build up the dopamine again. We can ride the dopamine train of pleasure.

If we focus on reaching this peak rather than the 'Peak peak, oh, we've gone over peak', then we can receive more, and if we are receiving more during sex, then we learn to receive more day to day, finding these dopamine hits elsewhere, riding the high for longer, engaging in the high for longer.

As we learn to work as a team with our body and cunt in this way, we learn how to live a more expansive life in general. We are learning how to ride the gentle waves of life rather than the 'go hard or go home' approach long sold to us.

And yet, sex is on the decline. Natsal-3 (the British National Surveys of Sexual Attitudes and Lifestyles) shows that in the UK, people have sex less than once a week. Many find that challenges with engaging in sex stem from feeling depressed, challenging relationships, poor health or finding it hard to chat sex through with their current partner. With sexual challenges lasting longer than three months: 34 percent of women shared that they lacked interest, 12 percent lacked enjoyment, and 13 percent felt uncomfortable due to dryness in the vagina (a lack of arousal may play a part here). In fact, 1 in 5 men and women in a relationship said their partner had experienced sexual difficulties in the past year.[4]

And so, onto the orgasm gap. Would a book about the vagina ever be complete without referring to the orgasm gap? The whole point of this book is for you, dear soul, to learn about your body in a way you likely have never learnt about your body.

This book is a tool I have birthed into the world to aid in closing this gap. One day you may feel ready to pass this book on to another. Buy it for your children. You may be in a relationship, so you can pass it on to them (or at least highlight the fuck out of the sections you want them to read, hun). Together, we work on making a massive difference to everyone living a less-than-orgasmic life.

Over 95 percent of women and men can orgasm through self-pleasure.[5] When men have sex with women, they also orgasm at an orgasm rate of 95 percent. When women have sex with men in a relationship, it drops to 65 percent.[6] When women have sex with men casually, it falls to a rate of 18 percent. Women having sex with women have an orgasm rate of 85 percent.[7]

Women report that the order of preference to achieve orgasm is self-pleasure, clitoral stimulation, oral sex, and (last and very much least) penetrative sex.

Men say that their top choice for that orgasmic experience is . . . penetrative sex.

Is this patriarchal conditioning, a lack of education, or a lack of care? Because I know many partners would love to learn more about their bodies and their partner's needs.

Here you all are, reading these pages, ready to close the gap.

We're replacing 'sex drive', like we're rabbits who have just had their Duracell battery changed, to 'desire'.

Desire is that almost intense feeling. You may have heard desire referred to as sexual drive, libido or being in the mood. I find all these terms problematic.

Arousal, however, is the physical sign of the sexual response. There may be lubrication in the vagina, the nipples may become erect, the clitoris and labia become engorged due to the blood supply, and the clitoris becomes sensitive, for example.

Understanding your own desire will support your journey. This will help everyone explore what sexual desire means to themselves, including those who are asexual. The problem is that life needs to consistently dance with pleasure and joy to understand daily desires. If we have an excellent grasp on daily desires, we can dance in our sexual desires more easily.

Consider what would happen if we understood how our body works, how we feel and where we feel these feelings. How we don't need to 'go over'. How we react to touch in various ways in and around our vulva. How we are all just on our own paths, removing expectations and the ego's grip on the narratives around how a life with sex included in it should be.

Well, things would be hella different for us all.

The Side Effect of Daily Joy

Is your life filled with joy, and do you truly understand what joy feels like for you? This is a long journey, one you may have already started exploring.

As a chronic people pleaser due to childhood challenges, I had zero clue about what a boundary looked like.

I have been working on boundaries for years. When we moved to Margate, I thought I was absolutely clear on my boundaries. I was ready to start afresh with new surroundings and new people.

Except, I fell into the same patterns. *Le sigh*.

I prioritised everyone else's needs before my own. It came to a head in January when I felt my usual middle-of-winter feels and could no longer 'keep it up'. I like to surrender to the darkness and cocoon fully. I suddenly realised that I was diminishing my own needs on a considerable level and pulled back. I communicated my needs poorly to friends.

In my time of need, there was tumbleweed in general. Maybe it was because I wasn't communicating my needs well, but I really wanted to be held in return for the support I had given in my time of need. Once I understood why I needed to step back from Margate busy-life for a while, I began to grieve for my inner child. Slowly, I established more gentle boundaries with clients, my social media followers and my husband. Every time I did these minor tweaks, I needed to return to my nervous system through the plethora of tools you continue to find in this book. On my thirty-fourth birthday, I was genuinely getting boundaries, something that felt alien to me for so long. But y'all gotta remember I am a water sign, Cancer, guilty, so I will still be learning about boundaries forever more. Who is with me?

I share this brief, more recent story on my own boundary work because as I have learnt more about boundaries, I have learnt more about what I need every day when it comes to finding joy. And the more I find daily joy, the more I soothe my nervous system. The more I make this nervous-system-led approach daily, the more I feel pleasure. The more I feel like engaging in sex.

You need to explore your daily pleasures cup. How full is your cup day-to-day? Sure, there will be days when you drop the cup, and it's empty. Life can quickly get in the way. But you need to make joy a priority. And the more you soothe yourself to activate the parasympathetic nervous system, the more you remind your body that you are safe, held and loved.

More joy = more safety = more pleasure = more sex.

The kind of formula we all needed to learn in our science lessons.

Key practice:
Find ritual in your day. This can be as short as five minutes if it needs to be, but begin to weave in ceremony into your day. This ritual could be anything that soothes you. This may be using face creams and making a big song and dance about it, using that crystal roller to reduce puffiness and playing your current favourite song to move your body simultaneously.

It could be sitting down to write your morning pages with a candle followed by a slow cat-cow on the mat.

This ritual could involve writing a list of things you are grateful for.

Whatever the ritual, it's got to feel good enough to come into your everyday. Yes, there will be days when it slips. But hold yourself accountable to make this ritual happen. As you feel into this ritual, where else could you add ceremony? When you think of life as a beautiful dance you may see on stage, you begin to slow into what was previously deemed the 'mundane'. Your cup of tea could become more than a cup of tea. How would your tea feel if you treated yourself to your favourite loose tea that you need to spoon into the strainer and leave for a specific time rather than just a tea bag? Then how could you make your tea in a particular mug that always feels more 'luxe' than the chipped Matalan one you know ain't the one. Then how could you enjoy that tea a little more within your day? You could take this tea outside to sit with the birds, feeling the warmth in your hand without your phone pinging. Even if for the initial ten minutes of the tea.

How can you dance with your life with a little more femininity just because?

Try this key:

Move into your day through your vagina. What does your pussy need to feel good today? You can check in with your womb, but you can also check in with your vagina. This is exceptionally useful for finding what you genuinely need/deserve/want daily. Make everything vagina-led. How can your day become a pussy-led vibe? Look, it's not going to be easy. It's not going to look like this every day. But the more you lead by your vagina, the more you will find pleasure.

Swap out your vibrators and start vibrating on a higher level yourself for a while.

What brings beauty into your everyday? Is it fresh flowers every week? Is it a particular brand of clothing that feels incredible? Is it a basic make-up application? Is it more houseplants? It could be a coffee from your local favourite café. Is it longer dog walks at a particular place you both enjoy?

When you invite in more beauty, you feel good; you are pussy-led. You feel like you can take on that meeting now, the text you've been meaning to send, or the job application you've been needing to finalise. You go get it, boo.

Team up pussy-led living with pleasure-based rituals, and you will be living an orgasmic life. Orgasmic lives mean not going 'over' regularly. They represent not riding a high and plummeting into despair with the 'Now what?' thoughts.

Orgasmic life is about riding the pleasure train—toot toot, all aboard.

Working with the First Gate of Your Vulva

Your clitoris and labia make up your first grail gateway into the centre of your womb.[8] There are eight grail gates to move through before you reach the centre of your womb. I have worked with many clients working with these gates. For some, there is a natural progression from one gate to the next within a short time frame. For others, navigating these gates will take many months or even years.

We take this journey through the first gate gently and with an inner knowing that there's no turning back once we have walked this path.

The gates have taught me much about the holding patterns within my pelvic bowl. We start this journey at the seat of sexual innocence, the entrance to all that is, the edge of all we are. As we dance at the gate, we dance once again with what love for ourselves truly means.

Your clitoris is twinned with your thymus gland because they act similarly. The thymus gland is sensitive to stress and can shrink to half its size in twenty-four hours following a stressful scenario or if we have been ill. The thymus also grows when we are happy. The thymus gland sits behind your breastbone (sternum) and between your lungs. Many of us understand what it means to put our shoulders back and feel our heart opening.

During yoga classes, we talk a lot about opening the heart. Relax the shoulders down and back, and open your chest. You are opening your chest and thymus gland to all the love in your day. How grateful your thymus is for this love, pleasure and joy. So thankful, in fact, that the gland opens and grows. This is the 'stress barometer' in your body. There are many of us with an underactive thyroid which we could, energetically, refer to as a direct link to a lack of life force energy.

The clitoris engorges and pulses in the same way. It also contracts and shrinks and numbs out if we do not honour the clitoris for all that it is. Just acknowledging its ten thousand nerve endings is a start, hunz. The clitoris may even throb or pulsate in response to something within your day. This may also be felt in the vagina through flutters. You've heard of tummy flutters; the root is filled with pussy flutters too. It's time to honour those if you haven't already. You and your pelvis deserve that.

For many of us, this first gate will have been through challenges. There may have been betrayals, forced entry, a lack of acknowledgement for all you are, and there may be fear held here due to experiences you have been through.

If there has been a lack of pleasure and joy, this area may feel numb to life. Is there any wonder you may feel numb to your own touch or others? This gate is linked to boundaries. All the times you consented when you wished you hadn't. When others have ignored your boundaries or needs. We can see again why boundaries are woven into experiencing joy and pleasure.

To move through this gate and the holding pattern there, we need to come into connection with our clitoris and labia in a way we may have never done before. We will continue to move through our days aware of this connection, this gate and the holding patterns that may be associated with it. As we feel into this space through breath and connection, we begin to soothe this area and allow ourselves to meet our deepest needs.

Unlock these answers:
· Where have you said yes when you wish you'd said no in general or during sex?
· What do you feel you need from this gateway of innocence and pleasure?
· Where in your life do you need more pleasure/joy?
· Do you feel respected day-to-day in your life?
· Where do you need more beauty in your life to feel as though you are more regularly dancing with the feminine?
· Placing one hand on your thymus (sternum) and one hand on your clitoris, what energy do you feel there as you connect the two?

Try this key:
Find yourself seated on the ground.

Bring your palms together at your chest and sternum, where your thymus sits. Inhale into this space.

Turn your palms upside down into the yoni mudra position, where your thumbs and first fingers touch.

Exhale down with your hands to your clitoris and lips, pausing at the end of your out breath.

Inhale, and as you do so, turn your hands around to point back up in a prayer position.

Continue to inhale until you reach the thymus (breastbone).

Turn your hands to the yoni mudra position and exhale to your lips/clitoris. (There's no need to touch your body during this; keep your hands at the distance you need to. Though you could begin to bring them closer as you feel safer.)

Continue this practice until you connect more with your clitoris and labia.

Pause and thank yourself, your thymus, your clitoris and your labia for the gift of joy and pleasure.

Choose something to do afterwards that will bring you joy, such as making that orgasmic cuppa.

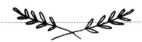

I pushed down my experience with my uncle,

Telling myself, it's OK.

Do you often ignore your feelings? I ask.

I do. She confirms through stories of heavy monthly bleeds

When your boundaries become stronger, your bleeds will become a little lighter,

I explain, with hope

—The 1980s

Sarah's Love Story to Her Womb

My periods were getting heavier and heavier, with alarming clots and debilitating abdominal cramps. I had started my womb/vulva healing independently but wanted to deepen my connection to my sacred feminine. I had done some mirror work and self-inquiry, so I was aware of the tension/trauma I was carrying in my sacral and root chakras. I had also become aware of trauma through the feminine line on which I felt called to do the more profound healing on.

I had neglected my cycle for decades and been pushing my body to the point of exhaustion; now, it was crying out for attention.

I was ready for more support and some bodywork. I could feel my body holding, so I wanted to offer it some healing touch. Naomi's vibe spoke to me.

I was bleeding so heavily that I couldn't continue with work/life as usual. As a yoga teacher, I bled through twice during one session. I didn't have the courage to stop the session, so I changed and continued, but this happened a few times.

I dreaded the next bleed as I struggled to cope with the pain.

When with Naomi, we spoke about everything flow-related, from practical things like smear tests and healthy products to use when bleeding to emotional work like boundary setting and ancestral trauma. Naomi even coached me when I felt guilty for taking this time for myself that I was a great role model for my niece and other women, modelling healthy cycles and self-care.

Now I understand my needs better, how to cycle sync and practice self-agency.

The cycle straight after my first session, I had a breakthrough. A night of HUGE healing. As my abdominal cramps got more intense and the bleeding heavier, I felt myself surrender to the experience; I held it and healed it. I had flashbacks and memories of past cycles where I had dishonoured my body and neglected myself. I saw and felt this for all womankind. I witnessed it and apologised, then set the intention to listen to and respect my cycles. Celebrate them, even!

After that night, my pain had reduced to the point where I barely noticed it, and my clots were nearly gone. I feel confident about how to look after myself.

After the sessions, I felt empowered and had a more profound awareness of practical tools to support myself. Plus, I now know Naomi can help if I need it.

It is your birthright as a woman to embrace the ebb and flow of your cycle and allow yourself the care you need. Honour your bleeds with as much rest as you feel you need. Don't feel pressured to stick a tampon up it, swallow a painkiller and get on as if nothing is happening, especially if you are suffering. Create boundaries that allow you to feel safe. You are valuable and deserving even if you are not outputting energy or constantly giving.

Slow down and look after yourself. Speak about your cycles to those in your life so they understand where you are at and can honour you in a way that feels right for you. Ask your friends and family how they find their cycles, and open up a dialogue that might help heal the collective. We hold so much creative potential, and women can harness this when they are in touch with their inner rhythms.

Step Five
It's All in Your Vagina

Botox

Your holding patterns can be found in your vagina. If you want answers, they lie in your vagina. If you truly want to move through the holding patterns binding you to the here and now, I am telling ya, they lie in your vagina. We've made it to step five and have done a lot of groundwork to get to this section. I advise that you do the previous key practices before engaging in the exercises in this section. Skipping the other parts is simply bypassing your deepest needs. You've gotta do the groundwork and lay the foundations before expecting to come into a relationship with your vagina through somatic touch. You've got to explore yourself a little more and get to know who you are on this journey. That's the magic of being on this path.

We've been taught that quick fixes are where it is at. I have been asked more than once what I feel about Botox for vulvodynia (pain in and around the vulva), for example. I share that if this is the route for you, then do you, boo, but Botox wears off in 3–6 months, placing you potentially back where you started. It may help at the time, and I am all for something that allows immediate relief when it feels too much. We know what we need. But my approach to everything is asking yourself, 'How long-term is that work?' What are you doing to support immediate relief at the same time?

For example, I was prescribed antidepressants at university when I was nineteen. I didn't enjoy taking them and, at the time, wondered what else I could do to support myself. I joined yoga classes every single week and got hooked on yoga workshops. After six months, I weaned myself off the antidepressants while falling into the arms of my regular yoga practice and breathwork to help me deal with my panic attacks more efficiently. Here I am at thirty-four, still having those dips here and there, but the difference is that I no longer fall back into despair for extended periods because I know I have the tools to support me. I have the net to catch me and understand more about why I may feel certain feelings. In time, the periods between feeling low also have extended.

I see how physical pain manifests from emotional challenges in this space with the pelvis. When we are aware of our emotional needs, the woundings we've been through, and the traumas we've endured, we can begin to physically move them through, rather than allowing them to sit in the body and cause further physical pain.

This section focuses on moving emotions through the body through somatic touch. 'Soma' means 'living body' in Greek. Neurobiology, psychoneuroimmunology and other medical fields have shown the connection between the body and the mind. During somatic touch, we remain present in the body, exploring any sensations that arise from pain, tension, tingles, movements, feelings and tears.

When we feel sadness in the mind, we know from our themes of consciousness that the mind could be feeling hopelessness, shame, guilt or judgement. When we feel sadness in the body, it can feel heavy, sharp and gritty; there may be aches and tears. When we marry the mind and body up this way, we garner much more guidance on moving through the emotion, challenge, wound or trauma.

We want to tune in to the symptoms arising for us so we can recognise our needs at any given time. Thus we will be able to flow with the responses, allowing ourselves to move the energy with intent. When the root tenses and closes due to the rising fear, we learn to soothe our nervous system and feel into what's needed. The impact of this will be to move from yet another emotionally and physically painful experience to one that gives us more hope and awareness around what we genuinely need to make these small steps to feeling whole once again. No, there aren't substantial quick fixes. But every single tiny adjustment and step . . . massive. They add up until you look back at the steps and realise you've taken one giant leap for you and us all. You absolute fucking hero, you.

The only issue: you've got to open your mind, body and heart to such an approach.

Sit Straight, Stand Tall

Your posture is important. Not only because it's going to help with all things breathing but because we are also aiming for the diaphragm to the line up.

The diaphragm is this giant parachute-like muscle that lines the ribcage. It separates the heart and lungs above from the rest of the body below. You can feel your diaphragm right underneath the bottom of the ribs. On inhalation, the diaphragm shortens and travels downwards. The diaphragm muscles attach to the ribcage and influence the ribcage movement.

As we breathe, the pelvic floor will move too. It will lengthen and move downwards as we inhale. This is because all the contents also have to go somewhere as the diaphragm moves down. The pelvic floor moves ever so slightly downwards. Then on the exhale, the pelvic floor moves back to the original position. Essentially the two are working together.

If your inhales aren't deep enough, then you aren't exerting this natural stretch with the pelvic floor muscles, thus weakening the pelvic floor over time, and if you are breathing too quickly, it means the stretch is more frequent, again causing issues with the pelvic floor.

What we also want is alignment. We can tune in to this alignment regularly. If we allow for our diaphragm to be stacked on top of our pelvic diaphragm, then this gentle teamwork continues with ease.

Learning to properly stand in tadasana is the perfect way to ensure you are stacking everything properly.

The steps to ensure you are 'stacking' correctly:

· Toes are pointing forward.
· Your ribcage is right on top of your pelvis.

- You are aligning the front of your ribcage with the front of your pelvis, your pubic bone.
- Breathe into this posture, considering a deeper breath.

There's a diaphragm at the bottom of your feet, which we are also aligning when standing in tadasana. Go to thisisnaomigale.co.uk/books and click 'how to stand in tadasana' for more support.

If we are out of alignment, we could unknowingly place pressure on the front of our abdomen, causing issues such as an inability to keep the front side of the body in integrity. Not utilising the natural stretch or tone of the pelvic floor can cause a failure to hold in ya wee or prolapse/prostate challenges, etc.

Regular gentle yoga practice can support moving into this gentle, necessary alignment. It really does pay to stand up for yourself, hun.

Your Vagina Holds a Grudge

Your vagina holds onto emotions, and those emotions are stored in the walls of the vagina, in the fascia.

I see many clients with vaginismus, vulvodynia or numbness in and around their vaginas. The people I see span the spectrum, from those who find it incredibly painful for themselves or others to touch their labia majora—I mean toe-curling cries of pain—to 'You could have been anywhere in my vagina and I wouldn't have known'.

Whatever happened to you happened. We know that. We know we cannot undo what occurred, but we can work on moving and unravelling the trauma challenges left in the mind, body and soul. Trauma takes pieces of you with it. We know by now from chapters in this book that our focus is to bring you back together a little more, in a way that is sustainable for you. Not with layers of tape, hoping for the best, but with tangible tools that allow you to make your small steps for long-lasting impact. These steps aren't linear. Though this book is five steps, these steps, in actual fact, overlap and cross over many times. You will be at one stage and then find that you need to focus back on a previous step. And so it is. Your healing journey.

The first thing we need to claim for ourselves, which is a big one for us, is our body back as ours. Your feelings, sensations and pain are valid. They always have been, and they always will be. You deserve, above all else, to come back into a relationship with your body, to feel the things you feel and step back from them, knowing that these feelings matter. Become aware of the emotions, no attachment, no chastising, no immediate need to change, but simply observe them as they are.

What I see is that there is a lot of pressure on vaginas. We already know there's a push in society to 'take cock', thanks to the orgasm gap stats. Yet we know our vaginas don't feel the same way about this.

Young people at university feel the pressure of one-night stands. Penetrative sex in marriages. Penetrative sex in abusive relationships. The list could go on. We then place a lot of pressure on ourselves to not react to impending fear.

If you've given birth recently and/or had an episiotomy, then a big cock wangled towards you with penetrative intent will feel challenging. If you have been raped, it may be challenging to have a one-night stand, even if the person is the nicest person you've met and you're both absolutely sober.

The issue is that thoughts arise, and we get angry. We find ourselves not simply observing but raging, crying or fearful. We land in one of those themes of consciousness but aren't truly aware of what is going on for us, or we find that we lose ourselves in the moment and don't take the time to observe what is arising. 'I should be able to have sex with my husband'. 'I am useless for not being able to just engage in sex with this nice person I met tonight'. 'The only way to make them happy is to have penetrative sex'. Your body may react to an impending cock with rapid heartbeats, defensiveness, anger, freezing, gut knots and shallow breath.

Your rational brain helps you identify where these feelings are arising from.

However, the more challenged we feel in a situation or about an impending situation, the more challenging we find the whole scenario. Our rational brains disappear out of touch while our emotions and ego run wild.

Yes, being aware of why we don't want sex with our partners doesn't change how we feel about it, but being aware of it allows you to make the choices you need to make, be gentle with yourself and pull on the tools you need to guide you.

We don't need to explore and dig up the trauma that occurred; we need to be checking in on the body in any given scenario. When a client comes to see me, we check in with the body and see where it needs more holding and love. When we work with our bodies, we need to find safety through touch. Finding someone who can gently touch your body, or learning to touch your own body so you can be with the parasympathetic nervous system, guides you into more safety. This will allow you to ground down through the root and thus explore how muscles in your root ebb and flow.

When we think about conditioning from society, we are often taught that during sex, we touch the vulva and then move fingers internally to the vagina for it to be deemed sex in the first place and to 'get the party started'. No. Absolutely not. We need safety first.

Key practice:

Before engaging in any touch with the body, your space must feel safe. What does a ceremonial space look like to you? Even on a one-night stand, you must consider whether the area around you feels nourishing. If you are someone who appreciates a candle, light one. Lights dimmed? Do that. New bedsheets? Sounds divine. A decluttered space? Makes sense. Your one-night stand should be no different to your long-term relationship or to a space for self-pleasure. The setting should always feel safe, nurturing, nourishing and grounding.

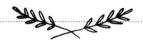

Fasciaaaaaaaaaahhhhh

Your vagina is a fibromuscular tube (fascia) covered with vaginal epithelium (skin). Think of your fascia as a support system for the vagina. Your vaginal fascia is suspended, elevated and attached to the muscles and ligaments of your pelvis. It's all very interconnected, hun.

Your fascia, however, is not just localised to your vagina. Nope. Your fascia was one weblike structure that began as a whole unified thang by the second week of your in-utero development as a foetus. This interconnected web will remain from top to toe for your entire life. It has been folded and refolded into this complex origami-like system, allowing you to do the basics all humans often take for granted, like eating, moving, standing and scrolling on ya phone. Fascia has been long ignored, cut through by surgeons to get to your muscles and bones. But your fascial system provides the environment for every cell in your body; it surrounds every single organ and then binds you to your shape, so you look like . . . a human being. Fascia, also known as connective tissue, is the largest organ in our body.[1] Before you @ me, it isn't the skin. This has been debunked, and you can thank me at your next pub quiz.

For a long time, fascia didn't seem to bring much to the table, so we all heard about bones, muscles, skin and organs instead. However, now we are aware that our fascia contributes to our well-being. Healthy fascia has a springy, resilient, hydrated texture and allows everything to function correctly.

Muscles, joints, organs and nerves will all function well, thanks to A-OK fascia. The most superficial layer of fascia lies directly beneath the skin.

If you press down on your arm now, you can press into the muscle; pressing hard enough you may feel your bone. Relax the touch enough to feel just under the skin so you aren't just touching your skin and you aren't pressing into your muscle. That's your fascia. Think of it like a webbing that your body is suspended in, like a bodysuit.

Fascia that needs more love will hold onto cellular waste, emotional stress and trauma. It creates toxic environments within the body, with stiffness, inflammation or disease. Fascia can become dry and brittle.

For example, when you feel an achy shoulder, as your whole body is linked, it may not be the shoulder that is the problem; the fascia may have become tight and meshed together further down your spine.

Think of your fascia like clingfilm (Saran wrap if you're American). Imagine it on top of water crumpled up. You want to begin to move it to become straight again without letting it sink. This is how it is to work with your fascia.

Your vagina is made up of fascia. Your vagina may have been through challenges such as painful penetration, childbirth, hundreds of tampons, cup insertion, dildos vibrating with strength, Gwyneth's special egg and more. Yet, when our shoulders feel tight, we stretch our backs, move our necks, and massage our shoulders. When our vaginas have lost all vitality and the fascia is screaming for some love, we don't bring in gentle touch as we would anywhere else.

We may feel enraged at the constant pain. We may buy dildos with more vibrational settings to actually feel something. We may ask for harder and deeper sex to feel some pleasure. We may use dilators and hope this opens up the root again. We may find ourselves with our third speculum inside our vagina within the last week while someone rustles around looking for a visible challenge.

I am here to remind you that your vagina deserves more.

Your vagina has always deserved more, and it's basic. It's not complicated. Humans still don't understand our bodies well enough because science is behind.

Fascia is 70 percent water with some proteins and proteoglycans. Water holds onto emotions, memories and experiences. Some scientists will say that's bullshit, but it's up to you what you choose to open your heart and mind to. There are plenty of scientists proving this is true. Your body holds onto emotions, challenges and traumas. This also has been proven many times. If water holds onto such memories and your fascia is 70 percent water, and your fascia is within your body, then it's up to you how you marry this information together.

Rape

I want to dedicate a whole section to rape. I talked about rape in the introduction, but I want to discuss this in a little more detail.

Based on stats in England and Wales, 1 in 4 women are raped, and 1 in 6 children are raped. These are just the cases that are reported. The highest-ever annual number of rape cases was recorded by police in the year ending in March 2022, at 70,330. In that same period, charges were brought to 2,223 rape cases.[2] So yes, a whole section on rape is necessary, especially when I see most of my clients have been through rape.

As you read this, if you feel triggered by the words on the page, then pause. Close the book. Come back to the section another time. Sometimes, I see people suddenly realise that they have been through rape but have avoided using the term or acknowledging that it was, in fact, this. You deserve to be held through whatever is arising. Seek that support. At the very least, send down your grounding cord to Mother Earth while reading this.

We are very aware of the connection between the pelvic bowl and our minds; therefore, when we go through trauma, we impact the mind-body connection through the damage done to our roots. When we go through trauma, it has implications for everyone differently, but the significance of vaginal trauma is more significant than we have been led to believe. Suffering with vulvodynia post-rape isn't just a physical response. Being unable to feel safe enough in a relationship to have sex with a loving partner isn't *just* a PTSD reaction. We are ignoring that rape harms the vagina and harms the person as a whole because it damages the source of someone's life-force energy.

Once a trauma occurs, it will always stay as something that happened in our lives. Though we move through trauma, allow it to be felt, and change how it sits on our body, we will still have been through the trauma. We all know that. After rape, no one will ever be the same as they were before. Society indeed ignores the impact rape has on a person. Rape is aimed at the brain and whole body, not just the pelvis.

A study on women who have been raped or sexually abused, especially in childhood, reveals that there are physical brain differences from those who have not been raped. The hippocampus's size and activation differ, as do cortisol levels.[3] Through sexual abuse, you are repatterning the body where there will be more fear and an easily triggered stress response, and someone will be more risk averse.

The point here is that we know the body remembers; we know experiences and challenges are woven into our being, held there to protect us. As a society, we have been ignoring the impact rape has on the body for potentially the rest of someone's life.

There's a ridiculous expectation placed on people to have penetrative sex when their vagina is left vulnerable and traumatised from assault or rape. The orgasm gap shows 95 percent of men engage in penetrative sex, and yet we know 1 in 4 people have experienced sexual abuse and 1 in 6 children have experienced sexual abuse[4]. There's a gap in society's understanding of what people need in general and particularly so for those who have been sexually abused. In my spaces, I see panic, fear and rage when it comes to the expectations placed on them to have penetrative sex. This expectation comes from those expecting that sex will end in penetration. Truly, deeply, what support and acknowledgement are we giving those who have been abused physically and emotionally sexually. Where people feel as though they can't even date because they worry the pain they are experiencing will upset the other person. Yet, if society placed more emphasise on the needs of a person sexually through reverence and deep holding, then someone who has experienced rape would feel more understood by society in general and would go into a date feeling as though there is a high chance the perspective partner will understand their needs.

Adding another layer here, statistics show that in 86 percent of cases of rape against women, the victim or survivor knows the perpetrator. In 50 percent of cases of rape against women, the perpetrator is a partner or ex-partner of the victim or survivor.[5]

On top of everything else we go through, including cycle shutdown; shame for menstruation; shame on vaginas; being shut down on social media for daring to use the word 'vulva'; and a lack of understanding of how the body even actually works, we are then expected to be raped and crack on with sex as we have before or as media shows sex *should* unfold.

This is why many vaginas are holding grudges, hunz. Studies show that 1 in 13 UK women find sex painful (dyspareunia),[6] and yet here we are going to the doctors with our legs spread to be mainly told it's all in our heads. Yes, babe, it's in our minds and our bodies, and the pain lives within us. Many, however, won't have the space or feel like they can tell the doctor currently pressing around the vulva, checking for pain spots, that they were raped as a child or more recently. It just doesn't come up. Or we don't feel safe bringing this up.

Everything neurological is very real and, of course, stays in the body. Stays in the vagina. Rape changes the body at an intimate level. We can move through our experience(s), but we need more than speculums, bright lights and blood pressure checks. Rape and early sexual abuse impact our parasympathetic nervous systems, repatterning our daily interactions. Long-term damage exists when we are unable to truly soothe our nervous system—we know that. It impacts our blood pressure, heart rate, breathing, our sudden reactions to things. Anything beyond our conscious control. One study confirmed that a history of sexual abuse can lead to the vagina responding differently overall. There may be less vitality. The vagina will engorge less and move less effectively. Even when viewing sexual material, for example. There is physical damage to the vagina, and sexual arousal is impacted even years after the trauma.

And here we are, discussing the need for more joy, pleasure and happiness, and you may be a rape survivor who has never been given the holding, love and understanding you need to find vitality again from the root up.

I am sorry, darling soul. I'm holding you on these pages. You are heard here.

PMSL: Pissed Myself Laughing

Post childbirth, I couldn't hold in a wee. Nope, I often had a little wee coming out while I ran to the toilet. And post-twin birth, I was fucked. I honestly shat myself more than once. Full shit, in my knickers, because I could do nothing. I'd tell my husband, 'Too late; I can't hold it'. He'd look at me reassuringly but with those sympathetic eyes. It got to the point where pissing and shitting myself was just a regular monthly occurrence, babe. Black knickers 4 life.

Farting, nah mate. I was buggered. For example, if I had eaten something that triggered my IBS at a party. Wow. I mean, it was next-level stress. I would literally hang my arse away from anyone and everyone. If someone wandered over mid-fart, I'd panic-walk towards them and hope the draft was enough to waft it in any direction but towards their nostrils. Life was genuinely challenging when I was loosey-goosey, letting everything just come and go as it pleased, with zero control in public. You know it's gone beyond when your son refuses an evening picture book with you because a little bit of fart came out in his room and, quite frankly, he'd rather forfeit the book than sit with his mother who cannot control her pelvic floor. He asked for Daddy instead. Tragic.

I downloaded the NHS's Squeezy app. But the issue was, I have never had a pelvic floor and, to be honest, have had a little bit of wee come out often, even as a child. I hated moving my pelvic floor. 'Do it every time you hit a red light in the car'. Trying to remember to do it wasn't the issue. The problem was that I felt sick whenever I wanted to engage it. It felt gross, and there was no way I would volunteer to squeeze when it made me feel nauseous. I paid £2.99 for that app and never once did a single squeeze.

Welcome to your pelvic floor.

Your pelvic floor muscles span the bottom of the pelvis. They support the pelvic organs, the bladder and bowel, the uterus and the vagina. When your pelvic floor muscles are weakened, it creates problems with bladder and bowel control. The pelvic muscles become too weak or too slow. They do not have the strength and quickness to do the job needed.

Muscular bands (sphincters) encircle the urethra, vagina and anus as they pass through the pelvic floor. When the pelvic floor muscles are contracted, the internal organs are lifted, and the sphincters tighten the openings of the vagina, anus and urethra. Relaxing the pelvic floor can allow for easy-breezy wee and poo movements. The pelvic floor muscles are essential for sex, with their relaxation and contraction combination, allowing for sex that is actually pleasurable.

The iliococcygeus, pubo-coccygeus and coccygeus most likely provide physical support or act as a 'floor'. While the puborectalis muscle provides the constrictor function to the anal canal, vagina and urethra. Based on the physiologic studies, the puborectalis muscle appears to be the third constrictor or the sphincter of the anal canal. Studies also show that the puborectalis muscle serves as the constrictor for the urethra as well. Meanwhile, the vagina has only one constrictor mechanism, solely provided by the puborectalis portion.

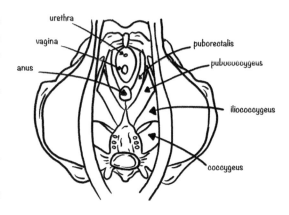

Your pelvic floor can be weakened by:
· Chronic constipation straining
· Pregnancy
· Childbirth
· Trauma
· Obesity
· Persistent coughs
· Surgery, such as an episiotomy
· Tension through painful periods or endo

These muscles form the base of the group of muscles called your 'core'. These muscles work with the deep abdominal muscles, back muscles and the diaphragm. They support the spine and control the pressure inside the abdomen.

The floor of the pelvis consists of layers of muscle and other tissue. These layers stretch like a hammock, from the front, at the pubic bone, to the coccyx, or tailbone, at the back, and from one ischial tuberosity (sitting bone) to the other (side to side). The pelvic floor muscles are normally firm and thick.

Some things that can improve as a result of working with your pelvic floor muscles:
· Bladder and bowel control

· The risk of prolapse
· Recovery after childbirth and surgery
· Sexual sensation
· Pain during sex

You'll also experience less frequent farting and fewer 'Oh, I have just shat myself' situations. (That's to say, it can improve your social life and the bond between you and your children at evening book times.)

Signs you may be having challenges with your pelvic floor muscles:

· A little bit of wee comes out when coughing, sneezing, laughing, bouncing on a bouncy castle or running
· Not making it to the toilet in time
· Anal farts or vaginal farts when bending over or lifting
· Lack of sensation in the vagina (numbness)
· Tampons that fall out or get lodged in too easily
· A distinct bulge at the vaginal opening
· General heavy sensations at the vagina
· A heaviness or dragging feeling in the pelvis or back
· Recurrent urinary tract infections (UTIs), or recurrent thrush
· Vulval pain
· Pain with sex
· Inability to reach orgasm (that peak one where you then go over)

Pelvic floor exercises are also called Kegels. Essentially you are squeezing your root, holding and letting go. But this isn't possible for everyone, and if you, like me, feel sick at the thought, you ain't going to engage with it either.

When I work with clients in a vaginal massage, I ask them to do their Kegel with my finger inside their roots. This is to check the holding pattern of their root overall. I commonly see that people think they are doing their Kegel and are simply tensing their abdomen, buttocks or thighs. The muscles inside the vagina do not move. This is common among all, not just those who have given birth or who are older.

The patterning of the root is one of the most fascinating parts of this work. The energy of the root and how the root adjusts after touch is incredible.

We've explored the fascia, we've explored how events will impact the body and change how it holds itself and we know how important it is to acknowledge the root for overall vitality in the body. Thus, working with our pelvic floor muscles is the missing key.

Finding your pelvic floor muscles:

Yes, everything is linked together. But to understand your muscles at your root, we are going to separate them and then bring them all back together to work as one. The sphincter muscles are quite circular, so it is helpful to think back to the water analogy when working with the fascia and imagine that as you release, they release like ripples in a pond.

To identify the sphincter muscles:

For the vagina, once you have sent down a grounding cord, if it feels safe to enter and pain-free enough, you can place one finger inside and squeeze the pelvic floor muscles around your finger. But we will explore this more later, so for now, it's plenty to just understand where the holding pattern for the vagina is without having to do anything just yet.

For the urethra, imagine you are having a wee, and you try stopping the flow in midstream. However, do not actually do this; you're aware of the difference between the spacing of the sphincters.

For the anus, pretend you are trying to stop a fart at a buffet and squeeze.

We all know that your diaphragm works with your pelvic floor a little like the movement of an undulating jellyfish; we also know that an orgasm, clinically speaking, is a series of involuntary muscle contractions. If your pelvic floor muscles are too tight or short, then when you orgasm and a contraction pulls on those repeatedly, it's gonna be painful. Or it may be painful post-orgasm—this I hear in this space often.

We've made it abundantly clear that you need a 'healthy' pelvic floor to live a life without hassle and full of vitality.

If you sit now and lift your shoulders around your ears, you'll feel them tightening and shortening. To find relief, you'll massage them back down and roll them over to get them to 'release'. You may rub them with your fingers or get someone else to.

When your pelvic floor muscles are tight, our automatic response isn't to massage them or bring in gentle touch and love as we do for the shoulders. And yet here we are, sitting on our pelvic muscles and expecting not to shit ourselves or experience existential orgasms like off of da telly. If your shoulders are tight, you'll do something proactive to help holistically aid the relief from them being this tight, especially if you end up with regular headaches or migraines.

Pelvic floor exercises aren't the answer.

Though you may be able to pull your muscles up and in every now and then, do not do Kegels every day. There aren't any golden stars for those who can lift pencils with their vaginas.

Likely, you aren't doing them right anyway. There's so much more to this than just doing your Kegels.

Try these keys

Yoga is a beautiful source for stretching your pelvic floor muscles. To move into the fascia, it's more beneficial to hold a pose for longer (3–11 minutes) and breathe into it gently. No pushing or pulling.

All these poses bring breath into the pelvic floor muscles. By breathing deeply through the nose, you are also activating the parasympathetic nerve response. Continue to breathe deeply into the pelvic floor muscles as you remain in the pose. Your breath aids the release of the muscles. Always exhale deeply and move slowly when coming back out of the pose, ideally doing a counter pose where necessary.

Tadasana (Mountain Pose)
- Stand with feet hip-width apart.
- Rest your hands at your sides.
- Line up your diaphragm.
- Lift your crown, with your chin slightly down to extend the back of the neck.
- Place a yoga brick between your thighs.
- Engage the inner thighs and imagine you are lifting the brick upwards.

Utkatasana (Chair Pose)
- Begin in tadasana.
- Bring your arms out in front of you, parallel to the floor.
- Bend your knees while pushing your hips back into a slight squat (hips no lower than your knees).

Setu Bandha Sarvangasana (Bridge Pose)
- Lie on your back with your knees bent, with your legs and feet parallel and hip-distance apart.
- Move your feet closer to your buttocks.
- Press down through your feet and inhale to raise your hips, lifting from the pubic bone rather than the navel.
- You can keep your hands by your side or bring them together under your back on the floor.

Baddha Konasana (Bound Angle Pose)
- Sit on your bottom, moving away fleshy bits.
- Bring feet flat to the floor and allow the knees to gently move outwards, bringing the soles of the feet together.
- You can use two blocks or a pillow to support the knees and gently push them away in time as the muscles relax.

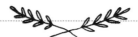

I Fell This One Time at Band Camp

'I did have this one fall when I was a child; I'd not really thought about it until now' is often the response I get from a client when I ask them about any injuries to their tailbone. We have this odd bit of tailbone, which you probably have never considered. The coccyx is at the base of your spine and is found directly above your buttocks. Of course, many ligaments and muscles attach to it, including your pelvic floor muscles.

The term 'coccydynia' describes pain around the coccyx area.

You may have had coccydynia if pain is worse:
- When sitting down or standing up

- When going for a poo
- When bending forward
- During sex
- During your menstrual cycle

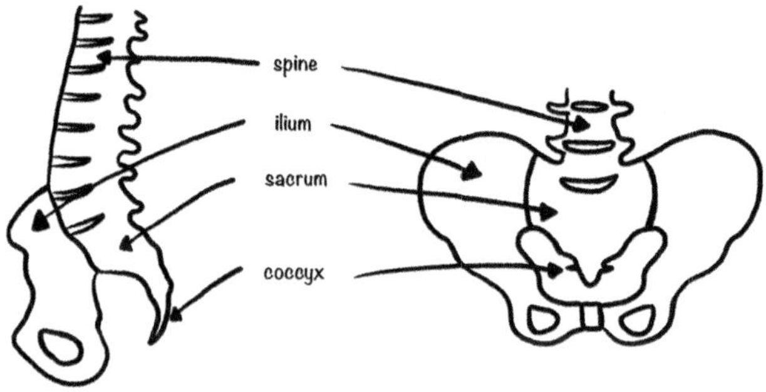

(Diagram labels: spine, ilium, sacrum, coccyx)

Some of the causes of coccydynia include:

- A fall directly onto your tailbone or a direct blow to the coccyx
- Pregnancy
- Giving birth
- Horse riding
- Previous injury
- A skiing, snowboarding or skating accident
- Hypermobility (increased movements at your joints)
- Prolonged pressure from poor sitting posture (for example, sitting, feeding a baby, driving, sitting at work and cycling)

Some of us may have had a fall when we were little and not even thought about it again. Except muscles remember, and if we have not spent time working with those muscles, then they may continue to be tight and in this protection mode until we work with them. There may not even be anything obvious to cause alarm. It could be as simple as struggling to engage in hip openers in a yoga class, sitting cross-legged, sitting for extended periods or not receiving much pleasure from sex.

We must work with our pelvic muscles and our coccyx to find release. I work with the coccyx with every client in ceremony. I mainly massage at the bottom of their back and under their coccyx into the ischiococcygeus (coccygeus). If the coccyx continues to cause challenges, then you can work with those previous pelvic-floor-focused exercises and try this key for yourself or someone else.

Try this key:

You can massage into this area deeply at the very base of the spine along the line of where your coccyx lies. It should feel gritty and like you are getting in there. I suggest working with this area to find more relief if it doesn't feel gritty. If you can feel the grittier parts, keep massaging them with your fingertips. You could ask a partner to help you with this, and they can use their thumbs and fingers to apply pressure and find a release here. This is a deeper touch than that of just working with your fascia.

Relieve the coccyx, and you may likely experience more pleasure daily and in sex.

It's Not about Gender, Hun

We are already very familiar with the left side and the right side of the brain. The left side of our brain is the masculine force. The right side of the brain is a feminine force.

The brain is shown to consist of two halves, a left hemisphere alongside a nearly symmetrical right hemisphere.

'Hemispheric lateralisation' is the idea that these hemispheres are functionally different. If we use this notion, the idea is that specific processes, behaviours and tasks are controlled mainly by one hemisphere. However, neuroimaging and other neuro-scientific methods show that both sides participate in most tasks, especially those involving creativity and logic.

Marrying up the two is the aim. However, it is helpful to be aware of the different energies within us. We never find balance as such but can learn to lean into the feminine and the masculine daily.

When we think of feminine energy, we think of 'be', which softens the masculine energy linked to 'do'.

What's important to note is that the left hemisphere controls the right-hand side of the body. It receives information from the right visual field controlling speech, language and recognition of words, letters and numbers.

The right hemisphere then controls the left-hand side of the body. It receives information from the left visual field controlling creativity, context and recognition of faces, places and objects.

According to the left-brain, right-brain dominance theory, the left side of the brain is considered to be all over logical, rational and calculating tasks. Therefore, the right side of the brain is best at artistic, creative and free-flowing tasks.[7] Utilising both sides for all tasks makes more sense when you think about it.

When we consider the yin and yang of Mother Earth. The feminine with the masculine. There's the sun and the moon. Light and dark. The day and the night. Our inhales and our exhales. Each one is essential for the flow of life. Without the exhale, there would be no room for the inhale. Without the darkness, there would be no found light.

Society has an uneven approach to the feminine and the masculine. It shows itself regularly through human behaviours such as men whose femininity is suppressed in favour of being more 'manly'. Young boys are conditioned to not feel emotions and 'grow a pair of balls'. And yet, for us to swan through life with more grace and less challenge, we need to dance in the duality of the feminine and the masculine energies. If one was to do this, there would be less struggle overall.

We favour masculine energies such as doing, reasoning and strength. We undervalue the necessity for nurturing, receiving and flowing with our emotions.

Some of us will express more femininity in our daily lives, while your work colleague, Tara, may express more masculinity in their life. Others may float between the two energies. Your overall identity and how you live your life through masculine and feminine expressions changes how you navigate your life. So much so that you may notice how Tara's relationship with work differs from yours.

We must open our minds and hearts to the presence of both energies. Be aware that these exist and how they can serve you daily. In doing so, you will find life to be a little more fluid.

People pick up on your vibe. We vibe with different people. We certainly only gel with some. We are instantly aware of people's energy. Their auras. Your vibe comes from within through your experience with life, the environment around you and those around you. Your first layer of consciousness.

Gender is a construct. Gender refers to the characteristics of women, men, girls and boys that are socially constructed. This includes norms, behaviours and roles associated with being a woman, man, girl or boy. As a social construct, gender varies from society to society and can change over time. We are highly aware of this when we walk into a nursery and watch the girls and boys interact with the given toys, or see how parents react to boys who want to play with dolls or who cry vs girls picking up dinosaurs and roaring.

Gender is how we express ourselves through appearance, behaviour and language within a culture. According to Dr Amanda Solomon Amorao, a lecturer exploring questions of cultural production, gender and decolonization, we live in a system where there are specific ideologies at any given point in history around gender, which then dictate what it means to be a woman or a man. Social institutions enforce dominant ideologies, which then shape a gender hierarchy. Gender formations justified by the reduction to whether you own a penis or vagina are enforced by institutions (the patriarchy), pushing the whole men-over-women dominance scenario.[8]

The expectations placed on people before they leave the womb are still rife. Think of gender-reveal parties and the expectations placed on the growing foetus around what they will be like and be interested in. These genuinely create challenging expectations for people and continue to cause issues in our society. We see violence against women, laws creating ridiculous challenges for LGBTQIA+ folk, unequal pay and pain in men who cannot express their emotions. Such experiences then form our identity and attitudes to such binary roles.

There's a lack of safety for us all when society focuses on a binary framework for sex. Sex equals gender, and that then equals sexuality. Cultural norms and societal expectations mould your life around gender, sex and sexuality. Cisgender women, cisgender men, intersex folks, transgender folks and nonbinary folks have different lived experiences when looking through the intersectionality lens. Gender and sexuality are social constructions (constrictions). Being aware of that is a start, hunz. This in itself begins to bring in more safety for us all.

But of course, we know only some are open to this.

However, the more we push 'divine feminine' vs the masculine on socials and daily life, the more we push social constructs onto people.

We can only be in our divine feminine if we are dancing in dresses while the wind blows through our hair with a beautiful backdrop. Though this is, of course, beautiful and necessary for many, it isn't what we mean by the divine feminine. Weaving in the divine feminine in our lives means being unapologetically you, using your intuition, being full of love, and embracing the beauty of nature and the universe. The divine feminine is about taking radical responsibility for ourselves.

We can only access our divine feminine energy by telling all men to go fuck themselves. Also not it, hun.

To live our lives to the fullest with freedom, we must know that there should be equal value placed on masculine and feminine energy. In the film *The Mask You Live In*, boys and men are faced with messages that encourage them to disconnect from their emotions, devalue authentic friendships, objectify women and deal with arguments through violence. Such gender stereotypes then interconnect with race, class and circumstance, creating a challenging web of identity issues boys and young men must try to navigate to become 'real' men.

Such messages perpetuate the idea that men who are indeed then masculine must be assertive (aggressive), physically strong and unemotional. They must remove themselves from anything remotely feminine so as not to be labelled as being anything like a woman. This eliminates the honour the feminine deserves. Men can then not tap into the feminine characteristics that exist within themselves or others.

Miss Representation is a film showing how the media sells the idea that a girl or woman's value is wrapped up simply in their beauty, sexuality and ability to remain youthful. It explores the underrepresentation of women in positions of power and influence. It highlights the media's limited portrayal of what it means to be a powerful woman.

These messages that women must dance in beauty only feed the statement that girls who speak up for themselves as powerful feminine beings are a pain in the arse. They are too much. Too mouthy. Should be seen and not heard. Women are here to dote on men and be good mothers. Women then have to turn their back on the masculine energy within them to not rock boats in the home environments or at work, for example.

My tantric-kundalini yoga training focused on the masculine and feminine qualities that exist within us all and within it all. We talk about father sky and Mother Earth. The shakti and shiva energies exist for everything to bloom. Only when shakti exists with shiva can we create. The humble female bumblebee worker busies from flower to flower while the flower blooms to reveal the pollen within its centre.

If we peel this back further and weave together the yin and the yang only, we remove the need to label anything as feminine and masculine. Shiva and shakti are one. We have both energies within us, and it's how we work with these energies to feel whole. How we navigate these within our cycle to find more ease as we jive with our hormone dance-off each month.

Key practice:

Create two columns for shakti and shiva energy. Add creative and destructive columns for shakti and creative and destructive columns for shiva. Write a list of the descriptions you resonate with the most without judgement. This would be a valuable activity to do in a relationship to create discussions around the energies in the partnership.

With creative shakti, you:
· Show vulnerability to others and yourself
· Are affectionate with others and yourself
· Are deeply authentic through an inner knowing of who you are
· Surrender into the flow of life
· Are compassionate with yourself and others
· Are playful, expressive and love to love
· Weave sensuality throughout your days
· Tune in to your body and trust what you hear
· Know what it means to feel grounded
· Tune in to energy and others' auras
· Are loving
· Understand what it means to be birthing and manifesting
· Feel a level of devotion to aspects of your life

With destructive shakti, you:
· Have people-pleaser vibes
· Find it hard to trust in the wisdom coming through the body
· Are unable to ground down and speak from the mind before checking into the body
· Lack boundaries for yourself or others
· Ask for validation from others a lot
· Are afraid of death (loss)
· Obsess over certain people or outcomes
· Are unable to allow others to be in flow for fear of something going wrong
· Manipulate outcomes
· Are insecure—seeking outside validation
· Put everyone else before yourself
· Lack safety within your body
· Find yourself behaving irrationally regularly

To twirl with more of a feminine balance through your days, be aware of the importance of reclaiming rest and sitting in the non-doing. This provides more focus and clarity overall. Remember, the journey is about flowing with the being rather than the doing. The universe has a plan, and you know you cannot control this plan entirely. You magnetically attract what you want. Loosen your grip just a little more. Look at the bigger picture and enjoy the process. Learn to say no more to the things that don't please you and will only ever please others. Find space on your own. Solo time allows you to hear the messages from within. You can also journal what comes through. Give yourself more love and more compassion. Look at the environment around you; how safe, loving and nourishing it feels. Continue to ground into Mother Earth. Move your body sensually through gentle movement, yoga, dance and running—whatever brings you joy during the movement. Find more pleasure through the items you wear and the things you buy for your space. Be more conscious and intentional with the beauty you create around you.

With creative shiva, you:
- Are responsive rather than reactive
- Are aware of death in a way that means you face fears
- Understand the need for support from others
- Encourage yourself and others
- Can find presence in life without pushing a goal
- Are grounded in the here and now
- Can hold space for yourself and others
- Bear witness to experiences without judgement
- Create safety around you
- Focus on what it means to be you (your personal truth)
- Listen to others
- Are supportive
- Guide and seek guides
- Respond to situations rather than react to situations
- Have an air of peacefulness around you

With destructive shiva, you:
- Ignore the wisdom of your emotional body
- Push on through without stepping back to look at the bigger picture
- Aren't connected to the wisdom that exists around you
- Push your own agenda
- Find yourself being aggressive often
- Have narcissistic tendencies
- Aren't able to be in the here and now
- Withdraw yourself from situations often
- Lack warmth
- Find yourself in the distance from scenarios
- Shame others or blame others instead of taking any responsibility
- Fear losing or failing
- Tend towards arrogant
- Think you are always right

To twirl with more of a masculine balance through your days, tune in to the way you hold your body. Is there an openness, or do you tend to lean over, round your shoulders or lean forward? Work on your tadasana. Connect with your primal energy by connecting back with nature and engaging in some primal kind of activities. Work with your inner desire for adventure by trying new things, meeting new people or going to new places. Find others to guide you, such as therapists or coaches. Find affirmations that support you in the here and now. Work on your boundaries for yourself and others. Be more willing to take risks but, of course, know what will be. List out your fears and where they stem from.

You need to prioritise yourself and learn more about your wounds, challenges and gifts.

One of the ways I love learning more about myself is through my root, through being in touch with my root. Once you have explored the above energies, you can bring yourself to your vagina and tune in to the holding pattern to reveal more and to tune in to yourself, your needs and the challenges you may still face. To bring the subconscious into consciousness. The above activities where you check in with your energies are all conscious. Working with our roots to excavate the subconscious while connecting with our pelvic bowl will give us so much more in our life. But first, you need to find more safety within your body before exploring the landscape of your vagina.

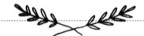

Feelin' Yo'self

Do you touch your body with gentle intention often enough? Do you massage your body with love with a moisturiser?

I ask clients this every time they work with me. Sometimes they retort, 'Of course!' Sometimes they go away and really think about it and realise their current version of a massage is equal to going in for a slap-dash massage that may exist in one of those pop-up chairs you see inside a shop offering you a ten-minute shoulder rub for a fiver. Slapping on moisturiser is not the same as giving your body a massage through loving touch.

As humans, we can really crave touch. If we aren't in a relationship (and sometimes when we are in a relationship), we can find this touch often enough. Learning more about your body and needs will only ever be of support when you expect touch from others.

Being able to bring in touch like this may feel alien, challenging or incomprehensible, and that's absolutely OK. This is you protecting yourself.

We are working on this resistance to meet it gently, lovingly and with honour so that you can find a release from it.

Your touch and anyone else's with you should be gentle but firm. The spaces you explore on the body should be met with the same energetic touch with no hesitation. This firm and equally energised touch throughout the body allows us to relax and release tension. The muscles relax a little more as the touch continues.

When mindful of our touch, we allow ourselves to ground into the body a little more. I often find myself bringing in this gentle but firm touch from the soles of my feet and along my legs whenever I can. Your feet connect to the ground, and your legs are attached to your feet like tuning forks. They are energetic prongs plugging you in, so bringing in form touch helps me to ground and feel loved.

We now can see how the body is restricted and bound by the emotions held within. When we release our shoulders, relax our jaw, allow ourselves to take in deep breaths and let out audible sighs, and cry those tears, we remove physical and emotional tension from within the body.

When we touch, somatically with this intention, we allow ourselves to unravel into the spaciousness created; our breath feels less laborious, movements less stilted, and life more free flowing. This kind of physical touch will enable us to find a home within our bodies that responds to finding a home in this way with the spaces and people around us.

Finding this level of safety allows us to feel our edges and boundaries. Imagine being aware of where your body ends in an energetic space, so you can explore your body with more rooted safety with others.

If you realise what brings you pleasure through this touch, you can verbalise what brings you joy with others. If you suddenly realise when you touch yourself that the soles of the feet feel incredible to be touched, then you can focus on this with others. (I'm not saying you've got a feet fetish, but if the shoe fits and you realise you're into it, then you do you, babe.) The point is that where you find an opening to more joy and pleasure is where you will feel more openings in life.

Key practice:

Engage in a full-body massage for yourself.

I've got an entire body massage playlist you can listen to, which takes you from an opening to a peak to an unwinding experience and can be found at thisisnaomigale.co.uk/books.

Set an intention for the ritual. An intention could be the questions:

'What am I looking to nurture right now?'

'Where do I need more love within my being right now?'

Make the environment yummy (safe): candles, post-bath or -shower, ya fave sheets, lamps. Use your best moisturiser or massage oil.

Find yourself wearing as many layers as you need, or be completely naked.

Play my playlist or one you have created. Make this a time when you won't be disturbed.

Remember to bring a firm and loving touch to every part of your body.

Direct your breath through deep inhales to each area of the body as you touch it. Allow the thoughts to flow in and out. Remain curious about these thoughts.

Start at the toes and move to the crown of your head. This process takes a minimum of fifteen minutes to an hour-ish.

As you move through each part of the body, you can say in a mantra for each body part to bring in gratefulness for being you.

Toes: 'I am rooted into Mother Earth through each and every toe'

Feet: 'I am rooted through each corner of my foot, knowing I take the steps I can take each day towards my most authentic, expansive life'

Ankles: 'I can surrender to the adjustments needed in life'

Knees: 'I can bend and adjust as I need to in life'

Legs: 'I am energetically connected to my feet and then to Mother Earth through each leg'

Hips: 'I feel the ease of life'

Coccyx: 'I feel the pleasures of life'

Stomach: 'I feel into my everyday needs for nourishment'

Womb: 'I feel the creativity that I birth everyday into this world'

Diaphragm (lower ribs): 'I do what I need to do for my needs'

Solar Plexus: 'I do know what I need for a more fulfilled life'

Breasts: 'I love to take time to connect in with my feminine self'

Shoulders: 'I love being in touch with my needs'

Elbows: 'I love flowing with life and adjusting with its course'

Wrists: 'I love to circle and dance though life with flowing ease'

Hands: 'I do know what I need to feel safe and held'

Throat and Neck: 'I speak up for my needs'

Jaw: 'I speak up to receive the honour I deserve'

Third Eye (between the eyebrows): 'I see where I need to gift myself more space and time'

Scalp: 'I understand that am safe, I am held, I am loved'

Once finished, you can bask in the joy and pleasure that touching your body in this way has given you.

As written in *The Gospel of Philip*: 'What you say, you say in a body; you can say nothing outside this body. You must awaken while in this body, for everything exists in it resurrect in this life'.[9] The body never lies and deserves to be held and respected.

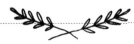

Your Vaginal Landscape

She lay there sobbing uncontrollably. The energy began to shift, and I spoke gently. 'What is arising for you?' Tears started to move through her body again. 'I have realised that no one has touched me in the way you are touching me right now'.

This isn't a unique experience. This is the experience of most of us who step into this work.

When we engage in a vagina massage, the touch can't be compared to any other touch. This is because the touch comes with no strings, ties, goals, intentions, or aims. The touch is healing, somatic, and gentle but with loving awareness. The touch from a vagina massage gives someone a starting point to what touching the vagina really needs to feel like for the vagina to unfurl petal by petal into any given sexual scenario. When the vagina feels safe, the vagina responds through opening, surrendering and expanding you likely have never experienced before.

A vagina massage is a missing link between you and any challenges currently rising for you in your root.

A vagina massage should be taught to everyone. If we all truly understood what it means to respect, love and honour the portal to all that is, we'd grow up with a very different understanding of what it means to house a pussy between our thighs.

Nope, we ain't fingering ourselves. And for anyone else reading this, guffawing and saying, 'I skipped to this page, and now she's saying we gotta massage our vagina'. Whatever you have to say on the matter, I've heard it before, because I have explained what this is on social media to millions of people. It's a snore-fest for me nowadays when people snigger or snort or avoid me at the school gates because they know what I do. I understand that this work is profound. But only those ready to open their hearts and minds to it will get it.

We aren't necessarily all ready for a vagina massage. It's a balance of understanding how to move through the edges that exist when you consider the idea of engaging in your own vagina massage.

Some practitioners offer vagina massage, including myself, of course. But there are considerable differences in what is available. I have had people travel from Scotland to Margate for a reason, hunz.

You only want to ever find someone who approaches a vagina massage from a non-goal-orientated stance and who works with vagina massage in ceremonies for healing and reclamation.

My roots for this work are in a holistic non-tantric approach. I work with the Metamorphosis Method, which you have been following this in the book. I find that the vagina often asks for you to work with it last because it wants you to be able to surrender into this space with ease. Clients will need to work with the rest of their body and pelvis before finding safety in working with the vagina.

The idea of this section is for you to explore your own vaginal landscape. I believe it is crucial to engage with this before going to a practitioner or while working with a vaginal-based practitioner. I often see those who have come to me for a massage leave and never try the process for themselves. This is a massive shame because the vagina massage should be revisited many times over. Every time you explore your landscape, you peel back another layer on your healing path to reclaim your cunt as yours.

This tool brings vitality back to the root, healing and reclamation. So if you have a loosey-goosey pelvic floor, this tool is for you. If you've been through rape, this tool is for you to bring in some of those pieces taken from you. For those with vaginismus or vulvodynia, this is THE number-one tool. Endo, painful periods—it's for you. Those who have said yes to sex and inwardly wished they'd said no, this tool is very much for you. Post-birth, miscarriage or abortion, you need to heal the portal that opened. It's for us all. There isn't a single vagina that doesn't need a vagina massage.

In a few years, we will seek a vagina massage the same as we have sought back massages. (In a ceremony, not in seedy back-end spaces.) There will be a change in the way we work with our wombs and vaginas. The generations here and coming through will understand the necessity to work with their roots in this way. I see you. I've got you. I am celebrating you. Thank YOU.

Key practice:

Before engaging in a vagina massage, the setting needs to be set. The area needs to feel nourishing, and safety needs to be found.

Go outside and connect with Mother Earth.

Connect with Mother Earth by grounding through the feet in the space.

You could start the ceremony off with a bath or a shower.

Know that you can switch to a full-body massage rather than a vagina massage at any point.

The most crucial aspect of all of this is that you feel invited in by the vagina to do this work, and the vagina will only do this when you are completely and utterly ready.

Stage 1: Send down your grounding cord

Once you have found yourself in a nourishing space, it's time to send down your grounding cord into Mother Earth. Your finger is simply the connection to Mother Earth; it's an extension of the grounding cord. Breathe into your belly, and as you have seen and read about previously, send down your grounding cord into Mother Earth, breathing with intention here. Do this before you engage in anything with the root.

Stage 2: Wait for your invite

Bring lubrication to your finger with an organic lubricant or coconut oil or almond oil. Your vagina will invite you in when the vagina is ready. Begin to touch from the top of your mons pubis down your labia majora and along the labia minora towards the anus and back up with intentional, firm, loving strokes. For some of us, we need to tune in to the wisdom of any pain; decide whether it feels so painful you find it unbearable or can be moved through with the touch.

The blood will move to the labia and engorge the labia. This increased blood flow helps to increase the production of vaginal lubrication. It causes swelling in the clitoris, labia minora, labia majora and vagina. Stroke enough for you to feel this adjustment occur in the root. So you feel you have surrendered a little more into the process. At some point, you will feel ready to pause at the entrance to your vagina. Place your finger inside the labia and begin to tune in to the vagina. By now, you'll see whether the vagina feels ready to invite you in. It's almost as though it surrenders, opens and allows the finger to be drawn inwards. A little 'Hello, I am ready for this honouring'. As you enter, do so millimetre by millimetre. Entering in ever so slowly to not startle the vagina, the complete opposite to when someone begins fingering you like they are rummaging for the last Pringle in the bottom of the tube. Niceeeee.

If you don't feel this opening, you can continue to touch the vulva until there is an invite. Or perhaps there isn't an invite, and now is not the time. Repeat the full-body massage and return to this step in the ceremony again.

Stage 3: Check in with your holding pattern

Your vagina and whole body have a left side (feminine, if you will) and a right side (masculine). We know how the right and left hemispheres work with the body, so you understand how your left and right sides are holding as a result of your experiences in life.

This means when you work with your root like this, you are simply surrendering with your Kegel. Ya ain't gonna be working towards pulling a truck with your vagina anytime soon. This is just for you.

Essentially, we are looking for the pelvic floor to be even and engaged all the way around. Imagine your vagina sucking gently on a straw, even all the way around and able to bring up the liquid gently. This is where it's at (and where most of us are not).

But in time, with this intentional touch, your holding pattern will shift and adjust to become more even.

Be here for a moment, tuning into the walls without movement.

(Post massage, you will notice the 'grip' almost feels lighter. That's great. You want a gentle pelvic floor that engages together.)

Stage 4: 'Testing' yours
·   Engage the muscles (do your Kegel).
·   Do this a couple of times as you try to tune in to what is happening, but not so much so that the muscles get too tired.

- When you have relaxed, ensure no engagement is still happening. We should have muscles that relax and then release. So bring in some breath to the area and direct it down if you still feel holding.
- You've completed the test. And with this test, we all pass. We pass because we all tried. And that's all anyone can ask for, loves. Do not do this test and chastise yourself for loose holding patterns. Your root is yours, and that's why you are here doing this work.
- What you are looking for here is where in the ring there was holding and where there wasn't. Was there more strength on one side than the other? Did one side come into the finger quicker than another? Tune in to this pattern around the ring, from twelve o'clock to six o'clock and then back to twelve o'clock. But don't worry about the holding at the urethra and anus specifically, just around each side of the clock.

Stage 5: Your first pilgrimage into the vagina

Your vagina's landscape will feel wild when you make your first pilgrimage. At the top of the vagina, you may feel your cervix; depending on your cycle, it will change how it feels. You do not need to touch your cervix. Remember that you do not need to touch the urethra or the anus. When exploring the landscape of your vagina, imagine it to be similar in layout to the inside of your mouth. This will give you more understanding of the layout of your vagina.

Some of us may not manage to get past the labia, and this is absolutely OK. For others, we will remain near the opening of the vagina, and for others, we will be exploring deeper into the vagina. Your finger will know where it is being called to tend, and the more you speak to this wisdom, the easier it will be to trust in this process. I often get asked, 'How do I know I am doing it right?' You are doing it perfectly. Trust, surrender and tune in.

Your touch needs to be a fascia-release touch. Refer to the fascia section to remind yourself of what this looks like and the reason we use the fascia here. But you are simply moving the fascia, which takes only a light touch. You're not pressing into the muscles but into the layer just above. As if you are moving that clingfilm on top of the water. There's no Swedish massage approach here, loves.

I remind clients and those in my vagina workshops to keep to one side and then switch to the other. It doesn't matter whether you start on the right or the left, but choose one. Explore one side fully before moving on to the other.

Between each side, we must pause, breathe and find ourselves simply bringing presence to the root. Your primary focus is to bring in a level of presence you may not have brought into the pelvis before. To find yourself breathing into your finger within your bowl and to remain with this presence. This unwavering presence brings love and support into the bowl in a way you may never have experienced before.

We choose one side over the other because the holding pattern is often very different and can bring up different emotions.

As you explore one side, feel into the holding pattern that exists. There may be a gritty-like feeling or pain. There may be numbness or very little cushioning, so there isn't much vitality within specific areas. Pause on any site that feels different. You can pause on the spot for as long as eleven minutes (though this is a very long time to hold the area for, so you may end up focusing on one place overall) or pause for a few seconds. But give your fascia time to move and release.

We can look into the energetics around the holding patterns, but as I say to all my clients, do not overthink these. Your holdings are yours, and you must tune in to what you think they may be first and foremost. You're excavating the subconscious, and it takes a lot to tune in to what may be coming up.

Wherever there is particular pain, tension or numbness, there are some questions to consider exploring post-massage.

Unlock your answers

The left side of the vagina (your left is your left-hand side):
- Where do you feel you lack devotion in your life?
- Are you giving yourself enough compassion?
- Do you feel like you receive enough mothering in your life?
- Where are you gripping too tightly in your life?
- Are you expressing yourself fully in your life?
- What are you holding back from yourself and your life?

The right side of the vagina (your right side is your right-hand side):
- Do you feel safe and held in your life by yourself and others?
- How present are you in your daily life?
- Do you cheerlead and encourage yourself enough to achieve your goals?
- Is there enough support around you from others?
- Are there any fears for the unknown right now in your life?
- Do you feel at peace with your daily life?
- Are you currently working on your goals, or have you paused on these for any reason?
- Are you seeking support, or do you have enough support?

Stage 6: Retesting yours

Once you have come to a close with your vaginal massage, you can pause back in the centre. Breathe into the centre and feel how the root has changed since you began this ceremonial practice. Breathe into your finger and redo your Kegel. See how the pattern changes around the finger. Do the muscles work more as one?

Stage 7: Exiting as you entered

After working with the vagina this way, the vagina opens up, surrenders and finds safety. The last thing we want to do is undo this process. Therefore, you must exit as you enter. Millimetre by millimetre. Once you leave, your root will likely feel very different to how you started because you have opened the petals of the vagina. The vagina is adjusting to this delicate expansion through the safety it has found. The other reason we exit slowly is that it can trigger an abandonment wound. It can feel like we are suddenly being abandoned if we leave the portal too quickly.

Stage 8: Lie back and think of England

Once done, it's the part we all wait for as soon as we enter a yoga class. The savasana. Integrating post-massage is the best bit. When you go for a massage, and the therapist says they'll leave you to get dressed—'No rush'—I dunno about you, but I lie there wondering what 'no rush' means because I could do with at least another hour. Give yourself as long as you need. Feel into the emotions that have arisen. Give yourself this time. It's a true gift. Journal afterwards if you feel called.

Babe, this is the most significant gift you could ever give yourself on this root-based journey.

FAQs about the vaginal massage

Q: What is the point of the massage?
A: There is no outcome here. The most minor changes add up to make the most significant impact. Isn't that great to know? You are simply soothing, guiding and bringing in more love. There's no outcome to the massage.

Q: What if I feel awkward?
A: That's OK. It is new, and this is a challenging task. Know that in time it eases. So keep easing into it. Finding new positions etc.

Q: How often and for how long?
A: To begin with, once every few days when you are called. Maybe two or three times a week if you are working with something specific like a childbirth trauma or a period of intense stress. How long depends on you. It may take a couple of minutes, five minutes, twenty minutes, or even half an hour. Your body will cue you when to stop. Don't engage for more than twenty minutes, as your root can tire quickly. And if it's your first time, I wouldn't go past ten minutes, ideally. For example, if you ache after or the next day, you should massage for less time in the next ceremony.

Q: What if I feel pain or aches after?
A: It's OK to feel something like this in the vagina. But it may be you need to take it easier or do it for less time next time.

Q: How far is my finger going?
A: It depends on you. Experiment up to the knuckle to down to the base. Move it into a hook position, or keep it straight. It's your body.

Q: What if my arm doesn't reach?
A: This is where you realise you may not be blessed with Mr Tickle's arms after all. So it would help if you kept adjusting to find as much comfort as possible. You may engage with the massage on your side or while lying on your back. Either way, to begin with, it may feel awkward, but you'll find more ease in time. Keep persevering. Remember to do so gently if you need to exit to move position.

Q: What if I am feeling nothing, not even numbness?
A: This may be because this is a more energetic experience for you. Bringing in visualisation and connection is powerful work. Don't underestimate that. Keep working with it, for sure.

Q: I am pregnant; can I do this?
A: It's best to leave the nest alone, so to speak. This includes if you are TTC (trying to conceive) and post-ovulation. You can, however, engage in visualisations with your vagina and womb—just no somatic touch internally.

Q: What if I feel the heat?
A: That's perfectly normal; this is just part of the muscles relaxing and releasing.

Q: Yeah, but will it feel sexual?
A: We should be utilising this work to connect and release through the fascia. This isn't sexual. Though you may feel more sexual energy or increased libido due to this work. It may even feel more accessible to orgasm, for example. Or after the massage, you may begin to feel aroused, but this varies. All is welcomed.

Q: There are so many spots to massage for me, though.
A: That's OK. Massage slowly; take your time. Come back to it again if you need more time.

Q: What if the tension comes back?
A: There are layers to this. You're like an onion. Keep peeling back the layers. In time, things will ease, and it will feel like you're making your way through those layers. Your shoulders spring back up around your ears, and your root is no different.

Q: What about scars?
A: Gently massage scars. Bring in more support to those areas. Scars love to be moved and massaged. They hold so much tension and so many memories.

No Need to Rummage for the Last Pringle

Once you have massaged your own vagina, you may like to ask a partner to massage your vagina. But only do so when you feel completely and utterly held for the experience. It took me around three years to ask my husband to massage my vagina in this way.

There have been many clients who attended my vagina workshop and went on to ask partners to create a ceremony.

A previous workshop goer commented on this on my socials one day, making my heart sing and making me realise we need a section on receiving this massage from a partner in this book. For them to read.

According to this follower, 'The workshop was life-changing. I just haven't been ready to express everything fully into words. It was a roller coaster of emotions afterwards that ended up with me standing in far more freedom and no shame! I taught my hubby what I knew from the workshop. Such a healing experience'.

When we work with the feminine, we work with all things receiving. How do you work on receiving in a way that brings healing, love and holding?

At school, we were shamed for wanting to receive love. We want to experience loving touch and pleasure to find more joy in our lives. But how can we do this if people are not shown what it means to touch and, more importantly, how to connect in this way. When we strip everything back and bring healing touch with no goals or aims, it changes the energy of our intimate experiences.

Being clear about the ceremony you are creating is the first step. You need to be in honour of this process for you both. The aim is to heal the vagina together. There is nothing sexual about this. We are not aiming for any pleasure in the patriarchal sense, and we are not aiming for orgasms.

You need to be clear on your boundaries and transparent with consent: 'I am giving you permission to massage my vagina for healing and reclamation, and at the end, we'll lie together to integrate with a cuddle'.

Or: 'I am giving you permission to massage my vagina for healing and reclamation through fascia-release touch. Afterwards, if this leads to sex, I would be OK with that, but I will let you know if I change my mind'.

We need to be super duper clear on our expectations.

Here are instructions for your partner. (They can also read the FAQs above, before or after reading the below stages.)

Key practice for a partner:

Stage 1: The grounding cord

Your partner will send down their grounding cord. They know what to do, but they are energetically plugging themselves into Mother Earth to ground into the experience. Ask them to let you know when they are ready for the next stage. You could ground with them by simply sitting next to them or on the bed, imagining yourself on the earth. This may feel wild or natural to you.

Stage 2: Wait for your invite

The vagina will invite you in when the vagina is ready. Begin to touch from the top of the mons pubis down the labia majora and along the labia minora towards the anus and back up with intentional, firm, loving strokes. For some partners, this will be incredibly painful. Check in with facial expressions and keep in touch by asking them if they are OK and how they are doing.

The blood will move to the labia and engorge the labia. This increased blood flow helps to increase the production of vaginal lubrication, as it causes swelling in the clitoris, labia minora, labia majora and vagina. Stroke enough for you to feel this adjustment occur in the root. At some point, you will feel ready to pause at the labia.

Begin to tune in to the vagina. By now, you'll see whether the vagina feels ready to invite you in. Place your finger at the entrance. It's almost as though the vagina surrenders, opens and allows the finger to be drawn inwards. Check in with your partner to be sure they are ready too.

As you enter, do so millimetre by millimetre. Entering in ever so slowly to not startle the vagina.

You ain't rummaging for nothing.

Once you enter, pause in the centre of the vagina. You're now in the centre of their pelvic bowl (it is everything within the pelvis, including the fallopian tubes, the womb, ovaries, etc.). If your partner does not house all of these organs, the energy of each one remains.

Check in with your partner again. How are they feeling? Allow them to bring in breath to your finger. You are their connection to their grounding cord. Feel how the walls of the vagina move and ripple around your finger without needing to move your finger. Find yourself tuning into the subtle changes.

Stage 3: Check in with their holding pattern

There is a right side and a left side to the vagina. You want to imagine the vagina as a clock, as you will be massaging from about twelve o'clock to six o'clock on each side. But you will be avoiding twelve o'clock and six o'clock, which is to say you won't be touching the urethra or the anus.

Ask them to do a Kegel around your finger. You will be tuning into the walls and how they 'come in' around your finger. Where do the walls come in quicker or slower? Where do the walls not move at all?

You are now tuning into the wisdom of your partner's root. Be with the walls around your finger. Nothing to do or change. Just tune in to the energy. You could close your eyes and follow your breath while remaining in the root.

But with this intentional touch, the holding pattern will shift and adjust to become more even.

Post-massage, you will notice their 'grip' almost feels lighter. That's great. You want a gentle pelvic floor that engages together.

Stage 4: 'Testing' theirs
·   Ask them to do a Kegel in their own time when they feel you have adjusted to the energy in the root.
·   Ask them to do this a couple of times or more as you try to tune in to what is happening. But not so much so that the root tires.
·   They should now have let go of the hold.
·   You've completed the test. Everyone passes.
·   What you are looking for here is where in the ring there was holding and where there wasn't. Was there more strength on one side than the other? Did one side come into the finger quicker than another? Tune in to this pattern around the ring, from twelve o'clock to six o'clock and then back to twelve o'clock. Don't worry about the holding at the urethra and the anus, just around each side of the clock.

Stage 5: Your first actual pilgrimage into the vagina
The vagina's landscape will feel wild when you make your first pilgrimage. You may be used to simply engaging with the vagina with pleasure. 'How can I touch the vagina so I am bringing in pleasure?' would be your usual approach.

Nope. This is different.

You may feel the cervix at the top of the vagina; depending on the cycle, it will change how it feels. You do not need to touch the cervix.

Imagine the layout of the vagina to be the same as the inside of our mouth and cheeks. This will help you get your bearings a little more when inside the vagina. The labia are like the lips of the mouth, and the walls of the vagina are similar to the cheeks inside the mouth.

You may find that you remain near the opening of the vagina. You will know what your partner needs because you are working together with the vagina.

You vagina-whispering hero you. The vagina knows you're loving, and you're holding them. They will open and surrender to your touch in a way you may never have experienced before.

'How do I know I am doing it right?' You are doing it perfectly. Trust, surrender and tune in.

Your touch needs to be a fascia-release touch. You're not pressing into the muscles but just above the layer. Imagine if you were to touch your arm with one finger, press into the muscles, release back up to the skin and then find yourself touching between your skin and the muscle. Here lies the fascia. This is the touch you will be bringing to the vagina. It feels incredibly light. It's as if you are moving that clingfilm (Saran wrap) on top of water.

Work around one side and then switch to the other. Pause between sides. You can check in as often as you need. Some question prompts:

- 'Is this OK for you?'
- 'Are any thoughts coming to you right now?'
- 'Is this touch OK for you?'
- 'Is there anything else you need right now?'
- 'Tell me if you need me to pause and return to the centre'.

As you explore one side, feel into the holding pattern that exists for your partner. There may be a gritty-like feeling or pain. There may be numbness or very little cushioning, so there isn't much vitality within specific areas. Pause on any site that feels different. You can pause on the spot for as long as eleven minutes (though this is a very long time to hold the area for, you may end up just focusing on one place) or as little as a few seconds. But give your partner's fascia time to move and release.

Stage 6: Retesting the Kegel

Once you have come to a close with the vaginal massage, you can pause back in the centre. Breathe into your own belly and remain with the energy in the vagina. How has the vagina changed? How has the atmosphere changed within the ceremony? How has your body changed? How has their body adjusted overall?

When you are both ready, ask your partner to redo the Kegel. See how the pattern changes around the finger. Do the muscles work more as one?

Stage 7: Exiting like you entered

After working with the vagina in this way, the vagina opens up, surrenders and finds safety. The last thing we want to do is undo this process. Therefore, you must exit as you entered. Millimetre by millimetre. Once you leave, the root will likely feel very different to how you started because you have opened the petals of the vagina. The vagina is adjusting to this delicate expansion through the safety they have found. The vagina is a portal; you have just opened this portal through your touch in this ceremony. Be gentle with your partner, and be gentle with yourself as you feel into this experience. It may well be a life-changing experience for you. You may never have touched the vagina in this way. And this is huge.

Stage 8: Lie back, and both think of England

Once done, lie down next to your partner. Don't rush off to wash your hands, for example. Don't check your phone for notifications. This can trigger the abandonment wound.

You could ask your partner how they'd like to be left. Perhaps stay in their space while you remain near them but not in their energy field. Maybe they'd like a cuddle. Perhaps they'd like their hand held.

Give yourself time. Give them time. This was a beautiful, healing experience for your relationship, for the vagina and for your sex life.

Fuck. I am celebrating you both on your journey together. What a gift you are to your partner. Thank you.

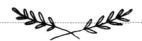

The masculine side feels so different to the feminine
she voices in a way that feels enlightened all of a sudden
goodness me how poetic
ain't it just

-leaning into the feminine

MC's Love Story with Her Vagina

I came across Naomi's work on TikTok and was taken in by how quirky yet serious she is about the work she does. Talking about the vagina is always tricky in public, and I admire how open and to the point she is in explaining that it holds so much of our power and trauma. So I took the plunge and reached out to her—and I am so glad I did!

I've been interested in bodywork and healing practices for almost two decades. I am familiar with the concept that trauma is stored in the body. The beauty of this work is that it can be done remotely—Naomi and I only ever saw each other on Zoom. It's gentle and sometimes unassuming. If you are open enough to work with yourself, it doesn't take much time, strain or pain—it's gentle work that somehow has magical results. Naomi has this unique mix of a super positive, supportive and funny disposition, intermixed with a deep knowledge, respect and mastery of her work. I can't think of anyone more suited to help newcomers and more experienced women on this journey. I felt safe and engaged every step of the way when working with her and realised that by gently and intuitively working with our fascia, a subtle yet potent shift happens.

At first, I thought nothing of it. Then I naturally felt more energised, grounded, empowered and optimistic about myself—tangible positive experiences seemingly out of nowhere reinforced that feeling.

Society's really done a number on us. They taught us that our feminine power is either scary, wrong, non-existent or the opposite of it—a weakness. The truth is, I really do believe it's the most powerful force on Earth.

It's our duty to ourselves and to each other to continue doing work like this. To help ourselves and each other reconnect with this power, get to know it and learn how to wield it. In doing so, I do believe we will heal ourselves and our lineages, past and future.

To my younger self or anyone unsure whether this work is safe or real, give it a try. It's so gentle; it's such a powerful entry to a whole world of positive transformation, which you can take one step at a time.

As an old teacher used to say: 'Remember, your pace is the pace'. And Naomi is the best ally you can hope for—as well as great fun!

The Key to Your Happiness

Moving on up and Fallin' Back Down

In the words of Primal Scream circa 1991, you may have been blind, but now you can see. You're likely feeling like a believer. Your light shines on. You may have been lost, but here you are completely and utterly found (held).

If you made it here reading this with a newfound belief in the power that lies between your thighs, well, babe, what an absolute root-loving, chain-breaking hero you are. I'm here with my pompoms out, and seriously, pop on Primal Scream's 'Movin' On Up' right now. Because you've made it to the end. The application of it all. The integration of all that we've discussed.

You may find yourself moving out of shame with your vagina. You finally feel as though you are glowing between your legs, and there's a big fuck you to the shackles holding you back from achieving all that you deserve in your life. However, you may be feeling grief. Grieving the loss of the years spent not believing in yourself enough or believing you weren't worthy. Or you may find yourself moving from hopelessness due to the tools you have been given in this book but landing in fear. It may feel overwhelming.

Find yourself lost in these pages where there is endless hope through key practices and questions. Remain here for as long as you need. Come back to these pages again and again.

Whenever your ego begins to remind you of stories, come back here; come back to the hope that lies in the stories, the poems, the tools, and the words of encouragement on these pages.

For it is this hope and holding that is missing in many pelvic consultations, assessments and appointments.

Healing is not linear. It can feel overwhelming. Like there is no way out of the current scenario. 'Will it always feel like THIS?'

There's a reason why 1 in 5 of us have suicidal thoughts.[1] It's easier at times to imagine the pain and challenge simply ending. Healing is really, really hard at times.

But healing is also the most incredible journey when you realise there's nothing to fix, heal or do.

Just be.

We may wish there was something that made this all quicker, easier and more immediate. But the truth is, healing is fluid.

Hope lies in everything you do; every small step brings a shift. Small shifts add up to big shifts. Big shifts make considerable differences in our lives.

We don't need to exhaust ourselves on a constant conveyor belt of healing to find more happiness. There's nothing in the search. Pull on the tools you love the most daily/weekly/monthly. Find joy with these, and it will all feel like less of an uphill battle.

Be nervous-system-led. Always tune back in with your body in the here and now. There's nowhere to go or be. Be in the present. There's less suffering, challenge and heartache in the present.

There will always be triggers from scenarios or people. These triggers keep you safe. Be aware of these triggers and be led by them.

You will have days where you feel a little bit or a lot shit and days where you float from space to space like the pussy-led wonder you are. All should be welcomed.

For when you fall into the velvety depths of the darkness, the light will always be found, and you will appear from these depths changed.

I've Got Gadgets and Gizmos Aplenty, Hun

Vibrator chat. I am not here to shame you for your love of a vibrator. Many of us own vibrators. I had long loved my Big Red Carl and silver bullets.

The thang is, we need to be more in tune with our self-pleasure tools, how we use them and what they give us in our lives.

Hear me out, and don't suddenly get your box of silicone lovers out to throw 'em in the bin. Not just because we can't be flinging them in our bins; according to UK law, sex toys that oscillate or vibrate are electrical items. This means all your sex toys are treated as other electrical waste, like toasters.

FYI, many local councils in the UK have disposal centres for said electrical items. You can search your local council's website to know if you can dispose of or recycle sex toys in your area.

Vibrators allow us to seek pleasure in the same way society depicts people seeking pleasure: hard, fast and quick.

Having sex with a vibrator can, for some, be the equivalent of choosing between buying their own ingredients for a meal in vs going to Five Guys. We love Five Guys as a treat, but we know we'd be more nourished through our home-cooked meal. We can't always be eating burgers.

Some of us find ourselves vibrating our way through pleasure. You may continue vibrating harder, faster and quicker to reach orgasm. Post-orgasm, the comedown can be even more significant because there isn't sustained pleasure from this approach.

For some of us, the only way to experience an orgasm is through a vibrator, meaning when you engage in touch through fingers or a non-vibrating penis, you feel very little.

Here's the key to all things silicone lovers.

We shouldn't be relying on a vibrator for pleasure. We also shouldn't rely on the same vibrator in the same place for pleasure.

If there's pain, the vibration can bring about some relief. You may be able to use a vibrator for a moment to de-armour the vulva and vagina to be able to bring in touch.

Begin to explore other vibrators, touch and places within the pelvis. Bring in a range of touch across the whole body, from firm massage touch to tickles with other tools.

Explore crystal pleasure wands, heating them under water or cooling them down. Find an excellent lubricant that's organic, and bring that into play.

As you continue to tune in to your root, touch yourself without a goal and bring in a relationship, you may find that what you need and want adjusts too.

Speak from Your Pussy

I was lying on my mat in my cabin in the middle of a solo circular breathwork journey, and the constriction around my throat was so tight I had to open my eyes to check there wasn't someone in the space holding me down by my throat.

My throat comes into most of my healing spaces. When you have been held back from speaking up for your needs as a child, you often feel as though your throat is restricted.

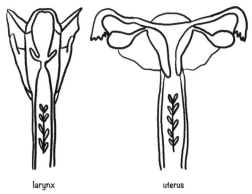

Singers trying to move into their most authentic spaces through their voices may find that they need to come into a connection with their roots. Your vagina is linked to your throat. Your larynx and your uterus behave similarly.

The neck is called the cervical spine, and the lower, narrow portion of the uterus is called the cervix (Latin for neck). In fact, the cervix and vocal fold tissue behave similarly when tested.

larynx   uterus

Open your vagina to open your throat.

One client came to me for a full metamorphosis retreat. During the opening ceremony, she mentioned her singing tutor had been telling her for months to work with her pussy. The day opened her vagina in a way she had never experienced before, naturally. During the massage, she explained there was tightness coming to her throat, which is common during a vagina massage. Through tears, she said it had changed her life before she'd even left the retreat day.

After her immersion, she began moving her body again. She came to me on a Friday, and she attended her first yoga class in months by Monday. She'd been stuck with movement, so going to a yoga class was an absolute win. At the end of her class, her teacher cracked out her ukulele and sang to the class. This client wouldn't normally do this kind of thang, but she felt a strong urge to ask her if the yoga teacher did singing coaching, as her current coach was based abroad, to which the yoga teacher replied yes. This client emotionally, physically and energetically opened her vagina and opened her voice in a way she had never experienced before.

How open your throat is. How relaxed your jaw is. How much you speak up for your needs is reflected in your root's holding patterns.

For years I have humorously used the phrase 'open throat, open vagina'—but there is truth to that statement. When the throat is open, this opening is reflected in the throat of the uterus, the cervix.

I don't know about you, but the car is one of the spaces where I find myself singing. I definitely sound like Shania Twain's twin. If going on the talent show *Stars in Their Eyes* was still an option, as long as I could drive into the studio and keep my windows up, I'd be there.

There's no judgement, worry, concern or stress while I drive monotonously accessing the subconscious, singing my heart out to 'That Don't Impress Me Much'. We know that the body tightens to stress, anxiety or fear.

When we are in danger, we either scream through a high-pitched shrill or cannot scream at all. Your voice reflects how you are emotionally, how deep your breath is and how tightly you are holding onto your body.

This is why hypnobirthing encourages you to loosen your jaw and be fluid with the sounds leaving your body. Gentle deep breaths, deep hums or sighs or aaaahhs. You'll be lengthening your breath, lowering the pitch and relaxing your root.

Singing, orgasming and childbirth all are moved through by rhythmic muscular pulses. If we shut down from the vagina, we shut down from our voice.

And yet, we must advocate for our needs and speak up for our wishes and our dreams. We need to be able to do this in a society that has shut down our inner power for so long through fear and shame tactics that have kept us held in spaces and places we no longer deserve to be tied to.

The vagus nerve is a physical thread between the throat and the vagina. The vagus nerve ('vagus' means 'wanderer') is the largest nerve in the body and wanders from the lowest part of the brainstem down into the pelvic floor, uterus, cervix and vagina. About 80 to 90 percent of the nerve fibres in this nerve are dedicated to communicating the state of your deep, inward feelings from your body up to your brain. This means it responds like our skin to movement and pressure-based stimulation. So not just electrical signals. And indeed, note the signals move from body to brain, not brain to the body.

The respiratory diaphragm actually massages the vagus nerve with each breath. When we discuss touch, it's a firm, intentional, loving touch that we need. Therefore the quality of the movements from within the diaphragm matter.

We want quality breath teamed with these wonderful strokes teamed with the vibration of our voice to stimulate the vagus nerve. Sending messages of safety to the nervous system.

Deep, steady, massage-led vocalisation, such as singing and hums, will soothe the nervous system. In fact, those who often work with their vagus nerve internally often end up speaking with a lower tone.

When we use vocal toning, we use our voice to balance our cells, open our energetic pathways and find more harmony. When we chant mantras or songs, we use rhythm. Both heal, open and harmonise us from within.

Key practice:

To vocally tone is to heal. It:
· Encourages deep breathing
· Creates vibration through your body to help relax your muscles
· Aids in relieving pain
· Opens the throat and the root
· Brings about relaxation

You may be thinking, 'Glad she wrote this towards the end of the book'. As you sit humming on your meditation cushion, the incense burning, opening your pelvis in your bedroom, what a journey you are on, hun. Here are a few breathing practices, called *pranayama* in yoga, that you might explore.

Bhramari Pranayama (humming bee breath)

Named after the female humming bee in India, it also seeks to open the heart space.

Sit rooted. Bring your eyes to a close if you feel safe to do so.

Bring your hands into your lap.

Breathe naturally and come to stillness.

Inhale deeply.

Exhale with a hum tone that feels natural for you. The intensity, pitch or frequency should not change. Hum for the entire exhale.

On each exhale, find a different tone to hum, whether this gets higher or lower.

Continue to do so for as long as you feel called.

Resume a natural breath and find stillness once again.

Vowels

When we bring in different vowel sounds, it tones other parts of the body.

EEE is for the head

EY is for the throat

AH is for the heart

OOH is for the solar plexus

OOO is for the sacral

UHH is for the pelvic region and lower spine

The idea is that you can send the vibration toning the sounds to the different areas of the body. You'll know when you've connected to specific areas because you'll feel the vibration in the space you aim for. Try making the sound tones change to 'reach' these spaces.

Repeat the same steps as the humming bee breathing, but replace the hum with the vowels. You could stick with one vowel or work through all five.

Bija mantras

Any sound in the universe is vibrational energy. Our words are a combination of sound waves at specific vibrational frequencies. Quantum physics describes how the universe was created through cosmic sound energy. Then there was heat and light, then, ya know—beings. Sound vibration is linked to our life-force energy.

So it all makes sense that the vagina is linked to the throat via the vagus nerve and gives birth to life.

Bija mantras were developed to create balance and harmony in the body and soul. The idea is each part of our body functions to the best of its ability when it vibrates to a specific rhythm. When we are balanced and in tune as one, we vibrate in harmony.

The root chakra mantra is 'LAM'.

Repeat the steps per the other practices, and bring the mantra 'LAM' to your root. Keep using 'LAM' until you find this connection and feel the vibration within the pelvic bowl.

And now, sweet soul, you are moving through the blockages to enable yourself to speak up for yourself and your deepest needs. So onto consent.

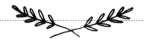

No Means No

I remember wandering the fresher fair and being given a sticker: 'No means, no'. Here we were in 2016 discussing how if we say no to sex, it actually means no. When my four-year-old says no, it means no, hunz. So we live in a society where still to this day consent is a challenging topic, one many of us are still trying to truly understand as we find our voices.

There we were on our holidays in Devon. I was holidaying out of a caravan with my school friends. It was my first holiday with friends, and it was going as I imagined it to go with six women in one caravan, all of us seventeen or eighteen years old.

We met a group of guys, obvs. We partied and hung out. One of the guys wrapped his arms around me, and seeded to like how I had no clue about my power as a woman. He preyed on me, as I was less sure of myself, insecure. At the time, I was seventeen, so to have a twenty-five-year-old man find me interesting was a coup I rolled with it.

When we were in his caravan one evening in bed together, he went to have penetrative sex with me. I told him I hadn't had penetrative sex before, and his eyes seemed to light up. No worries, he informed me, we don't need to engage in this right now.

Thank fuck, I thought. I wasn't ready for him to wang his wanger anywhere near my vagina.

Post-holidays, he kept in touch via MSN messenger. I was into it. So into it, I printed off his kind words so I could reread them again and again. *Le sigh*.

One day I saw him again. I wasn't really sure I wanted it, but I'd been primed for it by him via MSN.

We had penetrative sex, and it really, really hurt. I was not ready, but society tells you sex hurts, and your first time will obviously hurt. So I continued on with the throbbing pain.

After a while, he left and . . . I never heard from him again.

He came. He conquered. He disappeared.

I kept thinking about how a twenty-five-year-old took my first experience of any kind of sex with intent, and I won't ever get it back again.

I was in emotional agony. I didn't want to say yes, but I did.

My relationships continued this way: I said yes to sex when I really didn't want to, in order to people please. My childhood had primed me for such sexual relationships.

There was the time I had sex with a friend with a massive cock, when I kept saying I didn't want to, knowing full well he fancied me, and the friendship was very blurred.

The time I had sex and didn't want to with a guy I kinda dated on my gap year, who told me he probably fancied men but didn't want to. He was trying to reframe his thinking by having sex with me. Then he dropped me, then freaked out and picked me back up again on rotation for over a year.

The time I wore sexy lingerie when a long-term ex-boyfriend had cheated on me, left me and come back, and we had sex. I went into the bathroom and cried.

My point, sharing these sex stories, is that we often say yes while inwardly saying no to ourselves. Outwardly we do nothing more than go through the motions. We don't realise that we aren't giving explicit consent. The other person isn't obtaining clear consent, which continues to blur lines in 2022. I see you; I understand, darling soul.

My husband will continue to remind me during sex that 'we don't need to do anything you don't want to do'. We have been together for eleven years. It's still a conversation we have today, and we have been engaging with more the longer we are together because we've been working on our boundaries in general. It's important.

Consent in sex is getting more airtime. This is because as we learn more about what it means to have bodily autonomy, we begin to understand the importance of saying yes with clarity.

What is consent? It's where all the people involved in any sexual activity agree to engage by choice. Everyone will also have the capacity and the freedom to make a choice.

We do not have to kiss, be touched or perform a sexual act. We can change our minds at any time.

If there isn't consent and there's any kind of sexual activity, then this is sexual violence and is a criminal offence.

We live in a society where those who are victims are blamed for what happened. We then, as survivors, downplay what occurred. I see this again and again in my spaces. 'It was kinda my fault because . . .' 'It wasn't *that* bad, though'. 'My friend went through something way worse'. 'I've not told anyone because they wouldn't believe me'.

I want you to know here, potentially for the first time, that what happened to you was not OK, and you deserve to be heard.

The 2003 Sexual Offences Act confirms that someone consents when they agree by choice and when they have both the freedom and the capacity to agree.

Even if there isn't a clear no, this doesn't mean there is a yes.

But if someone doesn't say no out loud, that doesn't automatically mean they have agreed to it either.

If someone doesn't have the freedom or full capacity to agree to sexual activity, they:

·   are asleep or unconscious
·   are under the influence of alcohol or drugs
·   have been 'spiked'
·   are too young
·   have a mental health disorder or illness that means they cannot choose
·   are being pressured, bullied, manipulated, tricked or scared into saying yes
·   are experiencing physical force by the other person[2]

A yes does not always mean we are giving consent if we are saying yes because we are prioritising someone else's needs. A yes is certainly not giving consent if we are being bullied, bribed, coerced or made to feel like it's our only option. This means your freedom and capacity to say yes has been removed.

If you are sixteen, this is the age of consent. But there's extra protection for sixteen to seventeen-year-olds.

It is illegal to:

·   take a photo or video of someone aged eighteen or under engaging in sexual activity
·   pay for sexual services from someone under eighteen
·   take part in sexual activity with someone under eighteen if you are in a position of trust—for example if you are their teacher, social worker, doctor or care worker
·   take part in sexual activity with someone under eighteen if they are a member of your family

Smashing taboos together.

It's not just men who commit sexual assault. Though the stats show that most cases involve men, everyone should be heard.

Being pissed does not mean you deserved anything more than support to find a way home back to your own bed on your own.

The belief that people play hard to get and that when they say no it really means yes is a societal consent challenge we are navigating. The 'kiss chase in the playground' vibe.

Whether it's a partner or not makes no difference. Sexual assault is sexual assault.

Not hearing a no is not enough.

'If there's no screaming, shouting or hitting, then they wanted sex' really is a message we hear partly because people do not understand what the freeze or fawn response is and of course partly because they have no understanding around what consent looks like.

There's a belief that only certain types rape. Absolutely not.

If someone is a sex worker, they can't be raped? Now we understand what sexual abuse and consent are clearly; we know this is simply society shaming others.

'Those who walk home alone are asking for trouble' is something we often hear. Ridiculous.

In 86 percent of rape cases against women, the victim or survivor is raped by someone she knows. In 45 percent of cases, she is raped by a partner or ex-partner, and 1 in 3 adult survivors of rape experience it in their own home. Studies show that 1 in 4 women have been raped or sexually assaulted as adults, and 1 in 2 rapes against women are carried out by their partner or ex-partner [3].

If someone has been raped and takes a while to share, that's necessary for their processing. It doesn't invalidate the fact they were raped because it wasn't 'bad' enough for them to share at the time. FYI.

In terms of sexual violence against men, gender or sexual orientation makes no difference. All victims and survivors should be heard.

Consider that sometimes when someone shares that they were raped, friends believe they just regret having sex with them on a night out. We've got to listen to everyone's experience and understand what it took for them to share. No more shaming. Open, honest, frank and held conversations for all.

Key practice:

Many of us are not sure what consent sounds like with partners when engaging in sex. And we must remember that though we verbalised a yes or a no to begin with, we have the right to change our mind and speak this at anytime.

If you say no and someone continues, this is assault.

Consent sounds like this:

- 'YES. Yes I would absolutely love to engage in sex with you because you make me feel safe and held at the moment. It's a YES'.
- 'YES. I would love you to touch my body everywhere, but I ask you not to touch my inner thighs or my vulva. Everywhere else is in the green zone at this time, for sure'.
- 'YES. I would love to have sex with you. And yes, I would love penetrative sex if this is where we go. Ya know, it's a yes to your schlong in my vajayjay, your wand in my foof'. (Phrase as you feel the need, hun.)
- 'YES. I would like to have sex with you, but I would like to use my pleasure wand with you for penetration at this time'.

- 'NO. I do not feel safe enough right now to engage in sex with you. There's been a lot going on at work, and I feel ungrounded. But I would love a cuddle in bed'.
- 'NO. I am still struggling from our argument, and I do not feel held enough in our relationship to have sex. But I'd love us to have a grounded conversation about that'.
- 'NO. I feel like my nervous system is dysregulated because of the children being so challenging today. I was thinking I'd love a massage instead of sex tonight to help me regulate'.
- 'NO. I feel like the bedroom is too messy right now, and I just need to tidy this tomorrow to feel calmer to engage in sex another time'.

And if you would love something visual around consent, then there is an excellent video on consent by Thames Valley Police you can find by going to www.thisisnaomigale.co.uk/books.

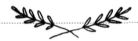

Consent with children

We need to get into the habit of teaching children consent. You don't need to be a parent to support this.

Flippant tickles without checking in first. Asking them to kiss Granny when they arrive. Getting them to say hello to someone new and telling them, 'It's polite to say hello to strangers'. The list could go on.

Someone will read this arguing it's rude.

Yet you wouldn't expect a young girl to say hello to someone they didn't feel 100 percent safe around on a night out, in case they ended up in an unsafe situation sexually. This is what you are teaching children. By teaching them to bypass their inner compass, you're conditioning them to do things they intuitively don't feel safe doing. You're raising 'polite' children who accept innuendos so as not to piss off their managers, leg strokes from uncles because they're the uncle and penetrative sex when they are asleep in relationships in their thirties because their body isn't theirs anymore.

Raising polite children ain't all that.

My husband used to slap me on the arse. I let him for years, and as I began to reclaim my body back, I one day voiced to him that it was too hard and triggered me with being hit as a child. Shit, he had no idea.

Teach your children consent at all times. Ask for consent and remind your children to ask for consent. They should use this word in their everyday.

I also want to include here that you should also approach any support with their vulva in the same way you would in the initial steps of a vagina massage. For example, my twins ask for cream when they get sore; now they are four and can verbalise their needs. We follow the same initial steps before the internal touch step, as per the vagina massage, before I place any cream on any part of their body.

It looks like this:

- I ask, 'Would you like to put your own cream on your body, or would you want me to? You can change your mind at any time'.
- I bring the cream on my finger to the area of the body to be in their energy field.
- I prompt them to bring in breath to the area, maybe closing their eyes if they feel safe enough.
- I watch their body soften.
- I ask them to tell me if they are still happy for me to place the cream on their body and let me know when it is a yes.
- Only then will I touch their body with the cream.

Ensure the children around you claim their bodies as theirs from the get-go.

Checking In

A full-bodied yes is always necessary, and when you check in for a full-bodied yes, it will bring you closer to your needs as a multidimensional being.

A whole-body yes means that you are fully aligned, and there's an overall sense of your well-being being considered within your choice.

Before making more significant or even smaller choices that impact your day-to-day life, check in.

You are tuning in for your whole being to be aligned with a yes.

Key practice:

When you are faced with a decision, pause. Tune in to your whole body. Move your body, stretch or breathe, and send down your grounding cord if necessary.

Check in with your head. Is there a yes?

Check in with your heart. Is there a yes?

Check in with your gut or womb. Is there a yes.

Check in with your pussy. Is there a yes?

When you have a full house of yes responses, you know this is a full-bodied yes. If there is a no in one of these spaces, then it is a no. You could explore where this no stems from and how this no feels in your body by breathing into this space and allowing yourself to hear the thoughts that arise. You may need to write these thoughts down to tune in to the no on a deeper level.

Just because it is a no right now doesn't mean it is a no always. Come back to the question again.

But the answer always needs to be a resounding yes.

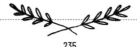

Your Liminal Space

As Heraclitus said, 'Change is the only constant in life'.

We often cling to the constants in life for fear of change or growth. To stay safe, we avoid expansion. We avoid expansion to avoid heartbreak. For if we are to remain exactly as we are, nothing and no one can let us down.

Liminality comes from the Latin word *limen*, meaning a threshold. Neither here nor there. The what was and what's to come. The space of the in between. We know that suffering comes from avoiding simply being here in the now. We must allow ourselves to sit in the present because the past and future will only bring suffering. However, not knowing where we are going is the hardest part of a healing journey. What will happen? What will become of us? What next? The discomfort of simply existing in the here and now is palpable for us all.

The caterpillar hatches from the egg and devours life. It eats the egg and then eats the most delicious leaves. It grows, flourishes, enjoys the adventure. The hungry caterpillar who eats his way through his Monday to Sunday, then suddenly finds itself with a gut feeling that something isn't quite right. This can't be all. But what is all? The caterpillar isn't sure what the next stages look like.

The bear caterpillar, all hairy and brown, being taunted by the other, more beautiful caterpillars. Not realising that they will turn into brown moths and the bear caterpillar will turn into a tiger moth, complete with the most incredible patterns. What if the caterpillars were aware of the impending change? Would this make their experience any less challenging?

Life changes, the fun ends, and the growth halts. It begins its descent into the unknown. Protecting itself from others through a cocoon. The caterpillar then pupates inside. The larval structures break down, and other structures appear, such as the wings.

During this process, they commit to being neither here nor there. They allow themselves to transform without realising how transformative the process is.

Once they are ready, they will emerge and cling to the now. The caterpillar experience is no more, and it's time to stretch their wings into the now. Except the now looks different.

In the story *Tadpole's Promise* by Jeanne Willis and Tony Ross, the tadpole loves his rainbow caterpillar friend. 'Promise me you'll never change', the tadpole says. However, every few weeks, the tadpole changes with new legs and arms. One day he comes to the surface looking for his rainbow friend, who he believes will never return. Except he does, as a butterfly. He stretches out his tongue and reaches for an incoming butterfly while mourning the loss of his best friend. He doesn't realise, however, that he just ate his friend because he resisted the inevitable changes they both needed to move through.

The liminal space is the here and now for those reading this book who feel as though life cannot be the same again. But what does life look like? What would life look like without panty liners everyday, without taking time off work for period pains, without pain in the vulva, without having to say yes when you really mean no, with orgasms, without antidepressants, with joy, with nourishing relationships?

It's a lot to imagine life with slightly fewer challenges. The challenges keep us safe.

Each and every page of this book was necessary but may also have felt like a lot.

The caterpillar was born with the potential to become the butterfly, but it isn't initially aware of this.

There's the deconstruction before the reconstruction.

What an overwhelming experience this is.

Except we often enter this liminal space either without realising it or while resisting it.

If we accepted that change was necessary, if we all accepted this, I'm not sure if it would make it easier. But at least we would have more permission from ourselves or others to build up our silk walls and pupate in our own space in our own time.

You deserve more happiness, joy, pleasure and contentment. You always have, and you always will.

Honouring you, holding you, loving you as you dance in your liminal space within your vagina.

Don't just peer inside your vagina; crawl all the way up inside, hun. It's your portal to it all, your portal home.

Eloina's Love Story with Her Decensored Vulva

Before embarking on this work with Naomi, I had, in some way, begun working with my root. I had been making feminist performance art to decensor bodies with vulvas for almost five years.

A huge part of the decensorship is by decensoring my body, so I mostly perform naked.

When I say I had 'begun working with my root' already, I mean literally. Like it felt like we were business partners. I would spend months carefully crafting one-woman shows, pulling poetry from my head and images from years of research, to reconnect others with all that we own: our bodies.

After months of making, I would be backstage, watching the room fill up with people, feeling their energy soak into my tingling nerves. When I can see everyone seated, I simply drop my dressing gown and enter the stage naked, as if I had been naked the whole time.

Yet the truth was, the one-woman show I'd carefully crafted had two of us in it. It was as if my yoni was a forgotten guest performer who turns up on the day, reads her lines and leaves once I leave the stage.

I'd spent years sharing her on stage, with my legs spread for hours on end to a room full of strangers as a reference for a vulva diverse to their own. As a scream for unity to not be ashamed. For others to learn from my vulva and for her to stay with them for years to come when their own judgement crept in. Yet I worked as if she wasn't even there. It was like I was using her to teach a lesson whilst I told the jokes.

My work, with the solitary goal to connect others with their own vulvas, had the foundations of a complete disconnect between myself and my own.

I realised this during one performance when I sat with my legs open and suddenly realised how vulnerable I was. How open she was. I thought, 'Most of these people haven't even said hello to me, yet they are seeing my most prized, intimate, beautiful thing'. Then I thought, 'I haven't even said hello to her today. I haven't even looked at her, yet I am putting her in front of others'.

After this, I attempted to connect to her through self-pleasure, and it actually made me feel like I was distracting myself from connecting wholeheartedly with her.

I had been sent Naomi's work and thought it may offer me the deeper, nonsexual connection I needed. That instinct was absolutely true.

I expected to work with Naomi and feel an overwhelming connection with my yoni. Yes, I did, but that was not all. In fact, it reminded me why I do my work. Through visualisations, I connected my root with my mother, my grandmother, her mother and all of my ancestors. Not only my ancestors who gave me this body and the energy that lives within my womb, but also, I connected with little me, little El.

It reminded me why I make my shows. I make my shows for ten-year-old me because that is when I started my period and my body started really communicating with me and others stopped communicating with me about my body.

During the yoni massage, I felt little El's innocence. Her love of joy and her resistance to judgement. I was reminded of mother nature's holding and nurturing space. It allowed my body and mind to feel safe, held. The freedom to be fun and explorative.

During Naomi's workshop, I was astounded by how the extremely gentle and slow touch within created such waves of pain, emotion and memories. I was reminded of moments which had definitely caused residual trauma, which I had decided to push out of my head. I hadn't realised I had pushed them out of my head until that moment; dismissive experiences with doctors after labial injury, aggressive experiences during colposcopies and smear tests. Uneasy, non-consensual experiences with partners. I felt all of this again, deeply. I realised that my vagina still held this. And all it took to unearth was the gentlest touch.

I thought about how we can be so quick and forceful with the things that go inside us that I sometimes don't even have the time to feel everything.

I realised how much I hold there. And I wondered if others could feel that too. Then I realised I am now in a community of people feeling and experiencing the exact same sensations. Even though these experiences cannot be changed, how oh so beautiful it is to feel them and give them space to speak to me alongside others doing the same.

This pain being remembered was heartbreaking and simultaneously brought out the most beautiful realisation: that I am held and can breathe through any pain and send it to Mother Earth. How else would we survive childbirth?

Here is a sharing from my journaling after the workshop:

My fleshy cord is rooted to the centre of the golden core. From my womb, through my cervix, my vagina and down into the earth's core. I am held and can breathe through any pain, sending it down to mother nature, the golden core below.
My yoni is not something to be used.
It is something to open up and to water with cherishing, golden, light touch.
I promise to never forget you again, yoni.
I promise to never stop watering you.

I left Naomi's workshop feeling like I had a new understanding of what my vulva needs and wants sexually. I developed a new language to communicate that. I left feeling like I could hear her speaking those needs to me and I could share back.

Before and after sharing her on stage, I now use Naomi's grounding meditation as a ritual to connect myself to my root and my root to Mother Earth. Sometimes that is in the form of a full meditation. Sometimes it's in the form of me looking at her in a mirror and saying, 'HEY BITCH, WE'RE GOING ON STAGE TOGETHER!!! I am honouring and loving you the whole time, and if you need to not be there at any point, you let me know because we're in it together! LET'S DO THISSSSSSS!'

My work, to me, is a true gift to myself that I share with others. Those others are those dedicated to connecting with themselves and their inner child. I believe this is the gift that I, in turn, received from Naomi and her work.

Empowered Vaginas Galore

I'd say there wouldn't be a single soul who hasn't felt shame around their vagina. To have picked up this book, you would have felt shame and allowed yourself to lean into your vulnerability with what may have arisen in the face of reading page after page, wanging on about your most shamed body part.

This season of your life, the one where you explored a deeper relationship with your vagina, will be one that may have cracked you open in unexpected ways. And for that, I am in awe of the strength it would have taken you to do the key practices and unlock the answers to the questions nestled within the education of this resource.

Whenever I was asked what I do for work at the beginning, ya know, working with others, their wombs and vaginas, I wouldn't share that I had people surrender into the bottom of my garden to engage in life-changing work with their pelvis. I felt palpable shame from society to share that this is my work. In time, I began openly sharing what I do with flippant strangers, which was regularly met with shame. Bashful looks, flushed cheeks, side-eyes, oohs, snorts, titters. It's rare to find someone who engages in the discussion but then doesn't begin to feel the emotions arising for them when talking to me about the vagina, suddenly realising the feelings arising when openly talking about what has been to them an intimate space no one opens up about. And this shame presents itself differently for different people. I have learnt.

Society wallows in shame because that feels safe, relatable and familiar. Having the courage to dance in the portal takes a level of vulnerability we don't find it easy to be with. Vulnerability brings up emotions of shame, guilt, judgement, hopelessness, grief, fear, desire and anger. To be able to dance with these emotions, cosy down with them and feel them within the body, is unfamiliar territory for us all. For we cannot move into a loud and proud relationship with our pelvis without feeling the emotions that arise at any given time.

You're not wallowing; you're feeling into the feelings pushed down within that have manifested into disconnect, pain and emotional turmoil.

You deserve much more than what has been given to you and the experiences you have landed in. But every experience will provide you with something to explore and work with.

To come back stronger, angrier and ready to feel the warm glow from coming home into the belly of your womb space, your hara, your centre.

My wish is that parents begin to work on their own shame, challenges and wounds so they can give their children the level of support needed. Thus parents begin to take note of the level of support, holding, love and education needed. Such holding encompasses the spectrum of emotions that arise, questions that need answering and depths that need dancing in for their children to truly leave the cocoons of home empowered, pussy-led and able to feel the joy, pleasure and happiness available from within and around them at every given moment.

My desire is that everyone begins to remove the shroud of shame that dangles, the X that has been placed between our thighs, and feels into the power, glory and love that exists from worshipping our flappy flaps—yes our hanging minoras and majoras in all their bloody glory, our wombs, our vaginas once again. Honouring us as sacred souls on this path to birth creativity and life every day. The remembrance of the womb comes back to all rather than just being lost in sacred language for the select few who find their spiritual path. My desire is that this becomes 'mainstream'.

My hope is that you read this book and took away something tangible for yourself first and foremost. You have been left feeling more love and power for who you are and your journey. You read these pages and tended to your needs at any given moment. You danced in your emotions, held yourself, hugged your pelvis, mothered yourself and spoke words of love to all you are—a soul navigating the ebbs and flows of the seasons of life. My hope is that this book remains somewhere safe, held and under-stood amongst the other self-help books that have shaped your life so you can return to these words at any time.

Celebrating you. Holding you. Always.

Remain open, curious and turned on.

From my empowered vagina to yours, Naomi xx

(Naomi's arm reaches through her flaps and gently waves to you.)

Sarah's Love Story with Finding Freedom from the Binds

I left home at eighteen with little exposure to the outside world. For the first eighteen years of my life, my only exposure to the outside world was church events and the grocery store, with just two years of school experience. Due to the frequent physical abuse at home, my nervous system defaulted to freeze in the flight/flight/freeze/fawn reaction we all have when facing danger. This default mode was part of the reason that, when I was sexually assaulted at six years old, I was able to continue for years without a fight.

The belief that I was inherently sinful came from my abusers' mouths and echoed the words I heard from my mother. I took on shame and, worse than that, blame. This paved the way for the freeze response to several sexual assaults, from eighteen to twenty. As a result of the trauma and my upbringing, I was totally disconnected from my body, especially my yoni.

I believe this disconnect added to my health issues, like heart problems, endometriosis, and multiple medical traumas to my yoni. I wasn't aware of my level of disassociation from my yoni or its block to discovering myself.

I was a brain walking around without a body, and a body without a brain.

I had first realised something needed to be healed after being in a loving and sexual relationship for three years. After our wedding, our sex life became increasingly stressful, and neither of us knew why. I subconsciously believed that I would no longer feel sinful or be afraid of being touched in marriage. It's as if the act of marriage would reverse the years of disconnection and trauma. This was purity culture rearing its ugly head and magical thinking, but I didn't find that out for several more years. I wanted to share the same openness and passion I once had with my now husband and search for a solution. I started somatic trauma therapy once I could afford it.

My husband introduced me to the book *Pure* by Linda Kay Klein a couple of years ago and started the journey that led me to Naomi and one of her workshops. I began with acts of love towards my yoni through books and educating myself on the basics of sex. I began pampering the yoni with herbal baths, sunbathing in the nude, spraying myself with rose water, buying flowers and focusing on sending love to my yoni regularly.

Masturbation became an act of self-love where I touched more than just my vagina; it was a full-body experience that was less outcome-based. I started processing sexual trauma experiences through somatic modalities with a therapist, and I realised that every time I checked in with my yoni, the muscles were tense and tight. Choosing the workshop was like finally asking to take my relationship with my yoni to the next level. My desire was to make the connection to my yoni stronger and release old beliefs/traumas.

The awareness that it is the connection to life and everything in it was the threshold for healing that gave me the bravery to work with Naomi. I first encountered Naomi on TikTok and felt so drawn to her no-shame approach to caring for your womb space and that she encouraged the type of connection I sought. This is incredibly scary work, and she felt safe to me.

My surgery to remove endometriosis made me really start considering my pelvic bowl and the connection I had to it because it was entirely covered in translucent endometriosis tissue. Through somatic healing and massage therapy school, I learned how to release trauma from the body and knew that massage/physical touch is one way of doing so. I chose this work mainly to build a connection to my yoni. I wanted to say, 'Hey yoni, I love you, and I want a relationship with you'. I wanted to build new neural pathways to check in with it and feel it, knowing it's there. So it's not a blank space in my mind anymore or one of tension. I tried the tools she taught independently, but I needed more. I wanted to release the fear and shame that I still struggled so much with but didn't have the words to describe yet, and I didn't know how to connect to my yoni in a safe way.

I wanted to build a connection to my womb space to feel fully connected to who I am as a being and to those around me. I would have sexual experiences that left me feeling shameful or bad, especially if I enjoyed them. I would feel shame if I felt sexy or not sexy enough. I felt ashamed if I went in public and forgot to shave my legs. I would be afraid to initiate sex or respond to my partner sensually. The shame was everywhere, there was no aspect of who I was that did not have some layer of shame on it. This created disconnection from who I am, my intuition and, of course, feelings of love, acceptance and compassion because those feelings dispel the sense of shame. I wanted a more vulnerable relationship with my husband, but I couldn't be vulnerable with myself.

It's been quite the rollercoaster. I was in the midst of realising that I had built a life that did not bring me satisfaction. I realised I was on a constant road to an unknown destination. One beautiful surprise from working with your pelvic bowl is that it has the answers you are seeking, and indeed I have been able to break this cycle in my life by creating a solid connection with my authentic self. I realise now that by not choosing to meet my needs and accept myself, I ended up expecting to find the answers outside myself. I ended up in a murky place, far from who I was. I saw all my dark parts for what they were, unhealed, fragmented versions of myself controlling the narrative of my life. I think because I was already in the midst of this significant work, I wasn't too afraid to take on this new level of work with my womb space in the workshop. It's as if I thought, 'How much worse could it get?'

Working with your womb space is the toughest and bravest of all my work. It is not for the faint of heart; you'll go to the ends of the earth to rescue yourself.

I had a significant response to the vagina timeline Naomi asked us to make because it pulled together all the parts of me I had fragmented. Choosing to work with your yoni in this way is really brave. The womb has been so traumatised by society, cultures and sexual assaults for many, many generations. This is big, difficult and brave work to choose to heal. I had repressed memories resurface because I was finally in a space where I could open up to more of my story. The new realisations took me a while to work through, but I had the tools to process them, and the outcome is truly remarkable, and this is only the beginning!

Following this work, I accepted myself as pansexual. It's like I decided to stop denying parts of who I was, and I knew with complete certainty I was not heterosexual. I had truly hidden an entire aspect from myself for thirty-five years! I had shamed myself from a young age because my first kiss was with a girl, and I was taught that a demonic spirit caused this. I had locked away a part of myself for nearly my entire life and told her she was bad. On the other side of processing everything, I rescued her and finally felt unconditional love and acceptance from myself.

I was creating a new, beautiful connection to my yoni. I came out to my husband and had the best day, full of joy, harmony, gratitude and five different rainbows! The feeling of shedding years of shame was so freeing and almost magical. I felt the difference instantly. It was when I fully accepted who I was by accepting that even if my partner didn't accept me, I had to be brave enough to not hide any parts of who I am. I noticed things, like I didn't second-guess an outfit or feel uncomfortable talking to the same sex. I was more open with my husband, and this new level of closeness led to him giving me a vaginal massage like the one Naomi taught me to give myself. I embraced being vulnerable and allowed him to show me kindness. I let him meet a yoni need that had nothing to do with sexual gratification. It was a loving and healing act that created a new layer of safety within our relationship.

I don't care as much anymore about what people think of me. I am far more accepting of myself in ways I know others won't accept. I am no longer in an overwhelming place but one of gratitude. I am going out in nature, making new connections with friends and blossoming.

I see now that the womb space is the seed of your soul essence, and when we cover it up to hide it or protect it, we doom it because it cannot bloom from the darkness. No matter how hard we try to push through and force growth, we will not reach the light of day until we can do the brave work of deconstructing everything we built on top of it for protection.

If you can commit to destroying everything you built, you will bloom into a beautiful flower that cannot be damaged or changed. Something that looks like you and feels like you. Then you get the fun work of discovering who you are.

I have done a lot to deconstruct beliefs, and the most significant changes were that first, I did not lose anything when I had sexual interactions with anyone, nor was who I am changed in any way. The second was I've learned there are so many sexualities and kinks in a consensual relationship; they are all beautiful and should be celebrated. There is not a one-size-fits-all solution to pleasure. What can be ticklish to one person can be pure ecstasy to another. Most importantly, I learned that accepting who you are means accepting the parts you are afraid nobody else will accept. I now believe I am worth it, and I trust myself to always be there for me, no matter how hard or scary.

At first, I felt like I was left with a mess, but now I feel like a beautiful butterfly after shedding the cocoon, but my wings are still drying. My whole house of cards came tumbling down with the workshop. It was such a catalyst for change because it pulled all the fragmented parts of me into one space. It was like I split off the traumatised parts and gave them their corners to sit in, but this work called them all to come forward.

Through the continued work, I now have a beautiful patchwork quilt of parts of me that are all coming together through the healing thread. I am left with hope, excitement and a true sense of who I am. I now have the connection I was seeking, the one to my authentic self that is pure love and unchanged by my life circumstances. It's a marvellous connection that I now can experience more fully and frequently. Life without this connection is like going to Disney World and leaving before the fireworks show on Main Street at the end of the day. I am eternally grateful for the space created to do this work and the gift of Naomi's guidance.

You are a gift, and the sensual part of you is a divine gift of creation. It is a beautiful part of life. It is vibrant and can feel loud, sometimes making people uncomfortable. That is because of who they are, not because of who you are. By letting your light shine from this place, you give people the freedom to be themselves and stand in their own light should they choose to accept it. I don't wish for you to exist from darkness because you are a beautiful prism of light, and I would never want you to hide any parts of that light but instead let it shine in its full spectrum of colours.

So please, as you go through life, remember that this is part of your divinity, an amazing piece of who you are. The more you love and protect and hold it sacred, the more you free yourself. Whether that is sharing it with thousands or a few, just embracing this part of you and knowing however it looks in your life, you are doing it right, and you are good.

Nothing has ever been taken from you; you haven't lost any part of who you are. Who you are is untouchable, unchangeable and unbreakable. It is brave work finding your way here, but you are worth it and will never be alone in this journey.

Embrace who you are and what you think may be wrong; embrace it all, be gentle with yourself and stay connected to your body. At times you may have to disconnect, but when it feels safe, don't hesitate to build that connection again to experience the joy, ecstasy and connection in fullness. Do not be afraid; you will not create a stronger relationship with the pain. That pain exists only in the dark, fragmented parts of your story. Don't try to control how you heal or how your story plays out. Follow your desires and what makes you feel good with gratitude for the easy and complex parts.

I know you will find your way, and when you do, you will be amazed at what is waiting for you. I am always so proud of you and love you so much.

There's a Dodo Bird in the Garden

I was on a trip to Copenhagen with my grandma in my early teens. We'd been exploring the city over a weekend.

She took tablets regularly, so I asked her what they were for. She said she was in pain, but everything was OK. She just needed to take some pain relief, and she could crack on with her day.

I knew something wasn't right, but no one was really telling me much.

My relationship with my grandma had been strained in the early years. It seemed to me she quite openly disliked me. She regularly visited, which I look back on fondly because it felt at times safer to have her around.

Over time we bonded. My grandma was visible in her immediate community, with such roles as the village hall key-holder, girl guides leader, and other responsibilities she took on.

If there was a gadget, she had it. When I struggled with a lack of breast growth, she bought me a blow-up bra with a mini pump. I'd go from zero to Pamela in seconds. It was a little too much, but the thought was everything, as I felt seen rather than ignored or downplayed, as I often did growing up.

I loved our time crafting together the most. If there was a craft she had yet to try, it was undoubtedly next on the list.

She also adored taking photographs. There were hundreds of printed photos around the house.

I'm pretty sure it was in her late fifties when she went on a round-the-world trip with her friend. Mainly in search of butterflies. She adored them. There were butterflies all over the house, from real framed ones to sculptures on the wall to painted eggs with tiny butterflies stuck on them on mini golden stands.

One of her favourite places was Stratford-upon-Avon butterfly farm. I grew up mainly near here, so we often went. She told me the park was the best place for butterflies, even after going around the world.

Soon after the Copenhagen trip, I learnt that my grandma had endometrial cancer, and it was terminal.

After this, I have very little clarity about what unfolded.

I have memories here and there. It felt like her life was slipping through my fingers, and there was nothing anyone could do.

She became very ill very quickly.

Or maybe she already knew she was very ill, and after the diagnosis, she could surrender into the process.

I remember one day, she stood with Cheltenham University's booklet in her kitchen. 'This looks like a great one to go to'. I was, like, fourteen at the time. But we'd long discussed my dreams of becoming a primary teacher, as I was already helping at many school clubs and felt I was destined for the classroom. She wholeheartedly supported this.

When I applied to all the universities that offered a Bachelor of Education degree specifically training teachers with five-to-eleven-year-olds for three years, there were few, and Cheltenham was one of them. I tried for them all. Cheltenham was at the bottom of my list. Guess where I ended up.

Another day, in her kitchen again, while she was in her bed facing the garden and looking through the glass patio doors she continuously told me not to dick around with as a child, she screamed out my name.

Hearing my grandma call my name in her liminal space was too much for me to bear. I left the house for a moment. Breathing into my own liminal space.

She called out that there was a dodo bird in the garden. She was on morphine, and I remember feeling so much light. She was absolutely convinced. I loved *Dodos Are Forever* by Dick King-Smith, so I was more than happy to roll with the idea that the dodo bird was alive and currently strutting through a garden in Leicestershire.

Before she was bed-bound, we took one last trip to Stratford Butterfly Farm. I have a photo of her on a bench with a butterfly on her finger. It is one of the last memories I have of us out together.

Losing my grandma to endometrial cancer in her early sixties was one of my most painful experiences. After she passed, I formed a strong relationship with my grandpa, who never overcame his loss. I often found him on the edge of his bed, looking down at his socks. He never left this liminal space and died a few years back; he gave up easily around ten years later. I know it was partly because he needed to be back with her.

He often told me how fond my grandma was of me. And when we spent time together, he said he understood why. I hold onto his words.

I'm not really sure how I ended up here, in a park in London, about to attend a show on labiaplasty, finishing the pages of a book on vaginas, vulvas and womb spaces.

I look back at my journey; it has been a wild, beautiful ride.

I was thinking about an afterword for this book. While in London today, I knew I needed to write the final words and walked past a cancer clinic. And so it was.

My grandma isn't often at the forefront of my mind when sharing this work.

However, she's part of my journey to this space.

I wonder, if she had been more in tune with her body, would she have lived longer? Would the cancer have been caught? Would she have been here to see the world change with even more gadgets? Would I have even started this journey?

Everything is meant.

Thanks, Grandma, for guiding me to write this book. You knew I was always destined to educate others. I miss you.

Nervous System Vaginal Toolkit
Regulated vaginas

A rooted toolkit for your nervous system
Emotions and thoughts affect our nervous system, affecting our muscles, fascia, circulation, lymphatic drainage, absorption, hormone balance and pelvic floor.

A grounding cord
A regulating tool that allows you to lean on support while gently coming back into self-presence. This allows us to find calm in the present moment. This can be used by itself or before any other regulating activity.
·   Sit comfortably, with shoulders relaxed, spine straight, crown and chin lifted
·   Begin to breathe consciously through the nose and into the belly
·   Exhale out of the mouth
·   Find your breath connecting to your womb space
·   Breathe into the darkness of the womb
·   Send down a thread of golden ribbon or a light or a root or a beanstalk image from the womb down out through the cervix, out of the vagina and into the earth below
·   Anchor into Mother Earth for as many breaths as you need
·   Allow the connection to fade when you are ready

Rooted Orientation
This allows you to focus on the environment you are in to begin to find safety within the immediate space around you so you can find presence in the now. It allows time to consider whether you feel safe in your current environment.
·   Begin by sitting comfortably, shoulders relaxed, spine straight, crown lifted, chin lifted.
·   Feel your perineum on the floor (the space between the anus and vagina), and feel into this connection.
·   Scan the room for a few moments, finding safety through any sighs or yawns. Rest your gaze on beautiful objects or objects that aren't as nice.
·   Become aware of every corner of the room, above you, behind and in front of you.
·   Set your gaze on something nourishing, pause for a moment and allow the feelings to land. As you look at this detail, ask yourself what the

colour is. Consider labelling the colour as if it were for a paint colour chart: 'Whisper White' or 'Glorious Yellow'.
· Continue to look around you for as long as you need while noticing your body adjusting in the space, noticing a surrender.
· When you feel you've landed fully in the here and now, you can gently close your eyes and breathe into the body.
· Place one hand on the heart and one hand on the womb, breathing deeply.

A conscious breathwork technique

Consciously controlling the breath can allow you to activate the sympathetic nervous system to physically calm the body down.
· Begin by sitting comfortably, shoulders relaxed, spine straight, crown lifted, chin lifted.
· Tune in to your natural breath
· Feel your perineum on the ground
· Slowly introduce a deeper exhale, almost as if you are gently pushing any 'leftover' air as you reach into a deeper exhale.
· As you breathe slowly, consciously, deeply and smoothly, think of a 2:1 ratio. Inhale for 2 and exhale for 4 counts, for example.
· You can slowly move on, inhaling for 3 and exhaling for 6.
· Be aware of your capacity here, as you want this to be easy-going to soothe the parasympathetic nervous system (the rest and restore system) and not the sympathetic nervous system (the fight or flight response).
· Ensure the transition between the inhale and the exhale remains smooth.

Heart/womb connection

When we allow for deeper harmony and embodiment in the body, we must allow ourselves to reconnect parts of us back as one.
· Find yourself in a seated or lying down position.
· Place one hand on the womb and one hand on the heart.
· Breathe through the heart into the womb.
· Feel the rise and fall of the belly as you do so.
· You could also bring in a count of breathing in for 4 and exhaling for 6.
· Imagine a golden thread or light connecting your heart and your womb together as you inhale light from your heart into your womb and then bounce the light back into your heart.

Soothe the vagus nerve

The vagus nerve wanders from the lowest part of the brainstem down into the pelvic floor, the cervix and the vagina. If we exhale longer than our inhale, we can trigger a relaxation response soothing the vagus nerve.

- Inhale in through the nose for a count of 4.
- Pause for a count of 7.
- Exhale through the mouth for a count of 8.

Visualisation

Our brains can't differentiate between reality and imagination, thus, a visualisation is an excellent tool for accessing our parasympathetic nervous system and finding more safety within the body.

- Imagine a peony or other flower of choice in your heart. Breathe into that flower, allowing the petals to unfurl one by one.
- After a while, you will find that the centre reveals itself in your heart space.
- Breathe into the golden nectar until it becomes a golden light.
- Allow the light to fill the heart space until it can no longer be contained and begins to flow down into the womb.
- The light swirls and whirls around the womb, touching the womb's edges and flowing to each fallopian tube, the right fallopian tube and then the left.
- It glows in the right ovary and the left ovary. As you breathe into the womb, the light continues to shine.
- When you feel the heart/womb connection has been fully formed, you can allow the light to fade and the flower to close petal by petal.

Sunshine-facing vulvas

This is something that many experts would say not to do. So do your own research on this before engaging in this regulation tool. The sun increases serotonin production, which acts as a mood stabiliser.

- Find a safe space to remove your bottom layers.
- Lie down somewhere in direct sunlight. This could be in a room where the sun streams in, your back garden, or a balcony, somewhere you know you can do this without any sudden onlookers.
- Remove the clothes shrouding your vulva.
- Place the soles of your feet together while lying down on your back or relaxing into pillows or a yoga bolster (reclined butterfly position). Make sure you protect your knees with blocks or pillows if you need them, and feel your knees just hanging in mid-air.
- Begin to feel the sunshine on your vulva.

- Breathe into the warmth landing at your root. If you feel safe enough to do so, close your eyes.
- Bring breath down into your root while sending your grounding cord into Mother Earth.
- Do this for 30 seconds to a minute.
- Feel this holding, love and warmth as if it's wrapping you in a cuddle.
- Finish by bringing your legs gently to a close.

Humming Bee Breath

To release cerebral tension, this is super helpful as a bedtime practice before sleep. Named after the female humming bee of India, it also seeks to open the heart space.

- Sit rooted. Bring your eyes to a close if you feel safe to do so.
- Bring your hands into your lap.
- Breathe naturally and come to stillness.
- Inhale deeply.
- Exhale with a hum tone that feels natural for you. The intensity, pitch or frequency should not change. Hum for the entire exhale.
- On each exhale, find a different tone to hum, whether this gets higher or lower.
- Continue to do so for as long as you feel called.
- Resume a natural breath and find stillness once again.

Sensations

Focus on your inner self in a non-judgemental way.

- Bring your eyes to a close when you feel safe enough to do so.
- Root down through the perineum.
- Tune in to your natural breathing through your nose.
- Nothing to change or do. Just be aware of the in breath and the out breath.
- In breath. Out breath. Without naming it as 'in and out'.
- Feel the different sensations of the in breath and the out breath.
- Now begin to scan your whole body for any sensations, slowly pausing from head to toe as you come across sensations. These could be anything from tingling, pain, or itches.
- Be here for as long as you need, checking into your body for any sensations as you do so.
- You don't need to tend to or label these sensations. Just be aware of them.
- Come back to the breath.

Dear Vagina

Dear Vagina,

Welcome to the agony aunt section of the book. This is a quick-reference guide to support you holistically with any physical manifestations of the pelvis.

Please note:

- This is to support you holistically, and any concerns should be brought to a competent medical practitioner with a clear list of questions before entering their space. Refer to the ending of Dr Sam's section to empower yourself.
- Vaginal steaming should be explored through a qualified practitioner such as myself.
- Labels can be a challenge to navigate, and often, I feel, we don't always need to label our experiences with our pelvis if we commit to working with our bodies. However, at times, labels are necessary.

Healing from	The physical challenges	Possible emotional challenges	Holistic support
Abortion	Also known as a termination of pregnancy. The pregnancy is ended either by taking medication or having a surgical procedure.	The context of the abortion will make a difference to the emotions post-abortion. It can take up to nine weeks for HCG levels to drop, so give yourself time to navigate the ebbs and flows emotionally. It can feel emotional for years afterwards. · 95 percent feel it was the right decision at the time and continue to do so five years after and beyond · Some feel they still need to process an abortion even if they know it was the right decision	Talk with close friends, family members or a therapist (those who ya know will hold space) to discuss any rising thoughts or feelings Come back to Mother Earth to feel mothered and held Create a ceremony to release the soul onwards in their journey Perform a post-bleed vaginal steam to cleanse and clear
Birth Trauma / Postnatal PTSD	Traumatic labour or birth can cause PTSD. This can be due to: · Painful birth · Unplanned or emergency treatment · Unplanned caesarean section · Traumatic experiences during or after birth. You may experience: · Vivid flashbacks · Intrusive thoughts and images · Nightmares · Intense distress at real or symbolic reminders of the trauma · Physical sensations such as pain, sweating, nausea or trembling	· Anger or sadness from a birth that didn't unfold as expected · Loss of bodily autonomy · Feeling a lack of control daily post losing all control of the birth · Loss of sense of self · Intense daily fear · Intense feelings of shame if you are judging yourself · Inability to express how you feel to yourself or others	· EMDR (eye movement desensitisation and reprocessing) · Close the birthing field through a ceremony · Do a rebirthing ceremony · Find support through others who have been through similar experiences · Meet your basic needs well through gentle exercise, a great diet and more sleep · Refer to the nervous system vaginal toolkit to soothe your nervous system daily · Get to know your triggers · Give yourself time · Mother yourself deeply · Ask for more support

Healing from	The physical challenges	Possible emotional challenges	Holistic support
Baby Loss	In some pregnancies, the baby dies before birth (stillbirth) or soon after (neonatal death)	· Anger for what unfolded · Loss of self · Disconnect from self and others · PTSD from the event (refer to postnatal PTSD section) · Shame if any self-blame is present · Loss of bodily autonomy	· Close the birthing field through ceremony · Work with the soul of the baby so they move through · Find support groups · Use helplines when needed · Refer to the nervous system vaginal toolkit to soothe your nervous system daily · Sands Memory Box (free) · EMDR (eye movement desensitisation and reprocessing) · Get to know your triggers · Give yourself time · Mother yourself deeply · Ask for more support
Bartholin's cyst	A fluid-filled sac inside the opening of the vagina caused by a blocked duct. If it grows too big, you may feel pain in the skin surrounding the vagina (vulva) while walking, sitting or during sex.	· Not feeling fully into your physical and energetic growth in life. · Feeling blocked in an aspect of your life. · Playing out painful experiences in your mind regularly.	· Perform vaginal steaming · Soak the cyst in warm water · Journal around what fears are arising for you · Journal with what hopes and dreams you have for yourself · Observe gratefulness · Use massage touch
Loss or Lack of Desire	Feeling a lack of desire for sex. It can be happen for several reasons, including: · The season of your life · Stress and anxiety · Tiredness · Ongoing pain in the pelvis · A challenging relationship with the self · Relational challenges with others · Hormone ebbs and flows · Not identifying daily joy	· Loss of joy and pleasure daily · Feeling disconnected from your body · Feeling disconnected from others · Lacklustre days · Hindered dreams	· Explore daily joy · Write in a gratitude journal · Go to bed earlier · Get more sleep (up your hours to 8 or 9 per night for a few weeks and see if it helps) · Change things around the bedroom · Keep phones out of the bedroom · Perform vaginal steaming · Seek body massage for reclamation and healing · Perform vaginal massage · Use organic lubricant (perhaps with CBD oil if I pain present too)

Healing from	The physical challenges	Possible emotional challenges	Holistic support
Ectopic Pregnancy	A fertilised egg implants itself outside of the womb, usually in one of the fallopian tubes. 1 in every 90 pregnancies is ectopic. This is around 11,000 pregnancies a year in the UK. Often there are no symptoms, but if there are, they develop between the fourth and twelfth weeks of the pregnancy. The symptoms could be akin to a stomach bug, so trust your instinct if you feel it doesn't feel right. It can be confirmed with an ultrasound. It can be very serious, so symptoms should always be checked.	• Anger or sadness from a pregnancy that didn't unfold as expected • Fear of future pregnancies • Feelings of shame for being pregnant but with the embryo not growing in the womb • Loss of bodily autonomy	• Perform vaginal steaming (post any bleeding) • Close the birthing field through ceremony • Work with the soul of the baby so they move on and through • Refer to the nervous system vaginal toolkit to soothe your nervous system daily • Get to know your triggers • Give yourself time • Mother yourself deeply • Ask for more support • Perform gentle womb massage
Endometriosis	Tissue similar to the lining of the womb grows in other places, such as the ovaries and fallopian tubes. The ONLY way to diagnose endo for sure is through a laparoscopy. Unless you have had this, it cannot be confirmed. Symptoms mirror challenges many of us have without endo: • Pelvic pain • Period pain • Pain in sex • Pain when peeing or having a poo • Infertility • Pain in lower back	• Eating feelings in the form of sugar • Feelings of disappointment in life • Shame of oneself or one's body • Disconnect from the pelvis - Insecure with oneself or others • Deflecting challenges onto others without taking radical responsibility	• Surgery isn't the way for most. Ongoing research is finding that surgery potentially does more harm than good. • Perform vaginal steaming • Do visualisations with the womb • Explore joy and pleasure daily • Perform womb massage • Perform vaginal massage • Use castor oil packs • Do self-pleasure • Explore ancestral trauma down the lineage • Cut down on or cut out sugar • Get acupuncture or reflexology support

Healing from	The physical challenges	Possible emotional challenges	Holistic support
Episiotomy and Perineal Tears	A cut in the area between the vagina and anus (perineum) during childbirth to make the opening wider. Other times a perineum may tear during childbirth. 1 in 7 births in the UK end in episiotomies. (It's problematic as they are performed unnecessarily often.)	- Emotionally unprepared for birth. - Previous birthing challenges in the lineage. - Medically induced/rushed - Labour rushing the process, thus unprepared physically or emotionally. - It can take much longer to heal from being cut than from a natural tear. A cut or tear can cause ongoing: - Struggle during exercise - Tight feelings around the pelvis - Pain in sex (years later). It cuts the energy and the physical space. - Feelings of frustration or being broken - Lack of pleasure - Disconnect from pelvis	- Initially after the tear, apply warm water when peeing - Perform post-bleed vaginal steaming - Use lubrication - Perform vaginal Massage - Use visualisations of light from the heart-womb-perineum - Explore pleasure around the body before touching the vulva
Gynaecologist Appointments	Appointments for long-standing non-urgent gynaecological problems including; - Heavy and/or painful periods - Pelvic pain - Ovarian cysts - Uterine fibroids and polyps - Infertility - Endometriosis - Suspected ovarian or womb (also known as uterine or endometrial) cancers Appointment Process: - Gynae will ask questions about symptoms The appointment could include: - Examination through feeling abdomen - Possible internal examination with a speculum - Potential for a scan externally or internally (with a dildo-style thang) - They may also take smears or biopsies, as necessary	- Previous appointments where there was gaslighting - Previous appointments where there was pain induced through the investigations - A continuation of appointments where questions aren't being answered - Survivors of rape may find these appointments challenging - Waiting rooms with bumps and babies can be triggering - Pain being ignored through use of incorrect-sized speculums or lack of gentle care	- Do your own research before going to the appointment and prepare your questions ahead of time in the notes on your phone or through printing off support - Join support groups to explore others' routes - Send down a grounding cord before and during the appointment - Come back to nervous system regulatory tools to pull on before, during and after - Cleanse an appointment through a vaginal steam - Refuse tests or investigations until you feel ready for them and understand it all from an empowered stance (consensual medical care)

Healing from	The physical challenges	Possible emotional challenges	Holistic support
Hypertonic Pelvic Floor Muscle Dysfunction	The muscles in your lower pelvis are in a spasm or constant contraction. This can be temporary or constant. They can't relax and coordinate the control of some bodily functions causing: · Pain · Peeing challenges · Bowel movement issues · Painful sex	· What are you holding onto in life that needs letting go of? · Playing out past issues and unable to move them through · A relationship that needs exploring so it nourishes you too or needs cutting completely · Trauma that is held in the body and needs moving through	· Perform vaginal massage · Perform vaginal steaming · Journal through current relationships and finding any challenges · Get somatic trauma support
Hysterectomy	Surgically removing the womb (uterus). There could be a number of reasons for this occurring, including: · Long-term pelvic pain · Womb cancer · Cancer of the fallopian tubes · Cervical cancer · To prevent cancer due to genetics With a total hysterectomy, the womb and cervix (neck of the womb) are removed; this is the most commonly performed operation. With a subtotal hysterectomy, the main body of the womb is removed, leaving the cervix in place. With a total hysterectomy, there is a bilateral salpingo-oophorectomy with the womb, cervix, fallopian tubes (salpingectomy) and ovaries (oophorectomy) removed With a radical hysterectomy, the womb and surrounding tissues are removed, including the fallopian tubes, part of the vagina, ovaries, lymph glands and fatty tissue.	· Feeling loss of organs or perhaps the chance of motherhood as you imagined · Being put into menopause and navigating the ebbs and flows of being menopausal suddenly · Shame due to having the womb removed · Fear of what life may look like after removal of these organs · Anger at what has had to unfold	· Explore darkness through dark goddess exploration · Light candles and bring light into the home · Connect to the energetic centre (Hara) and the energy of the womb space through visualisation · Connect with the joy of autumn and what that looks like for you · Take time to adjust to being without these organs · Connect into the body deeper through nervous-system-led tools in the vagina toolkit · Seek full-body massage with affirmations · Perform vaginal Steaming · Perform womb (Hara) massage · Seek out support groups to find support with similar stories

Healing from	The physical challenges	Possible emotional challenges	Holistic support
Irregular Periods or Hypothalamic Amenorrhea	The length of your cycle (the gap between your periods starting) becomes erratic. Your period maybe late or early. There may be more than two bleeds within one month. The average cycle is from 26–29 days, but if your cycle jumps around with missed bleeds and extra bleeds, then it is deemed irregular. A cycle that changes length-wise within reason each month isn't deemed irregular. Causes: · Puberty (being irregular for the first year or two is normal) · Perimenopause · Early pregnancy · Hormonal contraceptives (but this isn't a true period, and irregular bleeding should be investigated) · Extreme weight loss or weight gain · Excessive exercise · Stress or · medical conditions · PCOS · Thyroid challenges	· Thoughts of being worthy enough just as you are · Not being able to find a routine or rhythm within your daily life · You've lost sight of your needs, dreams, hopes or desires · Feeling shame for your body in some way · Feeling a loss of purpose in the world	· Track your cycle (work with a fertility awareness practitioner to check on ovulation) · Begin to understand your discharge · Come into a more dependable daily routine · Increase sleep up to 8–9 hours for 3 months Remember, any changes you implement will take 3 months to impact on a cycle · Up your glycinate magnesium intake and work with a nutritionist to support you with levels · Regulate how much exercise you are doing, and lessen HIIT training if this is potentially the cause · Consider re-evaluating your diet if this could be the cause · Perform vaginal steaming (if cycle is longer than 26 days and you've not had more than 2 per month in the last 12 months) · Perform womb massage
Self-love	Love of self or regard for one's own happiness. Often depletes over time or was never there in the first place from childhood conditioning	· Putting others before yourself (people-pleaser vibes) · Working too hard towards goals and ignoring the celebrations as you journey towards the goal · Being in shame and often putting yourself down · Remaining in the lower themes of consciousness, such as judgement	· Do mirror work · Do mirrovulva work · Do affirmation work · Explore the themes of consciousness · Mother yourself more · Only accept relationships that nourish

Healing from	The physical challenges	Possible emotional challenges	Holistic support
Miscarriage	A miscarriage is the loss of a pregnancy during the first 24 weeks.	Anger for what unfolded Loss of self Disconnect from self and others PTSD from the event (refer to postnatal PTSD section) Shame if there is any self-blame present Loss of bodily autonomy	Perform vaginal steaming (post bleed) Close the birthing field through ceremony Work with the soul of the baby so they move through Find support groups Refer to the nervous system vaginal toolkit to soothe your nervous system daily Get to know your triggers Give yourself time Mother yourself deeply Ask for more support
Numbness	A feeling of disconnect with the pelvis through neglect of oneself. Also could be compression of the pudendal nerve by nearby muscles or tissue, sometimes called pudendal nerve entrapment or Alcock canal syndrome. Caused by months/years of repeated minor damage to the pelvic area: Prolonged sitting Cycling Horse riding Constipation	Constant feelings of shame Anger towards oneself or others Putting others' needs before one's own Rape Sexual assault Consenting without wanting to truly consent Child loss Infertility challenges Miscarriage Abortion Lack of understanding of how the body works/needs of the body overall Guilt and judgement of oneself Life not unfolding as you hoped Loss of relationship(s)	Explore daily morning pages to explore current arising themes Perform vaginal steaming Perform full-body massage Perform vaginal massage Do visualisations with the womb Use nervous system toolkit support Connect to daily pleasure and joy Do mirrovulva work Express yourself through dance and free-flow movement Posture to deepen breath to the pelvis

Healing from	The physical challenges	Possible emotional challenges	Holistic support
Orgasms (Anorgasmia)	Delayed, infrequent or non-existent orgasms after feeling desire and then being aroused/stimulated	• Loss of joy and pleasure daily • Feeling disconnected from your body • Feeling disconnected from others • Lacklustre days • Hindered dreams	• Explore daily joy • Write in a gratitude journal • Go to bed earlier • Get more sleep (up your hours to 8 or 9 per night for a few weeks and see if it helps) • Find more safety in the partnership with yourself and/or others • Change things around the bedroom • Perform vaginal steaming • Perform body massage for reclamation and healing • Perform vaginal massage • Use organic lubricant (perhaps with CBD oil if there is pain present too) • Aim to curate an orgasmic life before focusing on your sexual orgasms
Ovarian cysts	Fluid-filled sac that develops on an ovary. They're common and mostly don't cause symptoms. However if it splits (ruptures), is super large or blocks the blood supply to the ovaries, you may end up with: • Pelvic pain, ranging from dull to heavy to a sudden, severe and sharp pain • Pain during sex • Difficulty emptying bowels • Frequent need to urinate • Heavy periods • Irregular periods • Lighter periods than normal • Bloating/swollen tummy • Feeling very full after only eating a little	• Ignoring the wonders of failures as well as growth • Not accessing the wisdom of your cycle • Not feeling into your physical and energetic growth in life • Feeling blocked in an aspect of your life • Playing out painful experiences in your mind regularly	• Perform vaginal steaming • Journal around what fears are arising for you • Journal with what hopes and dreams you have for yourself • Observe gratefulness • Perform massage touch • Perform womb massage • Do visualisations involving the ovaries • Understand how your cycle works fully

Healing from	The physical challenges	Possible emotional challenges	Holistic support
Partners Who Feel Lost	Those who are struggling to understand their partner or their partner's needs will need to come into relationship with the ANS and work on exploring a deeper understanding of the vagina	· Feeling bound to the current societal narratives around others' needs in sex or just generally · Feeling bound by previous lovers and what 'worked' for them · Feeling unsure of how the body responds to touch and what kind of touch will feel good, thus avoiding any kind of touch · Can occur post a trust challenge in the relationship and when there is confusion around what do to bring in repair	· Explore your love language and your partner's · Build an interest in a partner's state of mind, their stress levels and their need for relaxation · Drop all goals and simply work with areas of the body to explore the level of touch that creates holding and arousal · Explore the body without any penetration, and only explore this once the relationship and energy fields have been restored with each other · Understand consent fully · Be aware of how the body works through education on the menstrual cycle (engage in FAM together) · Follow the vagina massage section

Healing from	The physical challenges	Possible emotional challenges	Holistic support
PCOS	PCOS impacts how ovaries work. PCOS cannot be determined or ruled out via an ultrasound scan. It's an Androgen excess (high male hormones) when every other causes of androgen excess have been ruled out. It has nothing to do with cysts on the ovaries. If you have androgen excess as demonstrated by (1) high androgens (male hormones) measurable on a blood test, and/or (2) significant facial hair or jawline acne, PLUS other reasons for androgen excess have been ruled out, it's PCOS. The types of PCOS include: - Insulin-resistant PCOS · Post-pill PCOS · Inflammatory PCOS · Adrenal PCOS	· Where are you bypassing your needs? · Where are you leaning into your feminine flow of life? (Refer to the feminine/masculine energy list) · Are you placing others' needs before your own? · Who or what is toxic in your life? · How do you lean into the seasons of your life? · How does it feel to be a cyclical being?	· The pill does not treat PCOS · You will not necessarily struggle to get pregnant with PCOS once you understand your body a little more · Consider looking into natural support via a specialist nutritionist and/or do some research into your PCOS diagnosis type and the herbal remedies that would support · Reduce the amount of chemicals used in the home by switching to natural skin cream/hand soap/cleaning products, for example · There are several natural anti-androgen supplements to explore for facial hair (hirsutism) including zinc, reishi mushroom and agnus castus. Do some research on these. · Reduce stress levels · Incorporate more regular self-love classes such as yoga classes or sound baths to support with dropping into the body · Cycle track to check on ovulation · Perform vaginal steaming · Perform womb massage

Healing from	The physical challenges	Possible emotional challenges	Holistic support
Pelvic Floor Dysfunction (PFD)	This can include: · leakage when coughing, sneezing, running, jumping or bending · Passing urine frequently, needing to empty the bladder urgently · Bulge in the vagina due to descent of the bladder (cystocele), rectum (rectocele) or uterus (uterine prolapse) · Dyspareunia (pain on intercourse) · Urine leaking during sex · Pelvic pain including pudendal nerve irritation/damage · Scar tissue · Vaginal tissue · Hypersensitivity · Pelvic floor muscle spasm, · Obstetric trauma due to perineal tears, episiotomy or instrumental delivery	· Where do you need more mothering and support to unravel? · How mothered do you feel? · How nourishing do you find your relationship with yourself? · How nourishing is your relationship with others or a current partner? · What experiences are you holding onto? · How looked after do you feel by yourself and others? · Are you meeting your deepest needs? · Where do you feel you have let go in your life for fear of not achieving or gaining your original desires? · Where are you holding onto fear? · Where are you holding onto any shame?	· All these challenges can be supported with vaginal massage that integrates all the bodies including the physical and emotional bodies · Perform vaginal steaming · Give yourself deeper mothering
Perimenopause	Menopause is characterised by not having any periods for 12 months, usually post aged 45. Perimenopause occurs in the months or years before the menopause. Symptoms include: · Irregular cycles · Low mood · Anxiety · Mood swings · Low self-esteem · Memory challenges/brain fog · Hot flashes · Sleeping challenges · Dizziness · Headaches · UTIs · Aches · Weight challenges · Desire changes (. . . and more)	· Have there been any sudden changes in your life such as a child leaving home? · How does relaxing feel for you? · What are your feelings around darkness and death (raging fears)? · How much do you give to others before yourself (especially for those bleeding very heavily)? · Fears of no longer being needed or wanted · Shame for not achieving set goals or dreams by now · Worry about the impact on the world or those around you · Not feeling worthy	· Find a menopause specialist to support this transition · Do talk therapy to discuss current feelings around transitioning · Explore your autumn/winter needs · Get natural progesterone boosting support · Consider utilising Ashwagandha · Explore magnesium glycinate · Research taurine · Write in a gratitude journal · Make a vision board of your current hopes and dreams · Mother yourself deeply · Consider what your needs are as a priority

Healing from	The physical challenges	Possible emotional challenges	Holistic support
PMS (or PMDD)	Groups together symptoms we experience in the weeks or week before a period. Most have PMS at some point. Consider if it is impacting on your daily life. Symptoms include: · Mood swings · Anxiousness · Irritability · Exhaustion · Sleeping challenges · Bloating · Tummy pain · Breast tenderness · Headaches · Spotty skin/acne · Greasy hair · Changes in appetite · Desire changes (Note here that most of us would experience most of these within our cycles. Avoid jumping to the label of PMS if you feel you can explore holistic support to begin with)	· How do you lean into your feminine energy? · Resisting change · Finding life too confusing and not leaning into trust and surrender · Ignoring or resisting (pushing through) your daily protectors and triggers that show up · Allowing for everything outside of yourself to take precedence · Being unable to find light within darkness · Having poor boundaries with work or others	· Journal your cycle every day and commit to three months · Lean into what you love about autumn/winter · Track your cycle through FAM · How do you deeply mother yourself? · Create a period box · Acknowledge yourself as a cyclical being with ebbs and flows while exploring the ebbs and flows daily · Explore dark goddess work · Find your transition days with your seasons · Explore your seasonal mirrors · Explore daily nervous system tools from the vaginal toolkit · Research herbal support such as agnus castus, vitamin D and magnesium · Perform vaginal steaming · Perform womb massage · Use castor Oil packs · Do exercise that mirrors your cyclical needs · Get more sleep: up to 8 or 9 hours for 3 months and note the impact · Changes can take up to 3 months to make a difference · Seek acupuncture or reflexology

Healing from	The physical challenges	Possible emotional challenges	Holistic support
Pudendal Neuralgia	Long-term pelvic pain that originates from damage or irritation of the pudendal nerve—a main nerve in the pelvis. Areas include the lower buttocks, area between the buttocks and genitals (perineum), vulva, labia and clitoris. Feels like: · Burning · Crushing · Shooting · Prickling sensation · developing gradually or suddenly. · It can be constant or worse, or better at different times. It can: · Be worse or made better depending on whether you sit or stand. · Other symptoms can include: · Orgasm challenges · Pain in sex · Swelling in perineum · Numbness or pins/needles · Clothes touching the pelvis uncomfortable · Frequent need to pee	· Where are you feeling as though you want to have more impact in your life? · Where do you wish to expand more into all that you are? · Where do you feel trapped in your life? · How do you make time for yourself within your busy day? · Is your type of work aligning for you fully?	· Avoid activities that make the challenges with it worse (obvs) · Perform vaginal massage (consider also seeing a professional with this initially) · Sooth the nervous system through the vaginal toolkit daily · Do yoga practices to open the hips gently

Healing from	The physical challenges	Possible emotional challenges	Holistic support
Period Pains (Dysmenorrhea)	• Painful muscle cramps in the tummy, which can spread to the back and thighs, caused by gentle contractions in the uterus trying to expel the lining. • You could not have to suffer with period pains. Being in pain every cycle is unnecessary.	• What are you holding onto in your life that you are ready to move through? • Who in your life are you holding onto that you'd like to loosen the grip from? • Where in your life are you feeling guilt or judgement? • How does bleeding make you feel? • Where in your life do you feel a contraction rather than an expansion?	• Journal your cycle every day and commit to three months • Lean into what you love about your winter • Track your cycle through FAM • How do you deeply mother yourself? • Create a period box • Acknowledge yourself as a cyclical being with ebbs and flows while exploring the ebbs and flows daily • Explore dark goddess work • Explore your seasonal mirrors • Research herbal support such as agnus castus, vitamin D and magnesium • Do gentle hip openers during the bleed • Do free-flow movement through dance or stretching • Perform vaginal steaming • Perform womb massage • Use castor oil packs (not when bleeding but prior to) • Get more sleep, up to 8 or 9 hours for 3 months and note the impact • Change period wear to 100 percent organic • Do not use tampons anymore • Changes can take up to 3 months to make a difference • Seek acupuncture or reflexology

Healing from	The physical challenges	Possible emotional challenges	Holistic support
Sex (Dyspareunia)	Pain during or after sex (dyspareunia). Caused by: · Previous traumas/woundings · Infections · Physical challenges · How safe one feels during sex	· How safe do you feel in your own body? · How safe do you feel with others or with a current partner? · Where are you not meeting your needs daily? · How much pleasure or joy do you feel daily? · How have you grieved previous experiences?	· Explore daily joy · Gratitude journal · Find more safety in the partnership with yourself and/or others · Perform vaginal steaming · Perform body massage for reclamation and healing · Perform vaginal massage · Use organic lubricant (perhaps with CBD oil if there is pain present too) · Explore consent · Find what your love languages are daily and during sex · Work with somatic tools to move through previous holdings of trauma or wounds
Smear test	Cervical screening (a smear test) is checking for the health of your cervix. What happens: · A speculum will be inserted into your vagina · A soft brush is inserted through the speculum to the cervix · The brush rotates a few times to collect a sample · The speculum is removed Please go to your cervical screening checks as your medical practitioner invites you.	· How safe do you feel with consent in daily life? · How are you able to voice your needs and boundaries with others daily? · Knowing others' experiences are your experiences · Not all members of staff performing smear tests approach it the same; your concerns are warranted	· Ask for the smallest speculum first · If they can't find your cervix, this isn't your fault; try going when your cervix is at its lowest instead · Send down a grounding cord before the screening · Voice if you do not feel safe · Signal to stop at any time · Utilise the nervous system tools before and after · Cleanse the test through a vaginal steam · Visit https://mybodybackproject.com/ for cervical screening, contraceptive care, STI testing and maternity care information for people who've experienced sexual violence

Healing from	The physical challenges	Possible emotional challenges	Holistic support
STI	Sexually transmitted infections are common and nothing to be embarrassed about. Don't have sex, including oral sex, without using a condom until you've had a check-up. STIs can be present without us knowing. Symptoms can include: · Unusual discharge from the vagina · Pain when peeing · Lumps or skin growths around the genitals or bottom (anus) · A rash · Unusual vaginal bleeding · Itchy genitals or anus · Blisters and sores around your genitals or anus · Warts around your genitals or anus · Warts in your mouth or throat	· Where do you need more love for all that you are? · How do you feel about yourself as a whole? · What do you feel you deserve more of but aren't receiving from others or yourself?	· You can find free at-home testing kits online: https://sh24.org.uk/ is a great starting point if you are UK based · Perform vaginal steaming · Do visualisations of love to your pelvis · Understand consent fully · Work with nervous system tools to support you through the clearing-up · Work on your needs through deep mothering · Understand how worthy you are through affirmations and mirror work
UTI	Urinary tract infections affect the urinary tract, including your bladder (cystitis), urethra (urethritis) or kidneys (kidney infection). Some people have recurrent UTIs (1 in 5 people). Symptoms include: · Pain or a burning sensation when peeing (dysuria) · Needing to pee more often than usual during the night (nocturia) · Cloudy pee or strong smelling pee · Blood in your pee · Lower tummy pain or pain in your back, just under the ribs · High temperature, or feeling hot and shivery · A very low temperature below 36C	· Who is annoying you or aggravating you regularly? · Not taking radical responsibility for oneself, so blaming others or playing the victim regularly · How do you avoid looking after yourself? · Where do you feel like your life is currently hindered? · What relationships in your life don't align anymore and why?	· Perform vaginal massage to support pelvic floor, as it can be linked to a weak pelvic floor · Research D-mannose · Decrease sugar consumption · Avoid sex · Overusing antibiotics can increase risk of UTIs · Journal through your needs and work on meeting these more · Take a good probiotic for vaginal and urinary tract health · Research CranActin · Perform vaginal steaming · Use nervous system regulatory tools daily · Explore more joy and pleasure daily · Come back into the body through visualisation

Healing from	The physical challenges	Possible emotional challenges	Holistic support
Vaginismus	The automatic reaction to the fear of some or all types of vaginal penetration. The way the body braces itself. You may: · Find it hard inserting a tampon · Find pain with penetration during sex · Feel burning or stinging pain during sex	· How nourishing do you find your relationship with yourself? · How nourishing is your relationship with others or a current partner? · What experiences are you holding onto? · Where do you need more mothering and support to unravel? · How mothered do you feel? · Where in your life do you have to brace yourself, such as going into work or meeting up with someone in particular?	· Perform vaginal massage · Perform vaginal steaming · Do visualisation with your vagina · Get more support accessing your parasympathetic nervous system · Explore your needs through somatic therapy · Find more safety within your life and surroundings (and with others) · Work with crystal pleasure wands for de-armouring and don't use vibrators for a while · Use a vibrator just at the beginning of sex instead
Vaginitis	Soreness and/or swelling in and around the vagina. You may have all or some of these symptoms: · Itchy or sore vagina · Vaginal discharge that's a different colour, smell or thickness to usual · vaginal dryness · Pain when peeing · Pain in sex · Spotting Sore, swollen or cracked skin around your vagina. Caused by: · Thrush · STIs · Hormonal changes from perimenopause/menopause or breastfeeding · Skin changes from such things as thrush · Contraception, including copper coil	· Is there anyone frustrating you or annoying you? · How is the relationship with any current partner or with your mother? · How do you allow yourself to experience joy and pleasure daily? · Where do you cut yourself off from your needs?	· Support a healthy microbiome · Reduce or eliminate carbohydrates, sugars, and alcohol · Perform vaginal steaming (please ensure you seek a professional for your protocol) · Do not douche or use anything but water on your vulva/vagina · Wear 100 percent cotton underwear · Avoid tampons · Use 100 percent organic or reusable organic period wear · Air your vagina at night and in the day where possible · Take probiotics for vaginal health

Healing from	The physical challenges	Possible emotional challenges	Holistic support
Vulvodynia (Generalised or Localised)	Vulvodynia is persistent, unexplained pain in the vulva. Symptoms include: · Burning · Stinging · Throbbing · Soreness triggered by touch, such as during sex or when inserting a tampon · constantly in the background · Can be worse when sitting down · Limited to parts of the vulva or at the entrance · It can spread over genital area and the anus. · Generalised vulvodynia describes widespread pain throughout the vulvar region -Localised describes pain in just one area of the vulva, usually the opening of the vagina (vestibule)	· Where do you hold on tight to aspects of your life? · How much do you lean into the trust of life unravelling as it needs? · How do you lean into the ebbs and flows of your seasons? · How nourishing do you find your relationship with yourself? · How nourishing is your relationship with others or a current partner? · How safe do you feel in your own body? · Where are you holding onto shame in your life? · How much fear do you sit with? · How are you judging yourself? · What experiences are you holding onto? · Where do you need more mothering and support to unravel? · How mothered do you feel?	· Work with crystal pleasure wands for de-armouring and don't use vibrators for a while · Use a vibrator just at the beginning of sex instead · Perform vaginal massage · Perform vaginal steaming · Do visualisation with your vagina · Get more support accessing your parasympathetic nervous system · Explore your needs through somatic therapy · Find more safety within your life and surroundings (and with others)

Further Support from this Community

Welcome to the community. We're all working towards one goal: returning to a relationship with our pelvis for healing and reclamation.

I regularly share my musings and videos online by writing a regular newsletter which can be found on Substack: naomigale.substack.com where I can write freely. You can also join the conversation by finding me at @thisisnaomigale on Instagram or @thisisnaomigale_ on TikTok, with a backup account of @thisisnaomigale where I sometimes share posts, though less regularly nowadays due to being censored on social media

You can also find me chatting on my podcast, Fanny Chat, where we discuss anything that arises from pelvic-based chat with solo episodes and episodes with guests. I also have a YouTube account under @naomigale and an Insight Timer account under Naomi Gale.

For videos to support you with certain practices in this book, visit www.thisisnaomigale.co.uk/books.

Stepping inside a container to work with others on the same path can be one of the most empowering, healing and liberating experiences. It is a gift to hold these spaces. You can read more about these online or in-person opportunities for community, from workshops to sharing circles, on my website. To support the health of a cycle or physical manifestations, I offer vaginal steaming support. Learn more on my website.

Finally, I open my calendar for 1-on-1 support in Margate, UK, and online for those ready to be held, mothered and loved. You can read more about my 1-on-1 spaces, again, on my website.

I look forward to inviting you inside one of these spaces when they align.

Thank YOU for being part of this community and being part of the conversation. I look forward to seeing you around.

If you'd like to share how this book has supported you, my emails are always open. I'd so love to hear: hello@thisisnaomigale.co.uk.

Further Reading

Cancer
Gynae cancer support: https://eveappeal.org.uk/

How to check your breasts, and further support: https://coppafeel.org

Practical and social support programmes tailored to the needs of young adults, to give them a better chance of living well through and beyond cancer: https://www.trekstock.com

Children
Focuses on building up young people through focusing on the today's challenges such as body image from social media: https://www.girlguiding.org.uk/

FGC (FGM)
Working to end female genital cutting: https://www.orchidproject.org/

LGBTQ+
Fighting for the freedom, equity and potential of LGBTQ+ people everywhere: https://www.stonewall.org.uk/

Rape
A charity working to end sexual violence and abuse: https://rapecrisis.org.uk/

Support for young people on consent: https://www.childline.org.uk/info-advice/friends-relationships-sex/

Smear Tests
Cervical screening, contraceptive care, STI testing and maternity care for people who've experienced sexual violence: https://mybodybackproject.com/

Urgent Help
Free urgent mental health text line: https://giveusashout.org/

Other books from a range of authors and viewpoints:

Breath: The New Science of a Lost Art by James Nestor

Complex PTSD: From Surviving to Thriving by Pete Walker

Eastern Body, Western Mind by Anodea Judith

Invisible Women: Exposing Data Bias in a World Designed for Men by Caroline Criado Perez

Mind the Gap by Dr Karen Gurney

Mirror Work: 21 Days to Heal Your Life by Louise Hay

Period Power by Maisie Hill

Sexy but Psycho: How the Patriarchy Uses Women's Trauma Against Them by Dr Jessica Taylor

The Body Keeps the Score: Mind, Brain and Body in Transformation of Trauma by Bessel Van Der Kolk

The Inner Work: An Invitation to True Freedom and Lasting Happiness by Mathew Micheletti and Ashley Cottrell

The Trans-Gender Issue: Trans Justice Is Justice for All by Shon Faye

Vagina: A New Biography by Naomi Wolf

Waking the Tiger: Healing Trauma by Peter A. Levine

Womb Awakening: Initiatory Wisdom from the Creatrix of All Life by Azra Bertrand, M.D. and Seren Bertrand

Women Who Run with the Wolves: Contacting the Power of the Wild Woman by Clarissa Pinkola Estes

You are a Badass: How to Stop Doubting Your Greatness and Start Living an Awesome Life by Jen Sincero

References

Introduction: Not a Single Swimmer

[1] "Global and Multidisciplinary Perspectives on Unregulated Sperm Donation," *Frontiers* (online), www.frontiersin.org/research-topics/32271/global-and-multidisciplinary-perspectives-on-unregulated-sperm-donation.

[2] "Where Did the Concept of BMI Originate?" Gaspari Nutrition (online,) 2 December 2019, www.gasparinutrition.com/blogs/fitness-facts/where-did-the-concept-of-bmi-originate.

[1] "Educating Eve," Eve Appeal, https://eveappeal.org.uk/blog/educating-eve/.

[2] Sandee LaMotte, "Why Swearing Is a Sign of Intelligence, Helps Manage Pain and More," CNN Health, 21 April 2021, https://edition.cnn.com/2021/01/26/health/swearing-benefits-wellness/index.html.

[3] Ephrat Livni, "The Most Offensive Curse Word in English Has Powerful Feminist Origins," Quartz, 5 August 2017, www.qz.com/1045607/the-most-offensive-curse-word-in-english-has-powerful-feminist-origins/.

Step One: Holding onto the Cracks in Our Foundations

Your Metamorphosis Journey

[1] Hadley Freeman, "Why Is Gwyneth Paltrow Selling a Candle That Smells Like Her Vagina?" *Guardian* (UK Edition), https://www.theguardian.com/fashion/2020/jan/13/why-is-gwyneth-paltrow-selling-a-candle-that-smells-like-her-vagina-goop.

[2] "Gwyneth Paltrow Net Worth," Celebrity Net Worth, https://www.celebritynetworth.com/richest-celebrities/actors/gwyneth-paltrow-net-worth/.

[3] Janet B. Henrich and Catherine M. Viscoli, "What Do Medical Schools Teach about Women's Health and Gender Differences?" *Academic Medicine* 81, no. 5 (2006): 476–82, https://journals.lww.com/academicmedicine/Fulltext/2006/05000/What_Do_Medical_Schools_Teach_about_

WomensHealth.14.aspx.

4   Nicole Lock, "Clitoral History: A Tale of Love, Loss, and Discovery," Nursing Clio, March 25, 2014, https://nursingclio.org/2014/03/25/clitoral-history-a-tale-of-love-loss-and-discovery/.

5   Andreas Kalampalikis and Lina Michala, "Cosmetic Labiaplasty on Minors: A Review of Current Trends and Evidence," *International Journal of Impotence Research* (2018), https://www.nature.com/articles/s41443-021-00480-1.

6   Regina Nuzzo, "Pleasure at the Push of a Button, *Los Angeles Times*, 11 February 2008, https://www.latimes.com/archives/la-xpm-2008-feb-11-he-orside11-story.html.

7   "FAQs: What Is the Vaginal Biome and Why Is It Important?" Eve Appeal, https://eveappeal.org.uk/our-research/our-research-programmes/forecee/forcee-vaginal-microbiome-as-a-risk-indicator-for-ovarian-cancer/what-is-the-vaginal-biome-and-why-is-it-important-qa/.

8   Azra Bertrand, MD, and Seren Bertrand, *Womb Awakening* (Rochester, VT: Bear & Company, 2017).

9   Cathleen O'Grady, "COVID-19 Affects Men and Women Differently. So why don't clinical trials report gender data?" *Science*, 6 July 2021, https://www.science.org/content/article/covid-19-affects-men-and-women-differently-so-why-don-t-clinical-trials-report-gender.

10 Veronique M. M. M. Schiffer, Emma B. N. J. Janssen, Bas C. T. van Bussel, Laura L. M. Jorissen, Jeanette Tas, Jan-Willem E. M. Sels et al. "The 'Sex Gap' in COVID-19 Trials: A Scoping Review," *EClinicalMedicine* 29 (2020), https://www.thelancet.com/journals/eclinm/article/PIIS2589-5370(20)30396-5/fulltext.

11 "RCOG/FSRH Respond to Reports of 30,000 Women's Periods Affected after COVID-19 Vaccine," Royal College of Obstetricians & Gynaecologists, 16 September 2021, https://www.rcog.org.uk/news/rcogfsrh-respond-to-reports-of-30-000-women-s-periods-affected-after-covid-19-vaccine/.

12 Nicola Davis and Niamh McIntyre, "Revealed: Pill Still Most Popular Prescribed Contraceptive in England," Guardian (UK Edition), 7 March 2019, https://www.theguardian.com/uk-news/2019/mar/07/revealed-pill-still-most-popular-prescribed-contraceptive-in-england.

13 Anouk de Wit, Sanne Booji, Erik Giltay et al., "Association of Use of Oral Contraceptives with Depressive Symptoms among Adolescents and Young Women," *Jama Psychiatry* 77, no. 1 (2020): 52–59, https://jamanetwork.com/journals/jamapsychiatry/fullarticle/2751923.

14 Erin Blakemore, "The First Birth Control Pill Used Puerto Rican Women as Guinea Pigs," History, 11 March 2019, https://www.history.com/news/birth-

control-pill-history-puerto-rico-enovid.

15 "Eugenics and Scientific Racism," National Human Genome Research Institute, 18 May 2022, https://www.genome.gov/about-genomics/fact-sheets/Eugenics-and-Scientific-Racism.

16 Uma Dinsmore-Tuli, Yoni Shakti: *A Woman's Guide to Power and Freedom through Yoga and Tantra* (London: YogaWords, 2014).

17 Rachel Cohen, Jasmine Fardouly, Toby Newton-John and Amy Slater, "#BoPo on Instagram: An Experimental Investigation of the Effects of Viewing Body Positive Content on Young Women's Mood and Body Image," *New Media & Society* 21, no. 7 (2019): 1546–64.

18 Eleanor Cummins, "Bodies Are Canceled," *Wired*, 10 October 2021, https://www.wired.com/story/instagram-mental-health-psychology-body-image-science/.

19 Sarah Pruitt, "5 Notable Women Hanged in the Salem Witch Trials," History, 27 February 2019, https://www.history.com/news/notable-women-executed-salem-witch-trials.

20 "Witchcraft" UK Parliament website, https://www.parliament.uk/about/living-heritage/transformingsociety/private-lives/religion/overview/witchcraft/.

21 Libby Brookes, "Nicola Sturgeon Issues Apology for 'Historical Injustice' of Witch Hunts," *Guardian* (UK edition), 8 March 2022, https://www.theguardian.com/uk-news/2022/mar/08/nicola-sturgeon-issues-apology-for-historical-injustice-of-witch-hunts.

22 Shon Faye, *The Transgender Issue: An Argument for Justice* (Bristol: Allen Lane, 2021).

23 "Trans-gender Equality," UK Parliament website, 8 December 2015, https://publications.parliament.uk/pa/cm201516/cmselect/cmwomeq/390/390.pdf.

24 Zoe Williams, "Why, 50 Years after the Abortion Act, It's Time to Abolish the Law Altogether," *Guardian* (UK Edition), 25 October 2017, https://www.theguardian.com/world/2017/oct/25/abortion-act-law-50-years-terminations-criminal-stigmatised.

25 Beth Ashley, "Women Are Dating with Higher Standards and Demanding More from Their Relationships. Apparently, It's Hurting Men," *Glamour* (UK Edition), 20 August 2022, https://www.glamourmagazine.co.uk/article/women-dating-standards-higher-than-ever.

26 Robin Dembroff, "Trans Women Are Victims of Misogyny, Too—and All Feminists Must Recognize This," *Guardian* (UK edition), 19 May 2019, https://www.theguardian.com/commentisfree/2019/may/19/valerie-jackson-trans-women-misogyny-feminism.

27 Joan Harrigan-Farrelly, "For Black Women, Implicit Racial Bias in Medicine May Have Far-Reaching Effects," US Department of Labor blog, 7 February

2022, https://blog.dol.gov/2022/02/07/for-black-women-implicit-racial-bias-in-medicine-may-have-far-reaching-effects.

28 Anna Krist, "Please Stop Telling Women to Get an IUD," *DAME* 10 January 2017, https://www.damemagazine.com/2017/01/10/please-stop-telling-women-get-iud/.

29 Joan Harrigan-Farrelly, "For Black Women, Implicit Racial Bias in Medicine May Have Far-Reaching Effects," US Department of Labor blog, 7 February 2022, https://blog.dol.gov/2022/02/07/for-black-women-implicit-racial-bias-in-medicine-may-have-far-reaching-effects.

30 The Porn Conversation, https://thepornconversation.org/.

31 Léa Séguin, Carl Rodrigue and Julie Lavigne, "Consuming Ecstasy: Representations of Male and Female Orgasm in Mainstream Pornography," Taylor & Francis Online. [online]. 20 June 2017, *Journal of Sex Research* 55, no. 3 (2018), https://www.tandfonline.com/doi/abs/10.1080/00224499.2017.1332152?journalCode=hjsr20.

32 Susan Pollak, "Email Apnea: Breathing Meditations for the Workplace," *Psychology Today* online, 6 November 2014, https://www.psychologytoday.com/gb/blog/the-art-now/201411/email-apnea.

33 Jenny Pan, Holly Rhode, Bradley Undem and Allen Myers, "Neurotransmitters in Airway Parasympathetic Neurons Altered by Neurotrophin-3 and Repeated Allergen Challenge," *American Journal of Respiratory Cell and Molecular Biology* 43, no. 4 (2010): 452–57, https://www.ncbi.nlm.nih.gov/pmc/articles/PMC2951875/.

34 Peter A. Levine, *Waking the Tiger: Healing Trauma* (Berkeley, CA: North Atlantic Books, 1997).

35 Pete Walker, Complex PTSD: *From Surviving to Thriving* (Lafayette, CA: Azure Coyote, 2013).

36 Autumn Gentry, "Preventing and Healing Infant Birth Trauma," *Midwifery Today* 96 (2010): 48–9, https://pubmed.ncbi.nlm.nih.gov/21322456/#:~:text=Abstract,children%20heal%20from%20birth%20trauma.

37 Birth Trauma Association, https://www.birthtraumaassociation.org.uk/#.

38 "What Are Rape and Stealthing?" Rape Crisis, https://rapecrisis.org.uk/get-informed/types-of-sexual-violence/what-is-rape/.

39 "Sex and Consent," Brook, https://www.brook.org.uk/your-life/sex-and-consent/?gclid=CjwKCAjw9suYBhBIEiwA7iMhNC5gYmorD8rVAWtD06yoq0NHhL-KUduG0DxOufRD_9XWazqgjl-cAhoCr7YQAvD_BwE.

40 "Statistics about Sexual Violence and Abuse," Rape Crisis, https://rapecrisis.org.uk/get-informed/statistics-sexual-violence/.

41 "What is consent?" NHS website, https://www.nhs.uk/aboutNHSChoices/
    professionals/healthandcareprofessionals/child-sexual-exploitation/Documents/
    Consent-information-leaflet.pdf.

42 "Recovering from a Difficult Birth," Tommy's website, https://www.tommys.org/
    pregnancy-information/after-birth/recovering-difficult-birth.

43 "Intrauterine System (IUS)," NHS website, https://www.nhs.uk/conditions/
    contraception/ius-intrauterine-system/.

Step Two: You Deserve More Mothering, Babe

1   Melissa Hogenboom, "The Hidden Load: How 'Thinking of Everything'
    Holds Mums Back," BBC (online), 18 May 2021, https://www.bbc.com/
    worklife/article/20210518-the-hidden-load-how-thinking-of-everything-
    holds-mums-back.

2   "The Menstrual Cup Quiz (Find Your Best Fit!): We Know Your Perfect
    Menstrual Cup Based on 9 Questions!" Put a Cup in It, https://putacupinit.
    com/quiz/.

3   Dr Jessica Taylor, *Sexy but Psycho* (London: Constable, 2022).

4   Sanskriti Mishra, Harold Elliott, Raman Marwaha, "Premenstrual Dysphoric
    Disorder," National Library of Medicine, 5 May 2022. https://www.ncbi.nlm.
    nih.gov/books/NBK532307/.

5   Meggan Watterson, *Mary Magdalene Revealed* (Carlsbad, CA: Hay House, 2019).

6   Uma Dinsmore-Tuli, *Yoni Shakti: A Woman's Guide to Power and Freedom
    through Yoga and Tantra* (London: YogaWords, 2014).

7   Clare Shipman, Katty Kay, JillEllyn Riley, "How Puberty Kills Girls'
    Confidence," *Atlantic*, 20 September 2018, https://www.theatlantic.com/family/
    archive/2018/09/puberty-girls-confidence/563804/.

Step Three: Look Your Vulva in the Eye

1   Michael Magee, trans., *The Yoni Tantra*, Worldwide Tantra Project, 1995,
    accessible online at https://cleaves.lingama.net/news/attachments/sep2010/
    yoni.pdf.

2   Deborah Serani, "If It Bleeds, It Leads: Understanding Fear-Based Media,"
    Psychology Today 7 June 2011, https://www.psychologytoday.com/gb/blog/two-
    takes-depression/201106/if-it-bleeds-it-leads-understanding-fear-based-media.

3   Ashley Cottrell and Mathew Micheletti, *The Inner Work* (independently
    published, 2019).

4   Deborah Serani, "If It Bleeds, It Leads: Understanding Fear-Based Media,"
    Psychology Today 7 June 2011, https://www.psychologytoday.com/gb/blog/two-

takes-depression/201106/if-it-bleeds-it-leads-understanding-fear-based-media.

5   "Child Abuse in England and Wales: January 2020," Office for
    National Statistics, 14 January 2020, https://www.ons.gov.uk/
    peoplepopulationandcommunity/crimeandjustice/bulletins/
    childabuseinenglandandwales/january2020#:~:text=Around%20one%20in%20
    four%20women,where%20there%20was%20no%20difference.

6   Michael Magee, trans., *The Yoni Tantra*, Worldwide Tantra Project, 1995,
    accessible online at https://cleaves.lingama.net/news/attachments/sep2010/
    yoni.pdf.

7   Michael Magee, trans., *The Yoni Tantra*, Worldwide Tantra Project, 1995,
    accessible online at https://cleaves.lingama.net/news/attachments/sep2010/
    yoni.pdf.

8   Michael Magee, trans., *The Yoni Tantra*, Worldwide Tantra Project, 1995,
    accessible online at https://cleaves.lingama.net/news/attachments/sep2010/yoni.
    pdf.

9   Annemette Wildfang Lykkebo, Henrik Christian Drue, Janni Uyen Hoa
    Lam and Rikke Guldberg, "The Size of Labia Minora and Perception of
    Genital Appearance: A Cross-Sectional Study," *Journal of Lower Genital
    Tract Disease* 21, no. 3(2017): 198–203, https://pubmed.ncbi.nlm.nih.
    gov/28369012/#:~:text=The%20median%20width%20of%20labia,73.3%25%20
    had%20visible%20labia%20minora.

10 "Female Genital Mutilation (FGM)," UNICEF website, https://data.unicef.org/
    topic/child-protection/female-genital-mutilation/#_edn1.

Step Four: An Orgasmic Cup of Tea

1   Regena Thomashauer, *Pussy: A Reclamation* (Carlsbad, CA: Hay House, 2016).

2   Ben Taub, "Scientists Have Discovered how the Clitoris Generates so Much
    Pleasure," IFL Science, 28 October 2022, https://www.iflscience.com/scientists-
    have-discovered-how-the-clitoris-generates-so-much-pleasure-65967.

3   Linda Geddes, "Sex on the Brain: What Turns Women On, Mapped Out," *New
    Scientist*, 5 August 2011, https://www.newscientist.com/article/dn20770-sex-on-
    the-brain-what-turns-women-on-mapped-out/.

4   "Sexual Attitudes and Lifestyles in Britain: Highlights from Natsal-3,"
    Natsal, https://www.natsal.ac.uk/sites/default/files/2021-04/Natsal-3%20
    infographics.pdf.

5   Gayle Brewer and Colin Hendrie, "Evidence to Suggest that Copulatory
    Vocalizations in Women Are Not a Reflexive Consequence of Orgasm," *Archives
    of Sexual Behavior* 40 (2011): 559–64, https://link.springer.com/article/10.1007/

s10508-010-9632-1.

[6] David Frederick, H. Kate St. John, Justin Garcia and Elisabeth Lloyd, "Differences in Orgasm Frequency among Gay, Lesbian, Bisexual, and Heterosexual Men and Women in a U.S. National Sample," *Archives of Sexual Behavior* 47 (2018): 273–88, https://link.springer.com/article/10.1007/s10508-017-0939-z.

[7] Elizabeth Armstrong, Paula England and Alison Fogarty, "Accounting for Women's Orgasm and Sexual Enjoyment in College Hookups and Relationships," *American Sociological Review* 77, no. 3 (2012): 325–503, https://journals.sagepub.com/doi/full/10.1177/0003122412445802.

[8] Azra Bertrand, MD, and Seren Bertrand, *Womb Awakening* (Rochester, VT: Bear & Company, 2017).

Step Five: It's All in Your Vagina

[1] Petros Benias, Rebecca Wells, Bridget Sackey-Aboyagye, Heather Klavan, Jason Reidy, Darren Buonocore, Markus Miranda, Susan Kornacki, Michael Wayne, David Carr-Locke and Neil Theise, "Structure and Distribution of an Unrecognized Interstitium in Human Tissues," *Scientific Reports* 8 (2018), https://www.nature.com/articles/s41598-018-23062-6.

[2] "Statistics about Sexual Violence and Abuse," Rape Crisis, https://rapecrisis.org.uk/get-informed/statistics-sexual-violence/.

[3] J. Douglas Bremner, Penny Randall, Eric Vermetten, Lawrence Staib, Richard Bronen, Carolyn Mazure, Sandi Capelli, Gregory McCarthy, Robert Innis and Dennis Charney, "Magnetic Resonance Imaging-Based Measurement of Hippocampal Volume in Posttraumatic Stress Disorder Related to Childhood Physical and Sexual Abuse—A Preliminary Report," *Biological Psychiatry* 41, no. 1 (1997): 23–32, https://www.ncbi.nlm.nih.gov/pmc/articles/PMC3229101/.

[4] "Statistics about Sexual Violence and Abuse," Rape Crisis, https://rapecrisis.org.uk/get-informed/statistics-sexual-violence/.

[5] "Statistics about Sexual Violence and Abuse," Rape Crisis, https://rapecrisis.org.uk/get-informed/statistics-sexual-violence/.

[6] K. R. Mitchell, R. Geary, C. A. Graham, J. Datta, K. Wellings, P. Sonnenberg, N. Field, D. Nunns, J. Bancroft, K. G. Jones, A. M. Johnson and C. H. Mercer "Painful Sex (Dyspareunia) in Women: Prevalence and Associated Factors in a British Population Probability Survey," *BJOG: An International Journal of Obstetrics and Gynaecology* 124, no. 11 (2017) 1689–97, https://obgyn.onlinelibrary.wiley.com/doi/10.1111/1471-0528.14518.

[7] Eagle Gamma, "Left Brain vs. Right Brain," *Simply Psychology*, 18 May 2021,

https://www.simplypsychology.org/left-brain-vs-right-brain.html.

8   Lena Schmidt, ow to Find the Balance Between Your Masculine & Feminine Energy," Chopra, 31 May 2019, https://chopra.com/articles/how-to-find-the-balance-between-your-masculine-feminine-energy.

9   Meggan Watterson, *Mary Magdalene Reveale*d, (Carlsbad, CA: Hay House, 2019).

The Key to Your Happiness

1   "Mental Health Facts and Statistics," Mind, https://www.mind.org.uk/information-support/types-of-mental-health-problems/statistics-and-facts-about-mental-health/how-common-are-mental-health-problems/.

2   "What Is Sexual Consent?" Rape Crisis, https://rapecrisis.org.uk/get-informed/about-sexual-violence/sexual-consent/.

3   "What Is Sexual Consent?" Rape Crisis, https://rapecrisis.org.uk/get-informed/about-sexual-violence/sexual-consent/.

Acknowledgements

For my own womb, vagina and vulva, for continuing to guide me, hold me and remind me to take better care of myself. I wouldn't have been on this journey if you hadn't shown me that there is a better way of life.

Fully receiving the holding Mother Earth provided as I wrote these pages from early spring, summer, autumn, winter and then moving into spring again as I prepared for the book to be shared. How she held me in the cabin in the bottom of my garden through her seasonal changes reminding me to write to her rhythms.

Thank you to those who have messaged me in some way and told me that my support has given them some joy in their lives. Those words continue to keep me going.

To clients who have landed in my spaces one-on-one or in group settings. I continue to be in awe of the strength it takes to work with your pelvis in this way. Every single client has informed my spaces and the words in this book. I am so fucking grateful to you.

And those who saw the pre-orders and bought one of these books to support getting it out into the world. Thanks for believing in me and my words enough to do that.

This book wouldn't have been possible without my guides and teachers' guidance and wisdom. To name a few who have touched my soul: Clare Blake for holding me in your home while you showed me how spirituality isn't all white dresses, lip fillers and perfection. You remain one of my heroes. To Tami Lynn Kent, who reminded me of the importance of intuition and healing the whole person through energetic and physical touch in a way that continues to inform me every day. For Mat and Ash, who saved me at a time when I needed saving, guiding me through the most incredible year of yoga training. Ash, thank you for being on calls with me, reminding me of my worth, for inspiring me to write a book and for being your raw, vulnerable self. I love you and will always be unbelievably grateful to you.

For my talk therapist, Katharine, who held me and reminded me to tend back to the book when I dropped it for a moment as it was taking over my life. For also reminding me that I am worthy.

Thank you to my neighbour and friend Kat for taking me on long dog walks and voice noting me, reminding me how hard writing is and how it will all be OK whatever happens. Life can be really shit, hun, but I am so glad I can walk full of snot and bugs from our children by the sea here and there with you in Margate.

To Tamsin, who coached me through some of the harder months in this process, for reaching out to me and seeing that I was not OK at one point and for, in her own time, calling me to soothe my nervous system by the sea. I am grateful to you.

To my photographer, Artemis, for capturing me in my home just as I am and then for continuing to cheerlead the need for this book. To Pri for being patient with me while we changed the cover and created a cover fit for framing on the wall. Becky, I am so grateful to you for landing in my DMs and allowing me to whinge, moan, groan and perfect the cover and interiors of this book. Your eye for detail was a gift to me. Thank you for sitting with me in coffee shops and in my home while we went through my long 'don't like' lists. You were a gift from the universe in this process.

Thank you to my copy editor, Lindsey, for taking on this project and reading every single line before anyone else and not telling me it was a pile of wank. For your carefully considered emails and thoughtful edits as an American navigating my over-the-top Britishness.

To my cat Zuri, who sat by my side for twelve years where the process to coming home to myself began and while I wrote in my cabin for months on end, whose soul suddenly had to move on as this process came to a close. For sending me a new fluffy cat spirit who also sat with me and soothed me while I prepped the book for the final stage. I miss you endlessly, Zuri.

To the book's beta reader, Lou. Thank you for taking your time to go through every page and sending me feedback. You are an angel.

And to my children, Arlo, Paloma and Xanthe, who lacked mothering when I needed to write late into the evening, missing their bedtimes. Thank you for showing me the importance of play, slowing down and just being present. I will always be in awe of your zest for life. I wanted to show you that you can create whatever you want in life through the creation of this book. I hope your world is more pussy-led by the time you all transition through puberty.

Finally, to my husband, Ali. I don't have the words to describe your support for me as your wife, as a mother and as someone trying to pave the way. Your love is unwavering. Thanks for all the dinners and teas delivered to me in the cabin and for basically keeping me alive through Tesco shops and regular sustenance. I am so sorry I lost myself so many times in this process. We've been through so much together, and this was yet again another challenge for us to move through. If it wasn't for you, this book would never have got to this point, and it would never have been published. Your enthusiasm for the impact this work has on others is why I keep going. It has been the air I needed to breathe when I was crumbling in a heap. Thank you for being an incredible father when I cracked on. The children are so blessed to have you. I hope this book makes you proud as it lands in your hands for the first time, and it all felt worth it. I love you.

Book Cheerleading Squad

Everyone acknowledged below contributed financially to cheerlead/birth/encourage this book out into the world.

Kirsty Whitehead, Katie Allen, Vanessa Moody, Gracie Howells, Rachel Watson, Tamsin Crimmens, Annamaria Papayova, Lauren Pelham, Becca Barlow, Amy, Debi, Eve, Kats, Kat, Naomi, Rosa (the Vagsoc crew), Carlota Martinez, Anonymous, Shauni, Clare Sente, Natalie Payne, Sophie Neve, Lydia Mills, Jenny, Sitara Johns, Amy, Louise, Kate, Jo, Jenny Butterworth, Kristy Afrasiabi, Blanca, Zsófi Zádor, Helen Miller, Jade Wainwright, Hannah Carr, I+C+A, Laura McCrae, Sarah Gwilliam, Emily, Thatiane Benz Pisco, Fluffy Parrot, Kerri Tucker, Samuel Atherton, Melissa Rose Hirsch, Alexandra Peppitt, Emer Pearson, Leia Boote, Sarah King, Lesley Jepps, Belinda Knowler, Adina Oros, Lydia Reeves, Philomena Kurzawe, Frida Eliasson, Emma, Felitia de Baat, Ashley McMorrow, Eleanor Ashton, Frida Karlsson, Shannon Brown, Christine Drysdale, Kerry Lyons, Mollie Bylett, Rosie Spaughton, Aluna Francis, Kate Codrington, Jo Miller, Diane Salisbury, Natasha Cottrell, Anonymous, Marlene Alonso Gonzalez, Balca Balabaner, Sabrina Henrie, Rebecca Marshall, Jade Wadham-Powell, Emma Heideker, Amelia Griffiths, Jaimee Lee Elias, Ozlem Bektas, Grace Brickell, Chelsea Lillian Rogers, Julia Olah, Reka Vavrinecz, Carina Covella, Laura Wainwright, Karolina Siwik, Natasha Hurst, Tayla Courtice, Lily Summers, Eme Szelle Sido, Liz Hutchinson, Katrina Harradine, Chloe Lewis, Barbora Rybarova, Rebecca Harmer, Bethany Stewart, Nina Parmar, Yasmin Parmar, Livia Gibson, Simran Singhota, Sarah Burnett, Alice Wood, Nathalie Nguyen, Alida Urban, Monique Macfarlane, Eloina Haines, Jade O'Neill, Anna Grundy, Hannah Rzysko, Ciara, Sarah Gooslin, Sophie B, Vanessa Loibl, Carly, Kimberley Heavey, Lara Grum, Benita Nagra, Anja Summermatter, Lou Clarke, Ashleigh Luther, Theresa Hengerer, Sam Dawood, Ashley Pope, Emily Napier, Simone Campbell, Amy White, K Bishop, Alice Le Beau-Morley, Kate Dawson, Katya Blackledge, Lou Cowell, Kate OBrien, Katherine Louise Jessup, Imogen Povey, Charlie Amber Gunn, Molly Lewis, Charlotte Wright, Stevey, Katy Massey, Charlie Mankin, Folake Balogun, Charlotte Reddington, Joanna Colin, Maisy, Hannah Sutcliffe.

Your Fanny Notes

Printed in Great Britain
by Amazon

25817231R00172